MACROPHAGES AND LYMPHOCYTES

Nature, Functions, and Interaction

PART B

ADVANCES IN EXPERIMENTAL MEDICINE AND BIOLOGY

Recent Volumes in this Series

MACROPHAGES AND LYMPHOCYTES
Nature, Functions, and Interaction
PART B

Edited by

Mario R. Escobar
Medical College of Virginia
Richmond, Virginia

and

Herman Friedman
University of South Florida
Tampa, Florida

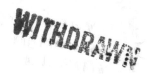

PLENUM PRESS • NEW YORK AND LONDON

Library of Congress Cataloging in Publication Data

Reticuloendothelial Society.
  Macrophages and lymphocytes, nature, functions, and interaction.
  (Advances in experimental medicine and biology; v. 121)
  "Proceedings of the eighth international congress of the Reticuloendothelial
Society, held in Jerusalem, Israel, June 18–23, 1978."
  Includes index.
  1. Macrophages — Congresses. 2. Lymphocytes — Congresses. 3. Reticulo-endo-
thelial system — Congresses. 4. Immune response — Congresses. I. Escobar, Mario
R. II. Friedman, Herman, 1931-   III. Title. IV. Series.
QR185.8.M3R47 1979   599'.02'9   79-9566
ISBN 0-306-40286-6 (Part B)

Proceedings of the Eighth International Congress of the Reticuloendothelial
Society, held in Jerusalem, Israel, June 18–23, 1978, of which this is part two.

© 1980 Plenum Press, New York
A Division of Plenum Publishing Corporation
227 West 17th Street, New York, N.Y. 10011

Printed in the United States of America

PROCEEDINGS OF THE

VIII INTERNATIONAL CONGRESS OF THE RETICULOENDOTHELIAL SOCIETY

Jerusalem, Israel   *June 18-23, 1978*

ORGANIZING AND PROGRAM COMMITTEE: M. Schlesinger, M. M. Sigel, H. Friedman and M. R. Escobar

ISRAELI HOST COMMITTEE: M. Schlesinger, M. Feldman, R. Gallily, C. Greenblatt, D. Pluznik and J. Yoffey

LIAISON MEMBERS: S. M. Reichard, W. Th. Daems, M. Kojima, M. G. Hanna, J. Harris and M. La Via

INTERNATIONAL REPRESENTATIVES: J. Babnik, L. A. Chedid, V. Esmann, K. Flemming, P. Garzon, J. Gras Riera, P. J. Jacques, D. Nelson, G. Nitulescu, F. Rossi, B. E. Schildt, O. Stendahl, A. E. Stuart, M. Timar and I. Toro

---

This meeting is dedicated
to the memory of
NEWTON B. EVERETT
May 12, 1916
May 23, 1979

---

v

Preface

The Reticuloendothelial (RE) Society, which is concerned with advancement of knowledge concerning the many diverse functions of RE cells, organizes national and international meetings and publishes a scientific journal. The VIII International Congress of the RE Society was held in Jerusalem, Israel, June 18-23, 1978. The Congress had as its scientific objective a wide range of subjects concerning the RE System, especially as related to macrophage function and interaction with lymphocytes. Emphasis of the Congress was placed on the nature and function of macrophages and other cells of the RE System with reference to immune responses, anti-infectious activity, tumor immunity, autoimmunity, and transplant rejection. The secretion of soluble factors by macrophages and lymphocytes and the mode of action of these factors on other cells was stressed. During the Congress some discussion was entertained concerning the controversy as to what constitutes the "RE System" per se. Some investigators feel that the phagocytic activity of macrophages is the most important aspect of the RE System playing also a major role in many parameters of immunity. Mononuclear phagocytes include tissue macrophages as well as circulating monocytes and their precursors. Although phagocytosis is a major functional activity of these cells, it is only one of several activities. The important role of mononuclear phagocytes and other mononuclear cells in immune responsiveness, - including humoral and cell mediated immunity, specific and nonspecific resistance to microorganisms and tumor cells, as well as homeostatic activities in general - has become the focus of attention of many investigators and served as a focal point for the exchange of scientific information during the Congress.

The Congress was immediately preceded by the 6th International Conference on Germinal Centers and Lymphatic Tissues in Immune Reactions being held in Kiel, Germany, June 11-16, 1978. The RES Congress was followed by the 12th International Leukocyte Culture Conference being held in Beersheba, Israel June 25-30, 1978. An attempt was made by the Organizing and Program Committees for the 3 conventions to interrelate the scientific topics planned for presentation. Thus, the RES Congress dealt mainly with

macrophage nature and functions whereas the Leukocyte Culture
Conference devoted much attention to the role and activities
of lymphocytes. The RES Congress was divided into symposia, con-
tributed papers, and workshop sessions. Five symposia were
held during each morning on the following topics: I. Regulatory
Functions of the RE System,   II. Enzymatic Activities of Macrophages,   III. Role of Macrophages in Tumor Activity,   IV. Environmental Factors Influencing the RES, and   V. Interactions
of Macrophages and Lymphocytes in the Immune Response.

Each afternoon was devoted to several simultaneous scientific
sessions with short papers presented on subjects of current
interest to the RE System. Although workshops devoted to particularly important areas of the RE System were useful and well-
attended, their publication is not included in these volumes because of the priority given to the large number of formal papers
selected for their high quality and relevance.

These volumes constitute the published records of the
proceedings of the Congress, including only the symposia and
selected proffered papers. However, the written contributions
are not arranged exactly as presented at the Congress but rather
they are interspersed according to the central theme of each of
the four sections for each volume. The first volume deals with
the enzymatic and metabolic activities of RE cells, the immuno-
pharmacology and regulatory functions of the RE System, as well
as with environmental factors influencing the latter. The second
volume includes papers concerned with immunity and infection,
interaction of cells in the RE System and immunomodulation in
cancer.

M. R. Escobar

H. Friedman

Acknowledgments

The editors are indebted to Drs. N. R. Di Luzio, K. B. P. Flemming, C. Greenblatt, M. G. Hanna, T. Mekori-Felsteiner, Q. N. Myrvik, D. Nachtigal, D. H. Pluznik, J. J. Oppenheim, M. Quastel, F. Rossi, J. B. Solomon, K. Stern and N. Trainin who chaired the Symposia. Many thanks to Drs. P. Abramoff, J. Battisto, T. K. Eisenstein, T. N. Harris, P. J. Jacques, A. M., Kaplan, M. Kojima, F. J. Lejeune, T. J. Linna, Q. N. Myrvik, S. J. Normann, P. Patriarca, J. Pitt, S. M. Reichard, B. V. Siegel, R. N. Taub, G. Wertheim and E. F. Wheelock who chaired the Short Paper Sessions. Gratitude is expressed to Drs. N. R. Di Luzio, T. K. Eisenstein, A. Ghaffar, C. Greenblatt, H. W. Holy, P. J. Jacques, H. Koren, P. Patriarca, W. Regelson, M. M. Sigel and others for their valuable assistance in preparing the workshops. This Congress could not have succeeded without the financial support of Accurate Chemical and Scientific Corporation; Battelle Memorial Institute; Dako of Denmark; Merck and Company; Nyegaard of Norway; Ortho Pharmaceutical Company; Owens-Illinois; The Upjohn Company; USV Pharmaceutical Company; and especially, the generous donation from the Fogharty International Center of the National Institutes of Health (USA). Recognition is extended to M. A. Dearing, I. Friedman and L. Sylte who shared in the monumental task of typing all the manuscripts; to the staff of Plenum Publishing Corporation for their expert assistance; and, to Mr. R. J. Burk, Jr. and his staff, from the Central Office of the Reticuloendothelial Society, for their advice and encouragement.

Contents of Part B

SECTION 1
THE RETICULOENDOTHELIAL SYSTEM AND IMMUNE
RESPONSES IN INFECTION

SECTION 2
NATURE, ACTIVATION AND INTERACTIONS
OF THE RETICULOENDOTHELIAL SYSTEM

SECTION 3
IMMUNOPATHOLOGY OF THE RETICULOENDOTHELIAL
SYSTEM

SECTION 4
THE RETICULOENDOTHELIAL SYSTEM
AND IMMUNOMODULATION IN CANCER

Contents of Part A

SECTION 1
ENZYMATIC AND METABOLIC ACTIVITIES OF THE
RETICULOENDOTHELIAL SYSTEM

SECTION 2
IMMUNOPHARMACOLOGY OF THE RETICULOENDOTHELIAL SYSTEM

SECTION 4
ENVIRONMENTAL FACTORS INFLUENCING THE RETICULOENDOTHELIAL
SYSTEM AND IMMUNE RESPONSES

Introduction

This volume deals mainly with the Reticuloendothelial (RE) System as related to immune responses in infections, tumor immunity and cells which interact in a wide variety of functions. The first section of this volume is concerned with immune responses in infections including genetic and nongenetic modification of macrophage functions as well as host immune system-parasite interactions with regard to either stimulation or depression of leukocyte and macrophage activities by microorganisms. The role of mononuclear cells in controlling infections by bacteria, viruses and fungi are also covered. The second section deals with the nature, activation and interaction of cells within the RE System. Dr. Joseph Yoffey, Distinguished Professor at the Hebrew University of Jerusalem, introduces this section with a conceptual paper dealing with lymphocytes and mononuclear phagocytes in the lymphomyeloid complex. Ultrastructural studies of lymphoid cells are also presented, as well as discussions of macrophage-lymphocyte interactions involving control mechanisms of immune responsiveness. The section on the immunopathology of the RE System introduces the interesting concept of immunosuppression as a homeostatic mechanism in disease and aging. Other chapters deal with the role of suppressor and phagocytic cells and humoral factors in various disease processes as well as RE System enhancement and autoimmunity.

The final section of this volume has as its central theme immunomodulation in cancer as related to the RE System. A review of the role of macrophages in tumor immunity and a discussion of macrophages as regulators of specific effectors of immunity against tumors are presented. The role of endotoxin in tumor resistance, as well as various factors related to RE cell activation in tumor resistance are described. A better understanding of the role of the RE System and its constituent cells in infectious diseases, tumor immunity and autoimmunity is certainly relevant to both conceptual and practical aspects of not only immunology in general, but also many areas of interest to medical and biological scientists. It is anticipated that this

record of the proceedings of the Congress will provide a cen-
tralized source of newer information concerning this rapidly
expanding field of biomedical research.

Part I
**Reticuloendothelial System and Immune Responses
in Infection**

It has been widely recognized for many decades that the RE System plays a vital role in infectious diseases. As long ago as the beginning of the century it was acknowledged that so-called "blockade" of the RE System with colloidal materials and non-viable particles such as carbon could interfere with immune resistance to many microbial infectious agents. However, the same agents used to induce RE System blockade often stimulated the immune system in regard to infectious diseases. Thus, it is quite evident that complex events occur when RE cells are either inhibited or activated in infectious processes. This section of the volume describes some of the complexities relative to the role of the RE System in infection and immunity. The genetic control of macrophage functions in relationship to antibody responsiveness and resistance is certainly an important concept which also is described in this section. The role of phagocytosis in antifungal as well as in bacterial host defenses and in immunity to tumor viruses is also important and is included in this section. Of special interest is a discussion of the relationship between protective immunity, mitogenicity and B-cell activation all of which may be induced by similar bacterial components. The effect of bacterial and viral agents on the functional activity of RE cells is equally relevant so that it is discussed in this section.

GENETIC MODIFICATION OF MACROPHAGE FUNCTIONS IN RELATION TO

ANTIBODY RESPONSIVENESS AND RESISTANCE TO INFECTION

C. STIFFEL, D. MOUTON, Y. BOUTHILLIER and G. BIOZZI

Institut Curie Section De Biologie
Paris (France)

The immunological defense of mammals against infections is due to the activities of 3 cell types: macrophages, T lymphocytes and B lymphocytes. The functions characteristic of these cells, in relation to immunity, are: phagocytosis and metabolic activity (microbicidal activity) for macrophages, cell mediated immunity for T lymphocytes and antibody synthesis for B lymphocytes. These 3 cell types have successively appeared during the phylogeny of the immune system. Phagocytosis being a nonspecific phenomenon was the most primitive function. Afterwards, cell mediated immunity which was the first specific response arose, followed by antibody production. In spite of their close functional cooperation these 3 cell types are in fact under distinct polygenetic regulation. This conclusion is illustrated by our studies on the genetic regulation of quantitative immune responsiveness.

A two-way selective breeding for maximal or minimal antibody response to heterologous erythrocytes has produced two lines of mice, a "high" (H) and a "low" (L) line for antibody responsiveness. In these two lines the immune response diverged progressively and the maximal interline separation was obtained after 16 generations of selective breeding. By that time, each line was considered homozygous at the level of all the loci controlling the character investigated (3,4,10). The immunological characteristics of these two lines were the following:

a) - Humoral response was always higher in the H than in the L line. A typical response of these two lines to an optimal dose of the selected antigen: sheep erythrocytes (SE) is presented in Fig. 1. Both, the level and the duration of the immune response, were very different in the H and L lines (5). This interline

difference was also evident for many unrelated immunogens: proteins (BSA, BCG, hen egg albumin (8,11,19), f and s antigens of
Salmonella (20), pneumococcus polysaccharide (12), T_4 bacteriophage
(13), picrylchloride (18), and histocompatibility antigens (15).

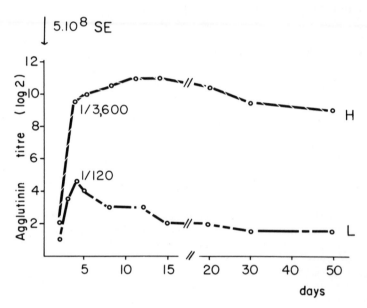

Fig. 1. Kinetics of anti-sheep erythrocyte (SE) agglutinins in
the H and L responder mice after i.v. injection of 5×10^8 SE.
(from ref 5)

     b) - Intensity of cell mediated immunity was similar in the
two lines. This was shown for skin graft rejection (15), graft
versus host reaction (7) delayed cutaneous hypersensivity (18)
and in vitro response of T lymphocytes to mitogenic activity of
Phytohemagglutinin (16).

     c) - Catabolism of ingested material was more intense in L
than in H macrophages. So, the rate of breakdown of ŞE antigens
was higher in L than in H macrophages (3,17). This was demonstrated by the following experiment (3). Random-bred mice preimmunized with a sub-immunogenic dose of SE received as a booster,
irradiated, homogenized spleens removed from H or L mice at
different times after i.v. immunization with an optimal dose of

SE. The persistence of the immunogenic form of SE in spleen macrophages of H and L donors was demonstrated by the antibody titers
found in recipients. Spleens of H and L mice removed 2 hr after
SE injection induced an equivalent antibody response in recipients.

Afterwards, the decrease in immunogenicity of the L spleen was
faster than that of the H spleen. No response was produced by the
L-line spleen removed 4 days after SE injection while the H-line
spleen still provoked an immune response 7 days after immunization.

TABLE I

Persistence of Sheep Erythrocytes (SE) Immunogenicity
in Spleen Macrophages of H and L Mice

Time After i.v. Injection of 2.10^9 SE	Anti-SE Agglutinin Titer[a] in Recipients of Spleen from	
	H line	L line
2 hr	1/1000	1/1280
2 days	1/640	1/ 480
4 days	1/480	1/ 20
7 days	1/120	<1/ 20

[a]Agglutinins were measured 12 days after spleen injection
(3).

The persistence of the antigen in its immunogenic form in
the macrophages induced a long lasting stimulation of lymphocytes,
then a high antibody response. In contrast, the poor response of
L mice is partially due to the rapid breakdown of the antigen by
the macrophage enzymatic equipment.

The higher bactericidal activity of L macrophages was demonstrated by the following experiment (R. Fauve, personal communication). At different times after the i.v. injection of live
Listeria monocytogenes, H and L mice were killed and the number
of bacteria in the spleen and liver were counted. The results
reported in Table II showed an equivalent multiplication of the
micro-organisms in the organs of H and L mice during the first
24 hr. Subsequently, the bacteria multiplication was stopped in
L mice whereas it progressed in H mice.

The bactericidal activity of macrophages on the ingested
living micro-organisms was a well-known component of host defense

against certain types of infection while the humoral antibody
response played an important role in the defense against other
types of infection.   Due to their immunological characteristics
summarized in Table III, H and L mice were useful to investigate
the relative importance of humoral response, cellular immunity
and macrophage activity in the natural defense against infections
or in the protective effect of vaccination.

TABLE II

Multiplication of Live Listeria monocytogenes
in Liver and Spleen of H and L Mice

Organ	Time After Injection[a] (hr)	Number of Listeria monocytogenes (10^6) H	L
Spleen	2	0.007	0.0055
	24	1.3	1.8
	48	15.0	2.8
Liver	2	0.180	0.330
	24	1.0	2.2
	48	54.0	2.4

[a]i.v. injection 7.4 x 10^5 Listeria monocytogenes (Fauve,
personal communication).

TABLE III

Schematic Comparison of Response of T, B Lymphocytes
or Macrophages Between H and L Mice[a]

Mouse Line	Antibody Response (B Lymphocytes)	Cellular Immunity (T Lymphocytes)	Enzymatic Activities of Macrophages
High	+++	++	+
Low	+	++	+++

[a]From ref. (2)

Salmonella typhimurium infection. The antibody response to f and s antigens of S. typhimurium is much higher in the H than in the L mouse line after immunization with an optimal dose of formalin killed S. typhimurium: 62-fold and 20-fold interline difference in antibody titers for f and s antigen, respectively (20).

A severe infection caused by i.p. injection of 1000 virulent S. typhimurium produces 100% mortality in the two lines; however, the mean survival time is longer in L than in H mice (Table IV). A less severe infection induced by intradermal injection of 5000 S. typhimurium also provokes 100% mortality in H mice whereas 55% of L mice survive.

TABLE IV

Natural Resistence and Protective Effect of Vaccination Against Salmonella typhimurium Infection in H and L Mouse Lines[a]

Host Mechanism	Challenge No. of S. typhimurium Injected	High Line		Low Line	
		Mortality %	Mean Survival Time (days)	Mortality %	Mean Survival Time (days)
Natural Resistance	1000 i.p.	100	5.4	100	8.7
	5000 i.d.	100	10.4	45	–
Vaccination with non-virulent S. typhimurium	1000 i.p.	100	8.6	10	–

[a]From ref. (9).

Vaccination with a nonvirulent strain of S. typhimurium increases the difference between the two lines. No protection is produced in the H line; whereas, 90% of L mice are efficiently protected (9).

These experiments confirm the fundamental importance of macrophages and the inefficiency of antibodies in anti-Salmonellae immunity.

Yersinia pestis infection. A severe infection (1000 Y. pestis
s.c.) produces 100% mortality in both lines with a longer survival
time in L mice than in H mice (7.7 days and 4.5 days, respectively).
Specific vaccination by an extract of Y. pestis totally protects
the L mice while no protection is produced in the H mice (1).

Leishmania tropica infection. Resistance of H and L mice to
this parasite has been investigated by Howard and Hale (personal
communication). L. tropica is a parasite of macrophages. Its
intradermal injection induces in the L line small skin lesions
which heal within 1-2 months. In the H line larger lesions are
produced and about 80% of H mice died. The different behavior of
macrophages in the two lines is demonstrated by the fact that the
parasites survive inside the H line macrophages; whereas, they
are killed by L line macrophages.

As expected, the antibody response to L. tropica antigens is
about 10-fold higher in the H than in the L line.

Plasmodium berghei infection. Natural resistance to infection
by merozoites of P berghei is similar in the two lines (Table V).
Vaccination by repeated injections of irradiated parasitized
erythrocytes produces in the H line a strong antibody synthesis and
a good protection against the infection. On the contrary, this
vaccination induces a low titer of antibody in the L line and
fails to protect these mice against infection. Hence the protection due to the vaccination is probably related to the level of
antibody (2).

Trypanosoma cruzi infection. Kierszenbaum and Howard (14)
have reported that L mice are highly susceptible to T. cruzi
infection (100% mortality) while H mice are relatively resistant
(12% mortality). No protection results from vaccination in the
L line; however, these mice can be effectively protected by passive antibody transfer: i.e. by administration of serum from
vaccinated H mice which are protected.

These data point out the important role of antibody in the
resistance against this infection.

Schistosoma mansoni infection. Blum and Cioli (6) studied
the role of innate and acquired immunity to S. mansoni infection
in the H and L lines. H mice produce higher antibody titers
than L mice; nevertheless, they were more susceptible to this infection. The number of worms recovered from the host and the
yield of schistosome eggs in the liver are higher in the H than
in the L mice. In addition, acquired resistance is identical or
even stronger in the L than in the H line. These findings rule

TABLE V

Natural Resistance and Protection Induced in the H and L Mouse Lines
by Irradiated Parasites Against Plasmodium berghei Infection[a]

Experimental Group	High Line			Low Line		
	Antibody Titer[b]	% Mortality	Mean Survival Time (days)	Antibody Titer[b]	%Mortality	Mean Survival Time (days)
Controls		83	16.6		92.5	17
Vaccinated mice[c]	1/10,800	5	-	1/1,000	83.6	19

[a]Infection: 10^7 parasitized mouse erythrocytes kept in liquid nitrogen 7 days after the last vaccination.

[b]Antibody titer measured by immunofluorescence (kindly performed by Dr. Monjour).

[c]Vaccination: 6 i.p. injections of 3.10^7 parasitized mouse erythrocytes irradiated with 60.000 r, a week apart.

out a protective role of humoral antibody and merely suggest the important role of macrophages. These cells may intervene by their intrinsic activity in the first infection and through their response to activating substances released from the sensitized T lymphocytes in the re-infection experiments.

The results reported above underline the interest of the two lines for investigating the role played by the different components of the host response in the mechanisms of natural or induced immunity against various infections.

ACKNOWLEDGEMENT

The study with the _Plasmodium_ _berghei_ model received financial support from the World Health Organization.

REFERENCES

1. Biozzi, G., In: Genetic Control of Immune Responsiveness (Ed. H. O. McDevitt and M. Landy), Academic Press, New York, London (1972) 317.
2. Biozzi, G., Mouton, D., Stiffel, C., Sant'Anna, O. A., and Bouthillier, Y., In: Parmacology of Immunoregulation (Ed. G. H. Werner and F. Floc'h), Academic Press (1978) in press.
3. Biozzi, G., Stiffel, C., Mouton, D., Bouthillier, Y., and Decreusefond, C., Ann. Immunol. 235C (1974) 107.
4. Biozzi, G., Stiffel, C., Mouton, D., and Bouthillier, Y., In: Immunogenetics and Immunodeficiency (Ed. B. Benacerraf), MTP Publishing Co. (1975) 179.
5. Biozzi, G., Stiffel, C., Mouton, D., Bouthillier, Y., and Decreusefond, C., In: Progress in Immunology, N. Y., Academic Press (1971) 529.
6. Blum, K., and Cioli, D., Eur. J. Immunol. 8 (1978) 52.
7. Byfield, P. E., and Howard, J. G., Transplantation 14 (1972) 133.
8. Del Guercio, P., and Zola, H., Immunochemistry, 9 (1972) 769.
9. Dodin, A., Wiart, J., Stiffel, C., Bouthillier, Y., Mouton, D., Decreusefond, C., and Biozzi, G., Ann. Inst. Pasteur, 1 23 (1972) 137.
10. Feingold, N., Feingold, J., Mouton, D., Bouthillier, Y., Stiffel, C., and Biozzi, G., Eur. J. Immunol. 6 (1976) 43.
11. Heumann, A. M. and Stiffel, C., Ann. Immunol. 129C (1978) 13.
12. Howard, J. G., Christie, G. H., Courtenay, B. M., and Biozzi, G., Eur. J. Immunol. 2 (1972) 269.
13. Howard, J. C., Courtenay, B. M., and Desaymard, C., Eur. J. Immunol. 4 (1974) 453.
14. Kierzenbaum and Howard, J. G., J. Immunol. 116 (1976) 208.

15. Liacopoulos-Briot, M., Bouthillier, Y., Mouton, D., Lambert, F., Decreusefond, C., Stiffel, C., and Biozzi, G., Transplantation 14 (1972) 590.

16. Liacopoulos-Briot, M., Mouton, D., Stiffel, C., Lambert, F., Decreusefond, C., Bouthillier, Y., and Biozzi, G., Ann. Immunol. 125C (1974) 26.

17. Mouton, D., Bouthillier, Y., Heumann, A. M., Stiffel, C. and Biozzi, G., In: The Reticuloendothelial system in Health and Disease: functions and characteristics (Ed. S. M. Reichard, M. R. Escobar and H. Friedman), Plenum Publishing Co., New York (1976) 225.

18. Mouton, D., Bouthillier, Y., Oriol, R., Decreusefond, C., Stiffel, C., and Biozzi, G., Ann. Immunol. 125C (1974) 581.

19. Prouvost-Danon, A., Mouton, D., Abadie, A., Mevel, J. C., and Biozzi, G., Eur. J. Immunol. 6 (1977) 342.

20. Sant'Anna, O. A., Bouthillier, Y., Siqueira, M., and Biozzi, G., in press.

THE CHEMOTACTIC, PHAGOCYTIC, AND MICROBIAL KILLING ABILITIES OF PRIMATE POLYMORPHONUCLEAR LEUKOCYTES (PML)

J. W. EICHBERG[1], S. S. KALTER[1], W. T. KNIKER[2], R. W. STEEL[3], and R. L. HEBERLING[1]
[1]Southwest Foundation for Research and Education, [2]The University of Texas Health Science Center at San Antonio, [3]Brooke Army Medical Center - San Antonio, Texas (USA)

Studies with nonhuman primates have demonstrated graded susceptibility to viral infections (especially by herpesviruses) and oncogenesis (1,3,6). Such differences have been related to variations in the degree of humoral and cell-mediated immune responsiveness (5,7,9,10,20,31). However, when somewhat primitive cellular responses, such as mixed lymphocyte response and skin graft rejection, of relatively immunodeficient cotton-top marmosets were compared to those of more immunocompetent baboons and cebus monkeys no significant differences were noticed (19).

The current study was conducted to establish a profile of nonspecific immune defenses in three nonhuman primate species and compare these to humans. Chemotactic, phagocytic, and killing functions of blood leukocytes, predominantly polymorphonuclear (PMN) leukocytes, were investigated.

MATERIALS AND METHODS

Animals. Normal adult baboons (Papio cynocephalus), cebus monkeys (Cebus apella), and cotton-top marsosets (Sanguinus oedipus) were studied. The animals were of approximately equal sex distribution. Seven animals of each species were used for the study of chemotaxis, and six for evaluation of phagocytosis and killing. Seven normal adult human volunteers were also studied for a comparison of results obtained from nonhuman primates.

Chemotaxis. To collect white blood cells, heparinized blood

(1,000 units of heparin per 2 ml of blood) was mixed with 6% dextran and allowed to sediment for 1 hr. The plasma containing the white blood cells was aspirated, diluted with an equal volume of RPMI 1640 medium, and adjusted to a pH of 7.4. After centrifugation at 160 g for 12 min, supernatants were discarded and cells were resuspended in medium containing Tween 80 (0.04%). Differential and total white blood cell counts were performed to determine percent and absolute numbers of neutrophils (PMNs) and lymphocytes present in the samples. Cells were adjusted to 2 x 10^6 neutrophils per ml.

Serum from each animal was "activated" by adding 150 μg of lipopolysaccharide (LPS from Serratia marcescens) to the clotted blood for 1 ½ hr at 37 C. Control serum from the same animal was incubated under the same conditions but not treated with LPS. After centrifugation at 500 x g for 15 min, the decanted serum was inactivated in a 56 C water bath for 30 min. A 20% serum dilution in RPMI, pH 7.4, was then prepared. Using a Boyden chamber, 0.5 ml (1 x 10^6 PMNs) were added to the inner chamber and 1 ml of activated or unactivated control serum was added to the outer chamber. After centrifugation at 90 x g, the chambers were incubated at 37 C for 3 hr. The filters were removed from the bottom of the inner chamber and stained with hematoxylin and eosin. Using a light microscope, the number of PMNs per high power field that had migrated to the bottom of the filters were counted. Every test was performed in duplicate and cells from normal healthy humans were included as controls. A chemotactic index (CI) was derived by dividing the number of PMNs that migrated to the bottom of the filter in the presence of activated serum by the number of PMNs that migrated in the presence of the control serum.

Phagocytic and microbiocidal assays. A fluorochrome microassay recently developed by Pantazis and Kniker was used (14,17); procedural details appear in the latter reference. Monolayers of leukocytes were prepared by placing five drops of fresh blood onto each of six flat, sterile glass coverslips per tested animal. The blood was allowed to clot while incubating at 37 C in humidified 5% CO_2 for 1 hr. Clots were removed by washing gently with prewarmed Hanks' Balanced Salt Solution (HESS), leaving behind a cellular film. Two drops of a standardized suspension of microorganisms were then placed onto the leukocyte monolayers. For E. coli, 2.5 x 10^6 organisms per ml were suspended in McCoy's 5A medium containing 10% fetal calf serum. For Staphylococcus aureus, 1.25 x 10^6 freshly prepared, viable organisms per ml were suspended in McCoy's 5A medium containing 10% autologous serum. For Candida albicans, yeast phase organisms were suspended in the same medium as for S. aureus, at a concentration of 2.5 x 10^6 organisms per ml.

During 90 min of incubation at 37 C, the coverslips were rotated at 60 rpm. Afterward, the monolayers were gently washed two

times with HBSS, then stained 1 min with acridine orange (3.3 x
10^{-5} M) dissolved in Gey's solution. Stained coverslips were
mounted face down and examined with an ultraviolet light microscope. Several fields of 100 cells each were counted and the
number of ingested organisms was recorded: green organisms were
considered viable and red organisms dead. Phagocytic capacity
was determined as the average number of organisms ingested by 100
neutrophils. Microbial killing was recorded as the percentage of
dead (red) organisms of the total phagocytosed (red plus green).
All tests were performed in duplicate, and normal human cells were
included as reference controls for the procedure.

Statistical analysis. The paired t-test and analysis of var-
iance were performed on a Compucorp 142E Statistician calculator
using the appropriate punch card program.

RESULTS

The chemotaxis data are presented in Table I. In all species,
numbers of migrating cells in control systems (unactivated serum)
were comparable in their marked variability. There were no statistically significant differences in chemotactic indices among the
three nonhuman primate species and man. In activated serum systems, the average number of cells migrating through the filter was
also not different among the four species investigated, with the
exception of the cebus monkey, whose numbers of migrating cells
were significantly lower than those of the baboon ($p<0.01$) and
marmoset monkey ($p<0.05$).

The capability of adherent blood leukocytes to ingest and
kill bacteria and fungi is presented in Table II. Total ingestion of candida was significantly reduced in the two relatively
primitive New World primate species, the cebus monkey and the
marmoset. As compared to humans, leukocytes from the three nonhuman primate species had a lower capacity for killing bacteria
and fungi which had been ingested. This difference in microbiocidal capacity between the human and the nonhuman primates was
statistically significant.

TABLE I

Average Chemotactic Response of Leukocytes from Four Primate Species

	Human (7)	Baboon (7)	Cebus (7)	Marmoset (7)
Unactivated serum	9.9 ± 6.1	29.3 ± 30.2	12.1 ± 9.4	23.8 ± 35.0
Activated serum	63.4 ± 32.8[a]	89.7 ± 27.7	43.3 ± 18.5[b]	79.2 ± 35.0
CI[c]	10.6 ± 11.6	5.4 ± 3.3	5.4 ± 3.7	8.9 ± 8.5

[a]Mean ± S. D.

[b]$p < 0.01$ when compared to baboon. $p < 0.05$ when compared to marmoset.

[c]CI = Chemotactic Index = $\dfrac{\text{Number of PMNs migrating through filters in activated serum}}{\text{Number of PMNs migrating through filter in unactivated serum}}$

TABLE II

Microbial Ingestion and Killing by Leukocytes from Four Primate Species

Source of Blood Leukocytes	E. coli		S. aureus		C. albicans		Total Ingested		Percent Killed	
	Total Ingested[a]	Percent Killed[b]	Total Ingested	Percent Killed	Total Ingested	Percent Killed	F	P	F	P
Human (6)	182 % 105	85 % 12	205 % 74	85 % 13	119 % 68	69 % 18	1.78	>0.1	2.08	>0.1
Baboon (6)	283 % 96	46 % 9	322 % 184	63 % 12	171 % 46	38 % 18	2.48	>0.1	6.40	<0.01
Cebus (6)	214 % 30	37 % 5	342 % 13	52 % 14	68 % 24	37 % 12	19.09	<0.005	3.44	>0.1
Marmoset (6)	152 % 70	45 % 17	427 % 283	50 % 13	69 % 14	28 % 13	7.39	<0.005	3.98	<0.05
F	2.99	18.56	1.42	8.75	7.66	7.36				
P	>0.005	<0.005	>0.1	<0.005	<0.005	<0.005				

[a]Ingested = Total number of red and green microorganisms per 100 adherent leukocytes.
[b]Killed = Number of red microorganisms per 100 adherent leukocytes divided by the total number ingested X 100.

DISCUSSION

Cell-mediated and humoral immune competence of the four primate species described herein have been assessed previously by a variety of in vivo and in vitro tests (7,10,19,20). Using humans as a reference, we found the immune competence of baboons to be similar to that of the humans, while the cebus monkey seemed to be less competent, and marmosets ranked last. These differences may be correlated with the degree of susceptibility of these species to certain viral infections and/or tumor induction by viruses (5,7,10,13,20,31). However, when compared by ontogenetically and phylogenetically more primitive immune responses, such as mixed lymphocyte reactivity in vitro and skin graft rejection in vivo (19), all three species have been shown to be similar to humans.

This report compares the response in primates of even more primitive defense mechanisms--the chemotactic, phagocytic, and microbial killing functions of blood leukocytes. There is general agreement that susceptibility to bacterial, and fungal illness is closely related to PMN function (8,11,15). Of three PMN functions, including phagocytosis, killing, and chemotaxis, the importance of the latter in inflammatory processes is least well defined (4,12). Directional migration is considered to be regulated by a very complex system (8), and the use of one particular cytotaxin (LPS) in our study might only partially reflect chemotactic capabilities of PMNs in the four species studied. Because of extensive variability, especially among the human chemotactic data, these higher chemotactic values of humans were not supported statistically. However, they tended to be higher than their nonhuman counterparts, which also did not differ significantly from each other.

Since its original introduction (21,22), acridine orange as a vital stain has been used to demonstrate dead or viable mammalian cells (23) or bacteria (2,16,18) and fungi (13). With a new fluorochrome microassay developed by Pantazis and Kniker (14), one can easily evaluate the viability of the blood leukocytes, as well as their ability to ingest and kill microorganisms. Phagocytic and microbiocidal data in the six humans employed in this study were comparable to those reported in the human controls reported in other studies (14,17), demonstrating the reproducibility and reliability of the method.

All nonhuman primate species exhibited poor killing of bacteria and candida in relation to man, although their phagocytic capacity for bacteria was comparable to or greater than that in humans. Since the nonhuman primates do not ordinarily suffer from serious recurrent bacterial infections, the significance of relatively poor in vitro bacterial killing is doubtful. On the other hand, cebus monkey and marmoset leukocytes exhibited poor phagocytosis and poor killing of candida organisms. Whether this impaired PMN function has any relationship to fungal ailments occasionally observed in these New World monkeys is unknown. Nevertheless, this report adds additional data to previous studies on the comparative immunocompetence of human and nonhuman primates.

SUMMARY

Functions of polymorphonuclear leukocytes including chemotaxis, phagocytosis, and microbial killing were investigated in baboons (<u>Papio cynocephalus</u>), cebus monkeys (<u>Cebus apella</u>), and marmosets (<u>Saguinus oedipus</u>). Cells from a group of normal adult human volunteers were also studied for comparison. Polymorphonuclear leukocytes from the three nonhuman primate species were comparable to each other and to humans in chemotactic activity using endotoxin activated serum. In addition, the ability of blood leukocytes to ingest and kill microorganisms was investigated using a new fluorochrome microassay. Leukocytes of all nonhuman primates were competent in phagocytosing bacteria, but leukocytes from cebus monkeys and marmosets ingested candida organisms poorly. Compared to humans, all nonhuman primates exhibited poor killing of the microbes.

ACKNOWLEDGEMENTS

This study was supported by USPHS Grant 5 RO1 CA15842. We appreciate the excellent technical assistance of Joyce McBride.

REFERENCES

1.   Barahona, H., Melendez, L. V., and Melnick, J. L., Intervirology, 3 (1974) 175.
2.   Casida, L. E., Jr., Can. J. Microbiol., 8 (1962) 115.
3.   Deinhardt, F. W., Falk, L. A., and Wolfe, L. G., Adv. Cancer Res., 19 (1974) 167.
4.   Harris, H., Physiol. Rev., 34 (1954) 529.
5.   Harvey, J. S., Jr., Felsburg, P. J., Heberling, R. L., Kniker, W. T., and Kalter, S. S., Clin. Exp. Immunol., 16 (1974) 267.
6.   Kalter, S. S., Felsburg, P. J., Heberling, R. L., Nahmias, A. J., and Brack, M., Proc. Soc. Exp. Biol. Med., 139 (1972) 964.
7.   Kalter, S. S., Heberling, R. L., Felsburg, P. J., McCullough, B., Eichberg, J. W., Kniker, W. T., Harvey, J. S., Jr., Macias, E. G., Eller, J. J., Rommel, F. A. and Steel, R. W., (Eds. de-Thé, M. A. Epstein and H. Zur Hausen), IARC Scientific Publications No. 11), Lyon, International Agency for Research on Cancer (1975) 133.

8. Keller, H. U., Hess, M. W., and Cottier, H., Semin. Hematol.,
    12 (1975) 47.
9. Klein, G., Pearson, G., Rabson, A., Ablashi, D. V., Falk, L.,
    Wolfe, L., Deinhardt, F., and Rabin, H., Int. J. Cancer, 12
    (1973) 270.
10. Kniker, W. T., Macias, E. G., Steele, R. W., Heberling, R.
    L. and Eller, J. J., Fed. Proc.; Fed. Am. Soc. Exp. Biol.,
    34 (1975) 824.
11. McCall, C., Caves, J., Cooper, R. and DeChatelet, L., J. Infect
    Dis., 124 (1971) 68.
12. Miller, M. E., Semin. Hematol., 12 (1975) 59.
13. Mote, R. F., Muhm, R. L., and Gistad, D. C., Stain Technol.,
    50 (1975) 5.
14. Pantazis, C. G., and Kniker, W. T., Clin. Res., 25 (1977) 76A.
15. Quie, P. G., Polymorphonuclear leukocyte dysfunction in
    patients with severe infections. In: "non-Specific" Factors
    Influencing Host Resistance; A Reexamination, (Eds. W. Braun
    and J. Ungar), Karger, Basel and New York, (1973) 68.
16. Ranade, S. S., Tatake, V. G., and Korgoankar, K. S., Nature
    (London), 189 (1961) 931.
17. Smith, D. L., and Rommel, F., J. Immunol. Methods, 17 (1977)
    241.
18. Silver, S., Levine, E., and Spielman, P. M., J. Bacteriol.,
    95 (1968) 333.
19. Steele, R. W., Eichberg, J. W., Heberling, R. L., Kalter, S.
    S., and Kniker, W. T., J. Med. Primatol., 6 (1977) 119.
20. Steele, R. W., Eichberg, J. W., Heberling, R. L., Eller, J.
    J., Goldstein, A. L., Kalter, S. S. and Kniker, W. T., J.
    Med. Primatol., 6 (1977) 163.
21. Strugger, S., Fluoreszenmikroskopie und Mikrobiologie, M &
    H, Schaper, Hannover, (1949) 194.
22. Strugger, S., Jena. Z. Naturw., 73 (1940) 97.
23. Wolf, M. K., and Aronson, S. B., J. Histochem. Cytochem.,
    9 (1961) 22.

PROTECTIVE EFFECT OF PSK, A PROTEIN-BOUND POLYSACCHARIDE PREPARA-

TION AGAINST CANDIDIASIS IN TUMOR-BEARING MICE

A. UETSUKA, S. SATOH and Y. OHNO

Laboratory of Medical Mycology, Dept. of Infectious
Diseases, Institute of Medical Science, University of
Tokyo, Tokyo, (JAPAN)

It is well known that the depression of the immune capacity in
cancer patients very often causes a variety of infectious diseases
by such opportunistic pathogens as Candida sp. (10). Recently, much
attention has been given to cancer immunotherapy, in which therapeutic effects can be brought by restoring or enhancing the
depressed immune capacity in cancer patients.

PSK, one of the immunostimulative anticancer agents is
extracted and purified from cultivated mycelia of a basidiomycete,
Coriolus versicolor, (CM-101. The preparation consists of protein
bound polysaccharide with a mean molecular weight of about 100,000
which contains about 18-38% of protein. The major polysaccharide
moiety of PSK is assumed to be $\beta 1 \rightarrow 4$ glucan which is branched at
3- and 6- positions at the rate of one per several glucose
residues (1,2). Acute toxicity is considerably low; for instance,
LD_{50} to mice and rats is more than 5 g/kg by intraperitoneal route
and 20 g/kg by oral route (6). There are no abnormal findings
due to oral administration of PSK at a dose of 1000 mg/kg/day for
180 consecutive days in mice, rats, dogs and monkeys. The
clinical application of PSK was already approved for stomach
cancer, esophagus cancer, rectum and colon cancer, lung cancer
and breast cancer by the Japanese Ministry of Welfare. PSK can
be expected to exert host-mediated protection against infectious
diseases as well as cancer. In the present paper, the protective
effect against experimental Candidiasis in tumor-bearing mice will
be discussed.

MATERIALS AND METHODS

Experimental candidiasis. About 15 of ddY mice (5 weeks old)
were used for each group in the experiments. A mouse was subcutaneously implanted with 2×10^6 cells of Sarcoma 180 solid
type. One day after tumor implantation, the mouse was inoculated
with 1×10^7 cells of Candida tropicalis ATCC 750 or Candida
albicans ATCC 752 intravenously. PSK supplied by Kureha Chem. Ind.
Co., Ltd. (Tokyo, Japan) was intraperitoneally administered at a
dose of 50 mg/kg every day 7 times before infection for the
pretreatment group, every other day 10 times before and after
infection for the pre- and post-treatment group; and every other
day 10 times after infection for the post-treatment group. Infected mice were fed for 3 weeks to examine mortality, viable fungal
cell count and histopathological feature of kidney, and tumor growth.

Clearance of C. Tropicalis from primary organs and blood. By
the same procedure as the experimental Candidiasis, tumor-bearing
mice were inoculated with C. tropicalis. Viable fungal counts from
liver, spleen, kidney and blood of survived mice were determined
at the appropriate intervals of time time during 3 weeks after
infection. One group of tumor-bearing mice was pre- and post-
treated with PSK.

Delayed-type hypersensitivity reaction. As an antigen, Candida
dead cells were applied for footpad reaction in tumor-bearing mice
infected with C. tropicalis or C. albicans. The same procedure
and schedule as those in the experimental candidiasis mentioned
before, was used for tumor implantation, Candida inoculation and
PSK administration. Candida heated cells (1×10^7) were injected
into the footpad of a mouse for immunization 7 days after infection
An increase of thickness in footpad was measured 24 hr after
immunization.

Peritoneal exudate cells (PEC). The effect of PSK administration on peritoneal exudate cells (PEC) in normal mice was examined
with 3% thioglycollate medium or C. tropicalis dead cells as an
irritant. Mice were intraperitoneally pretreated at a dose of
50 mg/kg of PSK every day 3 times. The irritants were intraperitoneally injected to mice after PSK pretreatment. Peritoneal
exudate cells were recovered on 1st and 4th day after irritation.
The total cell number was determined in a hemocytometer. The
numbers of macrophages and polymorphonuclear leukocytes were
microscopically examined by May-Grünwald staining.

Phagocytosis of C. tropicalis by peritoneal macrophages. The
effect of PSK administration on phagocytosis of C. tropicalis by
peritoneal macrophages from normal and tumor-bearing mice was
examined in vitro (8). PSK was intraperitoneally administered at
a dose of 100 mg/kg every day 5 times. Immediately after the

final administration of PSK, one ml of 0.1% glycogen was intraperitoneally injected to a mouse, and 3 days later, peritoneal
exudate cells were harvested with Eagle MEM medium.   Sarcoma
180 was subcutaneously implanted for the tumor-bearing goup one
day before the harvest. For comparison to PSK, a polysaccharide
(9) extracted from C. tropicalis by the Westphal method was applied
for a part of the experiment.

For in vitro phagocytosis, adherent cells which were separated
on coverslips were mixed with C. tropicalis viable cells (1:1 or
1:10) to incubate in Eagle MEM medium supplemented with 10% calf
serum at 37 C for 3 hr. At given intervals of time, coverslips
were taken out of culture bottles and double-stained with May-
Grünwald and Giemsa solutions. Phagocytic index was expressed as
percentage of phagocytized macrophages to total number of macrophages.

RESULTS

The results of experimental Candidiasis are shown in Fig. 1-4.
Pre- and post-treatment of PSK apparently prolonged the lifespan
of mice infected with C. tropicalis, as shown in Fig. 1. The period of time corresponding to 50% survival was 8 days for the control
group without PSK administration. PSK post-treatment, however,
brought about no prolongation of the lifespan. On the other hand,
any PSK administration did not affect the life prolongation of
infected nontumor-bearing mice, although the results are not shown.
The tumor growth was remarkably inhibited by PSK administration in
this experiment as well as other experiments. The mean tumor size
was 108 mm^2/mouse in the pre- and post-treatment group, 94 mm^2/mouse
in the post-treatment group and 233 mm^2/mouse in the control group
3 weeks after tumor implantation. It was preliminarily ascertained
that tumor-bearing mice never died of tumor proliferation within
3 weeks after tumor implantation, unless infected with Candida sp.

Against C. albicans infection, pre- and post-treatment of PSK
seemed to be more effective than post-treatment, although not
markedly (Fig. 2).

The protective effect of PSK pretreatment in tumor-bearing
mice inoculated with C. tropicalis or C. albicans was compared
to the pre- and post-treatment. As the results, a prolongation
of lifespan was observed in the pretreated mice as well (Figs. 3
and 4).

In comparison of mean viable fungal cell counts from kidneys
among three groups of tumor-bearing mice which survived 3 weeks
after infection, PSK treatment could restrain the counts to lower
levels than the control (Table I). Particularly the pre- and

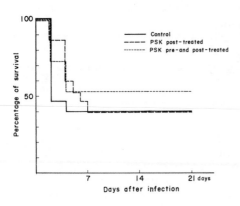

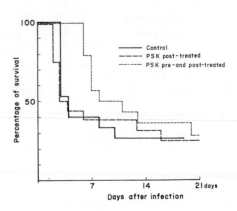

Fig. 1.   Effect of PSK on survival of tumor-bearing mice inoculated with C. tropicalis.

Fig. 2.   Effect of PSK on survival of tumor-bearing mice
inoculated with C. albicans.

post-treatment was most effective against fungal growth in kidney.

    Viable fungal counts of liver, spleen, kidney and blood in
infected mice were compared among three groups as shown in Fig. 5-
8.

    Among three groups of mice, there was no marked difference
in viable counts of liver and spleen. The viable count in kidney
of the tumor-bearing mice showed an increase from 1st to 3rd day
of infection, while such an increase was not found in other groups,
i.e., the nontumor-bearing mice and the tumor-bearing mice treated

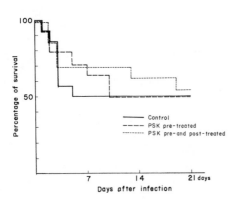

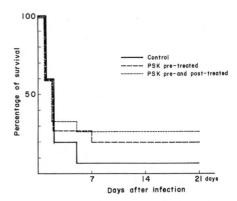

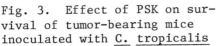

Fig. 3.   Effect of PSK on survival of tumor-bearing mice
inoculated with C. tropicalis

Fig. 4.   Effect of PSK on survival of tumor-bearing mice
inoculated with C. albicans.

TABLE I

Effect of PSK Viable Fungal Count from Kidney of Tumor-Bearing
Mice Survived 3 Weeks After Candidal Infection

Inoculum	PSK Administration	21 Days After Infection
C. tropical-	Control	3.8×10^5
is	Pretreated	2.4×10^5
	Pre- and post-treated	4.8×10^4
C. albicans	Control	4.8×10^5
	Pretreated	3.8×10^4
	Pre- and post-treated	1.0×10^4

with PSK. Viable fungal cells were cleared off out of the blood
of the tumor-bearing mice treated with PSK on the 7th day of infection or later, although fungal cells still remained in the blood
of other two groups.

In the delayed-type hypersensitivity reaction against Candida
dead cells as an antigen, there was a greater increase in thickness
of footpad of the tumor-bearing mice treated with PSK than the
control mice and the tumor-bearing mice without PSK administration
(Fig. 6).

The total number of peritoneal exudate cells (PEC) from both
normal mice and PSK-treated mice showed an increase over 10^7/ml on
1st day of irritation with 3% thioglycollate medium or C. tropicalis
dead cells. A decrease in total number of PEC occurred on 4th day
in the control, but the number of PEC from PSK-treated mice still
remained over 10^7/ml without showing such a decrease (Fig. 7).

The number of macrophages from PSK-treated mice was always
maintained from 1st to 4th day at a higher level than that from the
control, as shown in Fig. 8.

A rapid decrease of polymorphonuclear leukocyte counts was
found from 1st to 4th day. There was a discrepancy between the
control mice and PSK-treated mice, somewhat when using thioglycollate medium as an irritant (Fig. 9).

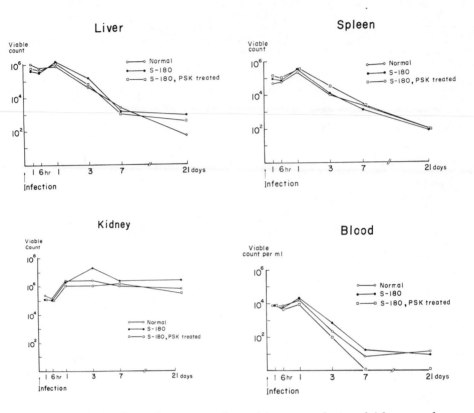

Fig. 5. Viable fungal counts from liver, spleen, kidney and blood of normal and tumor-bearing mice, treated with PSK and inoculated with C. tropicalis.

Phagocytosis of C. tropicalis viable cells by peritoneal macrophages (1:1) derived from normal mice treated with PSK or Candida polysaccharide was enhanced remarkably, particularly when mice were treated with PSK. Phagocytic index at 3 hr of incubation was 20% for the control, 50% for the mice treated with Candida polysaccharide and 80% for the PSK-treated mice (Fig. 10).

Phagocytosis by macrophages derived from tumor-bearing mice was suppressed to some extent, compared to macrophages from normal mice. The administration of PSK to tumor-bearing mice enhanced the suppressed phagocytic capacity over a restoration to normal level. In this case (Macrophages: Candida cells = 1:10), phagocytic index was 46% for the control (normal mice), 53% for the tumor-bearing mice and 72% for the PSK-treated tumor-bearing mice at 3 hr of incubation (Fig. 11).

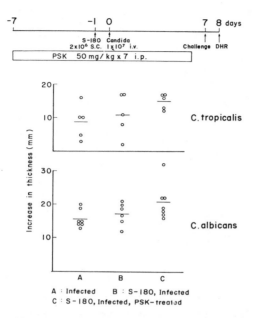

Fig. 6.   Effect of PSK administration on footpad reaction against Candida dead cells in tumor-bearing mice inoculated with C. tropicalis or C. albicans.

DISCUSSION

From the results of experimental Candidiasis in tumor-bearing mice, the PSK administration prior to infection was rather more effective on prolongation of lifespan than the administration after infection (Fig. 1-4). A prolongation of lifespan by PSK administration occurred within one week after infection. It suggests that at the early stage of infection, PSK takes part in restoration of host-protection which was depressed under the tumor-bearing condition. As a matter of fact, no enhancement of protection against infection by PSK administration was found in normal (non-tumor-bearing) mice.

Nomoto, K. et al. (5) reported that the capacities of mice to produce IgG antibody against sheep erythrocyte (SRBC), IgM antibody against hamster erythrocyte (HRBC), and IgG antibody against trinitrophenyl group (TNP) were depressed after implantation of Sarcoma 180 and were restored by intraperitoneal injection of PSK to the normal levels. In addition, Matsunaga, K. et al. (3) reported that resistance against the infection of Listeria monocytogenes in mice once depressed in the earlier period after Sarcoma 180 implantation was restored to the normal level by the

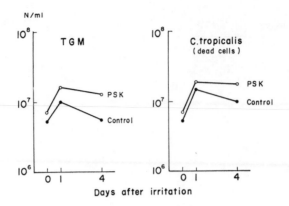

Fig. 7. Effect of PSK on PEC (peritoneal exudate cells) chemotaxis in vivo with thioglycollate medium or C. tropicallis dead
cells as irritant in normal mice.

combined therapy of PSK with operation. These immunological findings in the previous reports explains the results of experimental
Candidiasis shown in Fig. 1-4 so well.

The fact was reported by Nakano, Y. et al. (4) that the decrease of delayed-type skin reaction using hapten type antigen,
picryl chloride in Sarcoma 180-bearing mice was prevented by PSK
administration. In the present experiment with Candida dead cells
as antigen, such a prevention of decrease in footpad reaction of
tumor-bearing mice seemed to be brought about by PSK administration as well.

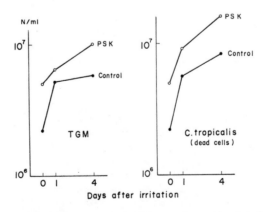

Fig. 8. Effect of PSK on macrophage chemotaxis in vivo with
thioglycollate medium or C. tropicalis dead cells as irritant
in normal mice.

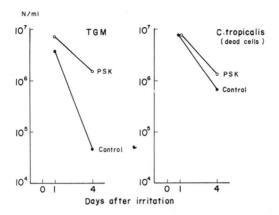

Fig. 9.   Effect of PSK on PMN (polymorphonuclear leukocyte) chemotaxis *in* *vivo* with thioglycollate medium or Candida dead cells
as irritant in normal mice.

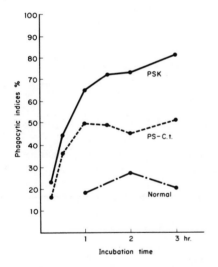

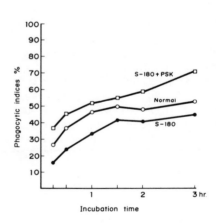

Fig. 10.   Phagocytosis of C.
tropicalis (viable cells) by
peritoneal macrophages from
normal mice treated with PSK or
PS-C.t. (C. tropicalis polysaccharide).

Fig. 11. Phagocytosis of C. tropicalis (viable cells) by peritoneal
macrophages from tumor-bearing mice
treated with PSK.

The viable fungal counts of kidneys which are primary target organs in Candidiasis, increased from 1st to 3rd day of infection in tumor-bearing mice, as shown in Fig. 7. On the other hand no increase occurred at all in tumor-bearing mice treated with PSK as well as normal mice. The prevention of fungal proliferation in kidneys by PSK administration accounts for the prolongation of life-span and implies a vigorous ingestion of Candida cells by phago-cytes during the earlier period of infection.

The experiments on chemotaxis and phagocytosis indicated that total PEC and peritoneal macrophages from PSK-treated mice increased in number on 1st and 4th day of irritation with Candida dead cells, and in vitro phagocytosis of Candida viable cells by peritoneal macrophages from both normal and tumor-bearing mice was definitely enhanced by PSK administration to mice in advance.

On the whole, these experimental results suggest that PSK administration restores the depressed protection of tumor-bearing mice against Candida infection, by enhancing the function of non-immune phagocytes, particularly macrophages.

SUMMARY

In an experimental Candidiasis of tumor-bearing mice, the administration of PSK resulted in a prolongation of lifespan when mice were treated with PSK before infection or before and after infection. The viable fungal counts in kidneys 3 weeks after infection was found to be less in PSK-treated mice than the control mice without PSK administration. The delayed-type hypersensitivity reaction in infected tumor-bearing mice against Candida dead cells were stimulated to some extent by PSK administration. The fungal proliferation in kidneys of tumor-bearing mice at the early stage of infection was prevented by PSK administration. The experimental results involving chemotaxis and phagocytosis suggest that PSK administration restores or enhances the depressed protection of tumor-bearing mice against Candida infection, mostly due to potentiating the phagocytic activity of macrophages.

REFERENCES

1. Hirase, S. et al. J. Pharmaceut. Soc. of Japan 96 (1976) (413.
2. Hirase, S. et al. J. Pharmaceut. Soc. of Japan 96 (1976) 419.
3. Matsunaga, K. et al. Proc. of 35th Ann. Meeting, Jap. Cancer Assoc., Abst. No. 486 (1976)
4. Nakano, Y. et al. Cancer and Chemotherap. 2 (1975) 13.
5. Nomoto, K. et al. GANN 66 (1975) 365.

6,   Tsukagoshi, S.   Cancer and Chemotherap. 1 (1974) 251.
7.   Uetsuka, A. et al. In: Chemotherapy (Eds. J. D. Williams
     and A. M. Geddes) Plenum Publishing Corp., New York 6 (1976)
     157.
8.   Uetsuka, A. et al. Proc. of 21st Ann. Mtg. The Jap. Soc. for
     Med. Mycol., Abstract No. 45 (1977)
9.   Uetsuka, A. et al. Proc. of 10th Intern. Cong. Chemotherapy,
     Abstract No. 101, Zürich (1977)
10. Young, R. C. et al. Ann. of Intern. Med. 80 (1974) 605.

PHAGOCYTOSIS OF CANDIDA ALBICANS BY POLYMORPHONUCLEAR LEUKOCYTES

FROM NORMAL AND DIABETIC SUBJECTS

R. A. JACKSON, C. S. BRYAN, and B. A. WEEKS

University of South Carolina School of Medicine
Columbia, South Carolina (USA)

Systemic candidiasis poses many diagnostic and therapeutic problems and is being encountered with increasing frequency in many medical centers. The basis for the pathogenicity of Candida albicans, and for the occurrence of invasive disease in some patients but not in most individuals colonized with this ubiquitous yeast, remains incompletely understood. Intact polymorphonuclear leukocyte (PMNL) function may be especially crucial for defense against invasive candidiasis (1).

Previous studies by one of us and co-authors (5) established that isolates of C. albicans vary considerably in virulence, in an avian model. The virulence of C. albicans for chickens, determined by morbidity and mortality, could be ranked systematically and could be shown to correlate with the mannan content of the yeast cell wall (5). The present studies extend these observations to man.

MATERIALS AND METHODS

Two isolates of C. albicans previously ranked for virulence in the avian model (5) were selected for these studies: strain 69 (virulent) and strain FBW (avirulent). These strains were allowed to grow overnight and were then suspended in Geys balanced salt solution.

Phagocytosis assays were done using a modification of the method of Leijh and colleagues (2). PMNL were obtained from EDTA-treated blood derived from normal and diseased individuals. A purified leukocyte suspension was obtained by placing blood on

33

Ficoll-Hypaque, centrifuging, and lysing the remaining red blood cells with distilled water.

The yeast suspension was adjusted to 1×10^7/ml, and the PMNL suspension was adjusted to 2×10^6/ml, by hemocytometer counts. Phagocytosis assays were performed by incubating 5×10^6 C. albicans with 2.5×10^6 PMNL to give a ratio of 2 yeast cells to 1 leukocyte in 0.1 ml of serum. The suspension was incubated at 37 C in a shaker bath. At 15 min intervals, 0.1 ml of the C. albicans leukocyte suspension was placed in formalin. The number of yeast cells lying completely free in the suspension was determined on a hemocytometer and taken as the measure of phagocytosis. Data were statistically evaluated by the Student's t-test.

RESULTS

Studies of phagocytosis in normal subjects revealed no difference in the ability of leukocytes to engulf the virulent (strain 69) as opposed to the avirulent (strain FBW) C. albicans.

Blood was obtained from five adult patients with diabetes mellitus in poor chemical control (mean fasting blood glucose value 331 mg/dl, range 271-400 mg/dl at the time of study) who were not in ketoacidosis. Their leukocytes showed no impairment of phagocytosis of the avirulent strain (FBW) compared to leukocytes from normal subjects. However, against the virulent strain (69), phagocytosis by the leukocytes from diabetic patients was impaired compared to leukocytes from normal subjects. The differences were statistically significant at 90 min only Table I).

Phagocytosis of the avirulent strain (FBW) by leukocytes from a diabetic patient with marked hyperglycemia (blood glucose 900 mg/dl) was also impaired, relative to phagocytosis by leukocytes from a normal subject studied simultaneously (Fig. 1).

An additional diabetic patient in ketoacidosis (blood glucose 471, CO_2 combining power 8, arterial pH 7.21) was studied. Compared to leukocytes from a normal subject, his leukocytes showed marked impairment of phagocytosis against the virulent strain (69) (Fig. 2).

DISCUSSION

We explored the possibility that strains of C. albicans with varying mannan content might differ in susceptibility to phagocytosis by human PMNL. When the leukocytes were obtained from normal subjects, no differences could be demonstrated.

TABLE I

Phagocytosis of C. Albicans by Leukocytes from Normal
Subjects and From Patients with Poorly-Controlled Diabetes

Group	Phagocytosis (Percent)[a]		
	15 min	30 min	90 min
Normal subjects	41.8 ± 7.3	59.2 ± 10.4	96.3 ± 5.6
Diabetes mellitus	39.2 ± 0.8[b]	54.2 ± 2.9[b]	86.6 ± 2.4[c]

[a]Values were mean ± S. D.
[b]These values do not differ (p>0.05) from the normal subjects.
[c]This value differs (p<0.001) from the normal subjects.

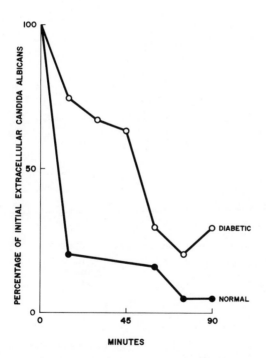

Fig. 1.   Phagocytosis of C. albicans strain FBW by leukocytes from
normal subject and from diabetic patient with marked hyperglycemia.

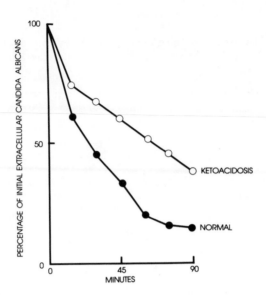

Fig. 2. Phagocytosis of C. albicans strain 69 by leukocytes from
normal subject and from patient with diabetic ketoacidosis.

However, significant impairment of phagocytosis of the virulent strain (69) of C. albicans by leukocytes from non-ketotic,
poorly-controlled diabetic patients was demonstrated, Impairment of phagocytosis of the avirulent strain (FBW) by leukocytes
from a patient with extreme hyperglycemia (blood glucose 900 mg/dl)
was also documented. Phagocytosis of the virulent strain was impaired in a patient with diabetic ketoacidosis.

Studies of phagocytosis of C albicans are given to problems
of interpretation (3), and previous investigations of leukocyte
function in diabetic patients have been conflicting (4). The present studies suggest that some of the discrepancies evident in the
literature might be explained by differences in strain virulence.
Thus, further characterization of these strains might be useful to
the study of both the epidemiology and the pathophysiology of
systemic candidiasis.

REFERENCES

1. Edwards, J. E., Jr., Lehrer, R. I., Steihmn, E. R., Fischer,
     T. J., and Young, L. S., Ann. Intern. Med., 89 (1978) 91.
2. Leijh, P. C. J., Van den Barselaar, M. T., and Van Furth, R.,

Infect. Immun., 17 (1977) 313.
3. Solomkin, J. S., Mills, E. L., Giebink, G. S., Nelson, R. D.,
   Simmons, R. L., and Quie, P. G., J. Infect. Dis., 137 (1978).
4. Tan, J. S., Anderson, J. L., Watanakunakorn, C., and Phair,
   J. P., J. Lab. Clin. Med. 85 (1975) 26.
5. Weeks, B. A., Escobar, M. R., Hamilton, P. B. and Fueston,
   V. M., Adv. Exp. Med. Biol., 73A (1976) 161.

RELATIONSHIP BETWEEN PROTECTIVE IMMUNITY, MITOGENICITY, AND B

CELL ACTIVATION BY SALMONELLA VACCINES

T. K. EISENSTEIN, C. R. ANGERMAN, S. O'DONNELL,
S. SPECTER, and H. FRIEDMAN
Department of Microbiology and Immunology, Temple
University School of Medicine and Albert Einstein
Medical Center, Philadelphia, Pennsylvania (USA) and
University of Southern Florida, Tampa, Florida (USA)

Factors involved in immunity to Salmonella infection have been extensively investigated over the past decades using a mouse model of experimental infection (4,10,11,22). It is clear that both humoral and cellular immunity contribute to the protection against this organism, but the relative contribution of each to the overall level of protection is still uncertain (2,23). The 0 antigens have been shown to be important in host defense, particularly via the humoral immune response (16,22), however, the antigens involved in protection via cellular immunity have not been elucidated.

A ribosome-rich fraction of certain species of Salmonella has also been shown to effectively vaccinate mice against experimental Salmonella infection. The nature of the protective immunogen in this vaccine is still unclear. Eisentein (6) and Angerman and Eisenstein (1) have found that 0 antigens are present in Salmonella ribosomes and ribosomal subfractions, and that they contribute to the immunity of these subcellular vaccines. Eisenstein (8) and Eisenstein and Angerman (7) showed that ribosomes or ribosomal RNA prepared from a mutant Salmonella strain which lacks the 0 antigenic determinants are not protective. Lin and Berry (18) and Misfeldt and Johnson (19) have reported similar results. Johnson has published evidence that the ribosomal fraction is protective because it contains a protein antigen (13).

The experiments reported in this paper were designed to investigate whether all of the protection of the ribosomal extracts is due to contamination 0 antigens, or whether the ribosomes contain additional antigens, or whether the ribosomes function as adjuvants for the 0 antigens. The results from both

in vivo and in vitro assays show that the ribosomal subcellular
fractions have activities that are different from those of
phenol-water purified LPS.

METHODS

   Animals. Female CD-1 mice, 18-21 g were purchased from
Charles River Mouse Farm, Wilmington, Mass. Female C3H/HeJ
mice were purchased from Jackson Laboratories, Bar Harbor, Me.
Inbred BALB/c mice were obtained from Cumberland View Farms,
Clinton, Tenn. They were housed in plastic disposable cages
with Absorb-Dri for bedding. Purina Mouse Chow was available ad
libitum, and fresh water was provided in plastic sterilizable
bottles. In each experiment, mice of the same age were used.

   Organisms. Salmonella typhimurium, strain W118-2, was
kindly provided by Samuel Formal, Walter Reed Army Institute of
Medical Research, Washington, D. C. and has been used previously
in our laboratory (1). This strain is strongly agglutinated
with 0:1,4,5,12 and H:i,1,2 antisera (Difco), and exhibits
typical biochemical reactions. The intraperitoneal lethal dose
(LD_{50}) is 1×10^{4} organisms for CD-1 mice and less than 6 cells
for C3H/HeJ mice.

   Bacterial storage and culture. Stock cultures were stored
lyophilized at -20 C. Organisms used for antigen preparation or
challenge were obtained from lyophils rehydrated with brain
heart infusion broth (BHI), and grown as previously described
(1). For challenge, the bacteria were counted in a Petroff-
Hausser chamber and the culture diluted in saline to the desired
concentration. The actual number of viable bacteria in the
culture was determined by duplicate plate counts.

   Preparation of vaccines. Phenol-water extracted lipopolysaccharide (PW-LPS) was prepared using the procedure of Westphal
and Luderitz as described by Nowotny (21). Thirty g of packed,
wet W118-2 cells were extracted with distilled water and 90%
aqueous phenol. After a series of cold methanol precipitations,
the concentrate was spun at 104,000 x g to sediment the LPS,
leaving the nucleic acid in the supernate. The pellet was suspended in distilled water and lyophilized. The purufied LPS had
a TD_{50} in CD-1 mice of 320 µg (1). As little as 0.0001 µg of
material was reactive in the Limulus Lysate Gelation Test. Phenol-
water extracted and TCA-extracted LPS of Serratia marcescens was
kindly supplied by Dr. A. Nowotny (University of Pennsylvania).

   Acetone-killed cells were prepared by the procedure of
Landy, as previously described (1). Ribosome-rich subcellular

extracts of strains W118-2 and TA1659 were prepared according to the method of Fogel and Sypherd, as previously described (1). Briefly, 50 g of bacteria were suspended in 200 ml of cold 0.01 $\underline{M}$ Tris buffer with 0.5% Brij 58 and deoxyribonuclease, and broken twice in a cold French pressure cell. After a series of ammonium sulfate precipitations and two ultracentrifugations, the pelleted ribosomes were dialyzed against Tris buffer with 10^{-2} M magnesium acetate and then against Tris buffer with 10^{-4} M magnesium acetate. The ribosomes were filtered through a .45 µm Millipore filter and either used immediately or stored at -20 C in small aliquots. "RNA" was prepared by 2-chloroethanol extractions of the ribosomes (8) and standardized by the $O.D._{260}$ (1 O.D. = 44 µg RNA (17)).

Sterility of all vaccines was insured by inoculating tubes of BHI broth and thioglycollate broth with either 5 mg of LPS, 5 mg of killed cells, or 1 ml of ribosomal vaccine. At 24 and 48 hr these tubes were subcultured to fresh broth and blood agar plates. If there was no growth at 72 hr, the vaccine was considered sterile.

Vaccine dosages were standarized on a dry weight basis. As LPS and acetone-killed cells were stored lyophilized, they were weighed out directly and diluted. One mg of acetone-killed cells contained 1×10^9 dead bacteria. An aliquot of ribosomes of strain W118-2 was desalted by dialysis and used for a dry weight determination (78 µg dry weight of ribosomes equaled 11 $O.D._{260}$ unit). For immunization, an appropriate volume of the vaccine was used based on the dry weight.

Immunization and challenge. Mice were immunized with one intraperitoneal injection of vaccine in a volume of 0.5 ml. When appropriate, vaccines were suspended or diluted with sterile, non-pyrogenic saline (Abbott Laboratories). Controls received saline. Three weeks after immunization, mice were challenged intraperitoneally with the desired dosage of live W118-2 in 0.5 ml saline. Cells were grown, and the inoculum standardized and verified, as described above. Protection was assessed by forty-day survival.

Serological studies. Serum was collected from groups of control or immunized mice 21 days post vaccination. Mice were anesthetized with chloroform and bled from the heart. Individual samples were clotted at room temperature for 1 hr and then kept overnight at 4 C. Equal amounts of serum from each mouse were pooled. To remove nonspecific agglutinins for passive hemagglutination titers, a portion of the pooled serum was absorbed twice at 36 C, for 30 min each time, with an equal volume of washed human erythrocytes. The serum was either used

immediately or stored in small aliquots at -20 C. To determine
hemagglutination titers, human Rh-negative, group 0 erythrocytes
were coated with W188-2, PW-LPS, according to the method of Neter
as described by Nowotny (21). In both the hemagglutination and
agglutination determinations, typing serum (0:1,4,5,12; Difco)
was used as a positive control. A standard, positive serum
sample raised against acetone-killed cells was also included in
each series of titrations in order to correlate the titers between experiments. Serum from control mice injected with saline
was also included.

Thymidine uptake procedure. Spleen cell suspensions were
obtained by teasing the cells apart in minimal essential medium
containing 10% fetal calf serum. The cell concentration was
adjusted to 1×10^7 per ml and 0.1 ml of the cell suspension was
added to the wells of Linbro plates containing 0.9 ml of RPMI,
1640 (Flow Laboratories) with 10% fetal calf serum. The cells
were incubated for 24 hr at 37 C alone or with the addition of
0.1 ml of the desired stimulator. Cultures were then pulsed
with 2 μCi of tritiated thymidine in 0.1 ml of medium. Eighteen
hr later the radioactivity was determined by standard scintillation counting. The Stimulation Index (ST) was calculated as the
ratio of CPM for treated versus untreated cultures.

In vitro antibody formation. Spleen cells were teased
apart in minimal essential medium containing 10% fetal calf serum
and adjusted to a concentration of 1×10^7 cells/ml. One-half
ml of the cell suspension was added to small glass vials as
described by Kamo et al. (15). In each vial was placed an additional 2 ml of medium and 0.5 ml of a standard nutrient cocktail
(18). The desired stimulator was added in a volume of 0.1 ml,
and where desired, 2×10^6 sheep red blood cells were also added.
The cells were incubated at 37 C in a humidified atmosphere of
83% N, 10% CO_2, and 7% O_2 for 5 days. The contents of the vials
were then harvested and centrifuged at 200 x g for 10 min at 5 C.
The upper 2 ml of supernatant was removed and the cell pellet was
resuspended in the remaining 1 ml of medium. The number of
direct hemolytic plaque-forming cells was determined using
localized hemolysis in gel as described by Jerne (12) using 0.1
ml of the cell suspension. The number of PFCs was calculated
per 10^6 viable spleen cells.

RESULTS

Protection studies. As shown in Table I, phenol-water extracted lipopolysaccharide, acetone-killed cells and ribosomes
protected mice equally well against a challenge of 100 LD_{50} doses
of strain W188-2. When the challenge dose was increased to 1000

LD_{50}s, lipopolysaccharide was found to be less effective than either acetone-killed cells or ribosomes. All three preparations also resulted in significant anti-0 titers as determined by passive hemagglutination.

The same vaccines were also tested for their immunogenicity and protective capacity in C3H/HeJ mice, a strain which has a genetic defect so that it gives no mitogenic response to phenol-water purified LPS, and only poor immune responses to this substance. As shown in Table II, the LPS, over a wide dosage range, was neither protective nor immunogenic in these mice when they were tested 21 days post vaccination. However, at certain doses, both the ribosomes and acetone-killed vaccine were protective and also resulted in an anti-0 response. Therefore, C3H/HeJ mice respond differently to 0 antigens present in whole cells or in ribosomal extracts than they do to 0 antigens present in phenol-water purified LPS.

TABLE I

Protection to Salmonella Infection in CD-1 Mice

Vaccine	Dose (μg)	Survival[a]		PHA Titer[b]
		1×10^6 Cells ($100\ LD_{50}$)	1×10^7 Cells ($1{,}000\ LD_{50}$)	
Saline	–	0% (0/10)	0% (0/10)	<1:2
LPS	10	100% (10/10)	0% (0/10)	1:32
	25	100% (10/10)	0% (0/10)	1:64
	100	100% (10/10)	0% (0/10)	1:512
	250	100% (10/10)	–	–
AKC	60	100% (10/10)	90% (9/10)	–
	100	100% (10/10)	100% (10/10)	1:256
	250	100% (10/10)	100% (10/10)	1:256
Ribosomes	100	100% (10/10)	80% (8/10)	1:64
	250	100% (10/10)	80% (8/10)	1:64

[a]Mice challenged i.p. 21 days post vaccination.
[b]Pooled sera of 2 mice.

TABLE II

Protection to Salmonella Infection in C3H/HeJ Mice

Vaccine	Dose (µg)	Survival[a]	MTD[b]	PHA Titer[c]	Aggl.Titer[c]
Saline	–	0% (0/9)	5	<1:2	<1:2
LPS	10	0% (0/10)	7	<1:2	<1:5
	25	0% (0/14)	7	<1:2	<1:2
	100	0% (0/10)	9	<1:4	<1:5
	250	0% (0/10)	9	<1:4	<1:5
AKC	60	57% (8/14)	26	1:64	1:64
	100	30% (3/10)	23	<1:4	<1:5
	250	0% (0/10)	19	<1:4	1:5
Ribosomes	100	30% (3/10)	26	<1:4	1:10
	250	50% (7/140)	29	1:64	1:64

[a]Mice challenged i.p. 21 days post vaccination with 55 cells
of Wl18-2.
[b]Mean time to death.
[c]Pooled sera of 5 mice.

Mitogenicity. Table III shows the results of an in vitro
mitogenicity assay using spleen cells of BALB/c mice. The data
show that of the Salmonella extracts, the "RNA" was the most
potent mitogen, giving stimulation indices of 9 to 15, comparable
to those of Serratia phenol-water extracted LPS. The ribosomes,
however, were only moderate mitogens with a maximum SI of 3.2.
The Salmonella LPS gave an intermediate response, greater than
the ribosomes, but not as great as that induced by the "RNA" or
the Serratia LPS.

Background PFC response. As shown in Table IV, both the
Salmonella "RNA" and ribosome fraction stimulated significant
increases in the background PFC response to sheep red blood cells.
In contrast, in this assay, the Salmonella PW-LPS fraction had
little effect, although the Serratia PW-LPS and TCA-LPS were both
active.

TABLE III

Mitogenicity of Bacterial LPS, RNA, and Ribosomal
Preparations for Normal BALB/c Spleen Cells

Concentration of Stimulator Added (μg/Culture)[a]	Material Added to Spleen Cell Cultures[b]				
	Salmonella			Serratia	
	PW–LPS	"RNA"	Ribosomes	PW–LPS	TCA–LPS
1.0	5.0	–	–	7.7	–
10.0	4.6	9.3	3.2	8.4	7.9
25.0	6.0	13.7	2.6	12.0	13.6
50.0	5.4	14.8	2.5	13.9	9.1
100.0	2.3	8.5	2.4	14.0	8.6

[a] Indicated extract, in 0.1 ml volumes, added on day of culture initiation.
[b] Stimulation indices for cultures of 1×10^6 cells after 2 days incubation; control cultures treated with 0.01 μg PHA gave an SI of 5.2.

Adjuvant activity. Table V shows the ability of the substances tested to act as adjuvants for the in vitro immune
response of spleen cells to sheep red blood cells. As is evident in Table V, both the phenol-water and TCA-extracted Serratia
LPS preparations gave generally similar stimulatory activity for
the antibody response to SRBC. Approximately a 2 to 3 fold increase in response occurred when 25 to 50 μg of these LPS preparations were added per culture. However, Salmonella LPS, in
the dose range of 5 to 50 μg, induced little if any significant
stimulation of the specific PFC response. Similarly, the ribosome-rich extracts also failed to result in a significant stimulation of the SRBC-induced PFC response, at least in the dose
range of 25 to 50 μg. In contrast, the Salmonella RNA preparation gave as good a stimulatory effect as the Serratia LPS, and
a much greater stimulation than did the Salmonella LPS or ribosomes in this assay.

TABLE IV

Comparative In Vitro Immunostimulation by Bacterial
Fractions on the Background-Induced PFC Response of
Normal BALB/c Spleen Cells

Material Added[a]	Dose (μg)	PFC/10^6 Spleen Cells[b]	% of Control
None (controls)	–	91 ± 18	–
Salmonella PW-LPS[c]	5	132 ± 23	145.1
	25	134 ± 37	147.3
	50	165 ± 46	181.3
"RNA"	25	476 ± 102	523.1
	50	419 ± 64	460.4
	100	398 ± 93	437.4
Ribosomes	25	361 ± 47	396.7
	50	320 ± 39	351.7
Serratia PW-LPS[c]	25	176 ± 43	193.4
	50	290 ± 59	318.7
TCA-LPS[d]	25	326 ± 40	358.3
	50	387 ± 62	425.3

[a]Indicated extracts added in 0.1-ml volumes to cultures of
5 x 10^6 normal spleen cells.
[b]Average PFC responses ± S. E. for 4-6 cultures assayed on day 5
after culture initiation.
[c]Prepared by phenol-water extraction method.
[d]Prepared by TCA extraction method.

    Range of activities. Table VI gives a qualitative summary
of the activities of the various preparations tested. The results show that each of the three Salmonella fractions had a
different spectrum of activity. The RNA fraction was active in
all three assays, whereas the Salmonella LPS was not active as
an adjuvant or as an enhancer of the background PFC response,
and less active than the RNA in the mitogenicity assay. The
ribosomes were the least active in the mitogenicity assay, inactive as adjuvants, but stimulatory of the background PFC
response. Taken together, the results suggest that in these

in vitro assays the activity of the ribosomal and RNA fractions
cannot be attributed solely to LPS contamination.

TABLE V

Comparative In Vitro Immunostimulation by Bacterial
Fractions on the SRBC-Induced PFC Response of Normal
BALB/c Spleen Cells

Material Added[a]		Dose (μg)	PFC/10^6 Spleen Cells[b]	% of Control
None (controls)		–	1,045 ± 227	–
Salmonella	PW–LPS[c]	5	988 ± 267	94.6
		25	840 ± 238	80.4
		50	1,160 ± 360	111.0
	"RNA"	25	2,270 ± 431	217.5
		50	2,340 ± 376	225.8
		100	2,215 ± 317	212.0
	Ribosomes	25	1,070 ± 292	98.8
		50	1,120 ± 236	107.2
Serratia	PW–LPS[c]	25	2,160 ± 430	206.7
		50	3,630 ± 470	347.4
	TCA–LPS[d]	25	1,930 ± 268	184.7
		50	2,340 ± 316	224.0

[a]Indicated extracts added to cultures of 5 x 10^6 normal spleen
cells incubated with 2 x 10^6 SRBC.
[b]Average PFC responses ± S. E. for 4-6 cultures assayed on day
5 after culture initiation.
[c]Prepared by phenol-water extraction method.
[d]Prepared by TCA extraction method.

TABLE VI

Qualitative Comparison of Mitogenic and
Immunostimulatory Activities of Salmonella
and Serratia Extracts

		Activity		
		Enhanced Back-Ground PFC Response to SRBC[a]	Adjuvant PFC Response to SRBC[a]	Mitogenicity
Material Added				
Salmonella	LPS-PW	−	−	+2
	"RNA"	+	+	+3
	Ribosomes	+	−	+1
Serratia	LPS-PW	+	+	+3
	LPS-TCA	+	+	+3

[a]These data do not permit further discrimination of positive
responses into categories from 1 to 3.

DISCUSSION

From the protection experiments in CD-1 mice it can be concluded that phenol-water extracted LPS is not as protective as
ribosomes or whole killed cells, even though vaccination with LPS
results in anti-0 titers that are as high as those engendered by
the other two vaccines. These results suggest that there is
either another protective antigen present in the acetone-killed
cells and the ribosomal extract, or that these more complex vaccines result in an immune response which is quantitatively different from that induced by LPS. For example, the passive hemagglutination assay detects primarily IgM, but the IgG titer may
correlate more closely with immunity. It is noteworthy, however,
that ribosomes or ribosomal "RNA" prepared from strains of Salmonella which lack 0 antigens, do not yield protective subcellular vaccines (6,7,18,19).

The results obtained using the C3H/HeJ mice also show that

ribosomes and acetone-killed cells have activities that cannot be duplicated by PW-LPS, since the latter resulted in no anti-0 antibody or protection 21 days post-vaccination, whereas the complex vaccines were immunogenic and protective. It is known that the spleen cells of this mouse strain do not give a mitogenic response to PW-LPS (27), although they will respond to LPS extracted by procedures which retain the LPS-associated protein (25). A small-molecular-weight polypeptide is apparently responsible for a mitogenicity of LPS in these mice (20,26). It is tempting to speculate that the reason the ribosomes and acetone-killed cells are immunogenic, while the PW-LPS is not, is because the former preparations contain mitogens. Preliminary results show that for C3H/HeJ spleen cells, the PW-LPS is not mitogenic, but that "RNA" ribosomes, and acetone-killed cells are.

In this project, vaccines were tested in BALB/c mice for their ability to stimulate cells of the immune system in various ways. The results show that the subcellular bacterial fractions which are rich in nucleic acid have activities which are not duplicated by phenol-water extracted LPS. The active factor(s) in these subcellular extracts might be the mitogenic protein described above, which may be preserved by the procedures used to obtain the ribosomal and RNA fractions. Alternatively, the nucleic acid itself may have immunostimulatory activity. Synthetic polynucleotides have been shown to be mitogens (24) and to act as adjuvants (3,14). There is, however, only one other report in which RNA from bacterial sources was tested and found to be mitogenic (5).

These studies, taken together, suggest that natural products of the bacterium, other than the molecule containing the antigenic determinant, may significantly affect the host immune responses. When a host is infected or vaccinated with whole microorganisms, it is possible that these natural products are released during bacterial degradation and become available to stimulate the immune system. Such natural products may be useful in combination with purified antigens in vaccines or as general immunostimulators in patients with depressed immune responses.

ACKNOWLEDGEMENTS

    This research was supported by Public Health Service grant AI-11860 from the National Institute of Allergy and Infectious Diseases, and by the Temple University Research Incentive Fund.

REFERENCES

1. Angerman, C. R. and Eisenstein, T. K., Infect. Immun., 19 (1978) 575.
2. Bladen, R. V., Mackaness, G. B. and Collins, F. M., J. Exp. Med., 124 (1966) 585.
3. Braun, W. and Nakano, M., Science 157 (1967) 819.
4. Collins, F. M., Mackaness, G. B. and Blanden, R. B., J. Exp. Med., 124 (1966) 601.
5. Dean, J. H., Wallen, W. C. and Lucas, D. O., Nature New Biol., 237 (1972) 154.
6. Eisenstein, T. K., Infect. Immun., 12 (1975) 364.
7. Eisenstein, T. K., and Angerman, C. R., J. Immunol., 121 (1978) 1010.
8. Fogel, S. and Sypherd, P. S., J. Bacteriol., 96 (1968) 358.
9. Frank, S., Specter, S., Nowotny, A., and Friedman, H., J. Immunol., 119 (1977) 855.
10. Herzberg, M., Nash, P. and Hino, S., Infect. Immun., 5 (1972) 83.
11. Jenkin, C. R., Rowley, D., and Auzins, I., J. Exp. Biol. Med. Sci., 42 (1964) 215.
12. Jerne, N. K., and Nordin, A. A., Science 140 (1963) 405.
13. Johnson, W., Infect. Immun., 8 (1973) 395.
14. Johnson, A. G., Schmidtke, J., Merritt, K. and Han, I., In: Nucleic Acids in Immun.,   (Ed. O. J. Plescia and W. Braun), Springer-Verlag, New York, (1968) 379.
15. Kamo, I., Pan, S-H., and Friedman, H., J. Immunol. Methods, 11 (1976) 55.
16. Kenny, K., and Herzberg, M., J. Bacteriol., 93 (1967) 773.
17. Kurland, C. G., J. Mol. Biol., 18 (1966) 90.
18. Lin, J-H., and Berry, L. J., J. Reticuloendothel. Soc., 23 (1978) 135.
19. Misfeldt, M. L. and Johnson, W., Infect. Immun., 17 (1977) 98.
20. Morrison, D. C., Betz, S. J. and Jacobs, D. M., J. Exp. Med., 144 (1976) 840.
21. Nowotny, A., Basic exercises in immunochemistry, Springer-Verlag, New York, (1969).
22. Ornellas, E. P., Roantree, R. J. and Steward, J. P., J. Infect. Dis., 112 (1970) 113.
23. Rowley, D., Auzins, I. and Jenkin, C. R., Aust. J. Exp. Biol. Med. Sci., 46 (1968) 447.
24. Scher, I., Strong, D. M., Ahmed, A., Knudsen, R. C., Sell, K. W., J. Exp. Med. 138 (1973) 1545.
25. Skidmore, B. J., Morrison, D. C., Chiller, J. M. and Weigle, W. O., J. Exp. Med., 142 (1975) 1488.
26. Sultzer, B. M. and Goodman, G.W., J. Exp. Med., 144 (1976) 821.
27. Watson, J. and Riblet, R., J. Exp. Med., 140 (1974) 1147.

EFFECTS OF BACTERIAL PRODUCTS ON GRANULOPOIESIS

R. URBASCHEK

Department of Immunology and Serology
Institute for Hygiene and Med. Microbiology
of the University of Heidelberg
Mannheim (West Germany)

Cell wall components of gram-negative bacteria - in particular the lipopolysaccharides or endotoxins - have potent effects on many biological systems. Their interaction with granulocytes and macrophages seems to be most directly related to host defense mechanisms during gram-negative bacterial infections. It is becoming more apparent that endotoxins influence host defenses by virtue of their ability to stimulate hematopoiesis, in particular granulopoiesis, probably through the release of endogenous mediators and regulators. The hemapoietic system is characterized by remarkable stability in the unperturbed state while it is highly responsive in terms of increased output on demand, such as in infectious diseases and in endotoxemia.

Our interest has focussed on the stimulation of granulopoiesis by gram-negative bacterial cell wall products and on the question of whether a relationship exists between the effect of these bacterial products on granulopoiesis and their ability to stimulate the colony stimulating factor.

The technique for the culture of granulocytic committed stem cells to form colonies of granulocytes and macrophages was introduced by Pluznik and Sachs (22) and Bradley and Metcalf (4). This opened a new era for the study of the kinetics of granulopoiesis and of the regulatory factors involved. Proliferation and differentiation of these stem cells along the granulocyte and macrophage pathway in vitro is dependent upon the presence of a humoral mediator, termed colony stimulating factor, CSF, the major source of which is the blood monocyte and the macrophage (6,9,10).

The effects of methylated endotoxin. It was found that an
endotoxin preparation with toxicity reduced by treatment with
potassium methylate, as described by Nowotny (19), induced nonspecific tolerance against lethal doses of endotoxin (32,33) and protected mice against lethal X-irradiation (32,34). Since Smith (29)
and Hanks (12) reported that early recovery of the hematopoietic
system is responsible for the increased survival of endotoxin-
pretreated animals following X-irradiation, the effect of methylated endotoxin on the hematopoietic stem cell compartments was
studied, following the observation that it caused elevated serum
CSF levels and an increase in endogenous CFU (35).

The number of pluripotent stem cells, CFUs, of bone marrow,
spleen and blood was determined as described by Till and McCulloch
(30) in the spleen of lethally irradiated NMRI mice seven days
after an intravenous injection. They were measured at intervals of
6, 24, 48, and 72 hr after injection of methylated endotoxin. At
the same times the granulocytic committed stem cells, CFUc, of
bone marrow and spleen were determined in a semisolid agar culture
in the presence of a standard CSF serum (two hr post-endotoxin).

As illustrated in Fig. 1, the femoral CFUs decrease at all
times tested whereas the splenic CFUs show significantly elevated
levels at 72 hr. At this time, the blood CFUs are also increased,
and show a considerable elevation as early as six hr after injection. The results of femoral and splenic CFUc are illustrated in
Fig. 2. The splenic CFUc increase continuously from six hr and
reach a peak at 72 hr. The femoral CFUc are only slightly elevated
above the control.

The kinetics of the hematopoietic stem cell population was
studied using hydroxyurea which is known to be selectively lethal
for cells in the phase of DNA-synthesis during the cell cycle (18,
28). It has been shown that a high proportion of CFUc is in active cycle, while most CFUs are quiescent, either in G_0 or in
prolonged G_1. These relationships as well as an increase in
number of cells entering into active cell cycle following an injection of methylated endotoxin are shown in Fig. 3 and Fig. 4.

From these results it is evident that this preparation of
methylated endotoxin has a marked effect on hematopoiesis. The
decrease in femoral CFUs might be due to an early emigration of
these cells from the marrow to the blood, and to an increased
differentiation of CFUs to CFUc. Both the splenic CFUs and CFUc
are significantly elevated at 72 hr, the latter to a much higher
degree indicating the marked stimulation of granulopoiesis. Until
this time the CFUc of spleen and bone marrow are triggered at all
times tested from a resting state into a state of active proliferation.

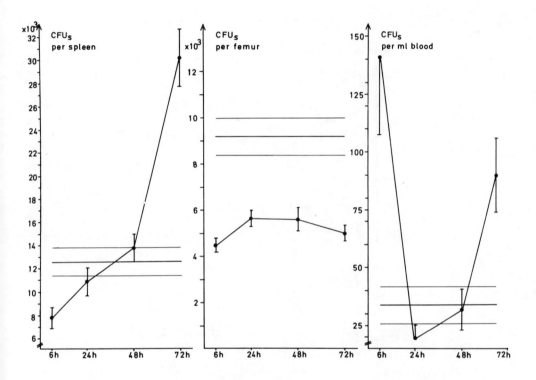

Fig. 1.   Femoral, splenic, and blood CFUs in NMRI mice at different times after intravenous injection of 50 µg of methylated endotoxin.   The vertical bars represent ± SEM and the parallel lines represent the mean and ± SEM for 4 control groups.

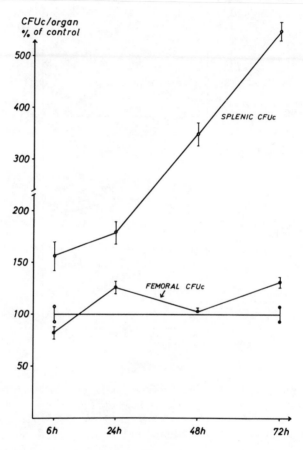

Fig. 2. Femoral and splenic CFUc at different times after intravenous injection of 50 µg of methylated endotoxin expressed as
percent of control, (± SEM).

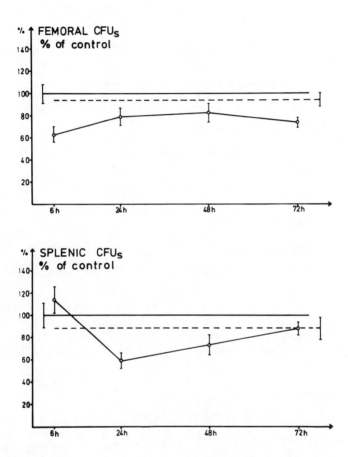

Fig. 3. Femoral and splenic CFUs at different times after intra-venous injection with 50 μg of methylated endotoxin in NMRI mice after _in vitro_ incubation of the cell suspensions with 2×10^{-3} M hydroxyurea for 2.5 hr, (± SEM).

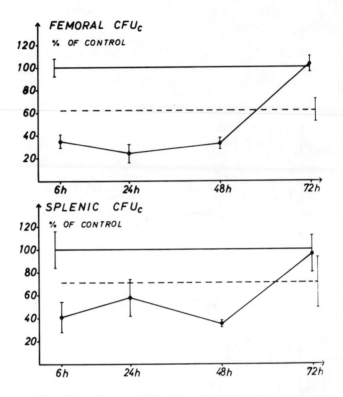

Fig. 4.   Femoral and splenic CFUc at different times after
intravenous injection with 50 μg of methylated endotoxin in NMRI
mice after _in vitro_ incubation of the cell suspensions with
2×10^{-3} M hydroxyurea for 2.5 hr, (± SEM).

The role of CSF in stimulating granulopoiesis in vivo.   The
question as to whether CSF which has been shown to increase after
endotoxin administration (5,16,23) is of significance in stimulating
granulopoiesis _in vivo_ remains to be answered.   Although it is
evident that CSF is necessary for proliferation and differentiation of CFUc _in vitro_, there is little direct evidence for the regulatory or stimulatory effect of CSF _in vivo_.   In this context
the results of Pachman (21) are of interest.   He was able to
demonstrate a beneficial effect of CSF-rich plasma that was induced in volunteers after an injection of thyphoid vaccine.   The
plasma was infused into a patient who suffered from chronic neu-
tropenia and repeated infections.   The patient recovered and
showed an increase in maturation of the myeloid compartment into
mature granulocytes.

That CSF may be essential to in vivo granulocytic stem cell proliferation and differentiation was shown also by Shadduck et al. (25). They noted that the number of granulocytic cells and of bone marrow CFUc were markedly reduced in diffusion chambers implanted into recipients that were treated with anti-CSF prepared in rabbits by injection of CSF obtained from L cell conditioned media (26).

In order to study whether anti-CSF has an influence on the increase in granulocyte precursors after endotoxin administration, antiserum to partially purified CSF from L cells - kindly provided by Dr. R. K. Shadduck, University of Pittsburgh - was injected into mice one hr before the injection of endotoxin. Table I shows that the number of stem cells in the spleen, which is highly elevated three days after endotoxin administration (148 colonies), is diminished to 48 colonies in mice treated with anti-CSF. This emphasizes the essential relationship between CSF and the stimulation of granulopoiesis in vivo.

TABLE I

Splenic CFUc (± SEM) in NMRI Mice Three Days
After Intravenous Injection of 5 μg of Endotoxin
(E. coli 0 111, TCA Extract)

Injection	CFUc/10^6 Spleen Cells
Endotoxin	148.0 (6.6)
Anti-CSF plus endotoxin	47.7 (0.6)
Control serum plus endotoxin	129.7 (9.1)
Saline	31.0 (3.0)

[a]Mice were injected with anti-CSF (0.5 ml), prepared in rabbits with L-cell conditioned medium CSF, or with normal rabbit serum (0.5 ml) one hr before the injection of endotoxin.

CSF levels following injection of gram-negative bacterial cell wall components. In addition to methylated endotoxin, other gram-negative bacterial cell wall components were tested for their ability to increase serum CSF levels. These included a phenol water extract (LSP P/W) and a lipid A preparation from E. coli K 235 as well as a lipid A protein provided by Dr. David Rosenstreich (NIH); a Freeman-type polysaccharide (8) from S. typhimurium and a peptidoglycan obtained from Dr. C. Bona* (Institut Pasteur, Paris, France) and a trichloroacetic acid extract

(LPS TCA) from E. coli 0 111 that was prepared in our laboratory,
were tested two hr after intravenous injection at several dose
levels (Fig. 5). The comparison of these preparations at 5 μg is
summarized in Table II.

It is of interest that except for the peptidoglycan all components were similarly active. One of them, the Freeman-type
polysaccharide, is nontoxic, nonmitogenic and nonpyrogenic, as
shown by Bona (3).

TABLE II

Serum CSF Levels in Mice Injected with Cell
Wall Components of Gram-Negative Bacteria (± SEM).

2 hr After I.V. Injection	Colonies/10^5 Bone Marrow Cells
LPS P/W	97.5 (5.0)
LPS TCA	132.0 (5.4)
Lipid A	107.2 (14.4)
Lipid A protein	172.2 (8.2)
Freeman PS	106.9 (9.1)
Peptidoglycan	0
Saline	4.9 (2.5)

The effects of the Freeman-type polysaccharide. If CSF
activity is related in a major way to nonspecific resistance it
should be possible to protect mice against irradiation using the
Freeman-type polysaccharide. Table III shows that as little as
25 μg of this preparation did indeed protect mice against lethal
irradiation.

As a sequel to these results it was of great interest to
study the effect of the polysaccharide on the stem cell compartment. Three days after injection, the splenic CFUc increased
significantly as illustrated in Fig. 6.

Studies in progress are designed to determine the effect of
this polysaccharide on the status of decreased ganulopoiesis
following cytostatic treatment.

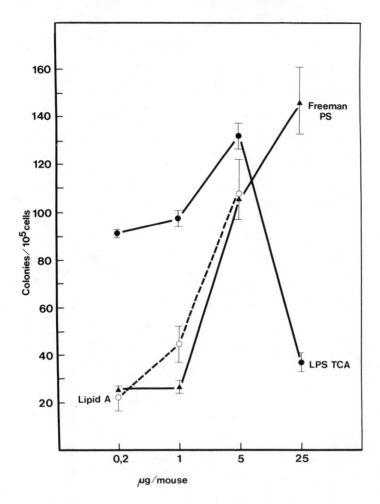

Fig. 5. CSF levels two hr after intravenous injection of different doses of lipid A, a trichloroacetic acid extract (LPS TCA) and a Freeman-type polysaccharide (Freeman PS).

In 1975, Nowotny (20) demonstrated a radioprotective effect of a polysaccharide-rich, water soluble fraction obtained by acid hydrolysis from endotoxin lipopolysaccharide. This polysaccharide preparation had a marked CSF-inducing activity (20), whereas Apte and Pluznik (2) reported that a polysaccharide preparation also obtained from endotoxin lipopolysaccharide had no CSF activity.

TABLE III

Survival Rate of Mice Following 650 R Whole Body Irradiation
After Intravenous Pretreatment with Freeman-Type-Polysaccharide
(FPS) from S. typhimurium 24 hr Before Irradiation

FPS	Dead/Total	Survival Rate
100.0 µg	4/15	73%
50.0 µg	7/15	53%
25.0 µg	8/15	47%
12.5 µg	13/15	13%
Control	15/15	0%

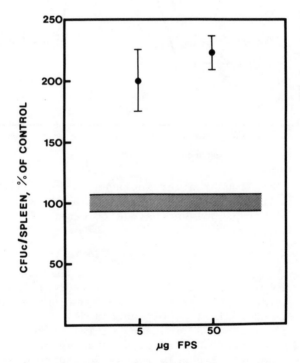

Fig. 6.   Splenic CFUc three days after injection of Freeman-type
polysaccharide (FPS) in NMRI mice expressed as percent of control
(± SEM).

The mouse strain, C3H/HeJ, which is known to be inherently nonresponsive to many of the biological effects of endotoxin, especially those related to the reticuloendothelial system, cannot be protected against lethal irradiation by endotoxin (34). An obvious reason why endotoxin might not protect these mice against irradiation would be their inability to produce elevated levels of serum CSF. That this occurs was observed first by Apte and Pluznik (2), who also found that the stem cells of these mice respond to CSF from an exogenous source. Their inability to generate CSF after endotoxin administration was shown to be under the control of a single autosomal gene (1).

As shown in Fig. 7, Freeman-type polysaccharide was unable to induce elevated CSF levels in low responder mice, while a TCA extract of E. coli 0 111 did. A genetically similar mouse strain, C3HeB/FeJ, which is susceptible to endotoxins, responded normally to both preparations. These findings suggest that C3H/HeJ mice respond to endotoxin which contains a cell wall protein that is known to be present in a TCA extract.

DISCUSSION

Despite the attempts of several workers to identify the cell wall component of gram-negative bacteria responsible for the appearance of CSF in blood or for the stimulation of granulopoiesis, the answer remains elusive. It is clear, however, that these changes occur whether the factor responsible is administered after it is separated from the microorganisms or is present as a result of an infection naturally or experimentally induced (31), including infections arising after irradiation (11,17). The final consequences in all situations are the same. In fact, the elevated rate of granulopoiesis may result in an increase in early nonspecific resistance which, in turn, may be more important to the host than specific immunity under some conditions.

Negative feed-back mechanisms of CSF activity or inhibitors of colony formation studied in vitro, such as chalones (14,24), interferon (7,15), prostaglandin (13) or tumor necrotizing factor (27) not discussed here, may play a role in the regulation of granulopoiesis, and in the breakdown of host defense during the course of infection. The activity of these inhibitors in vivo has still to be proven.

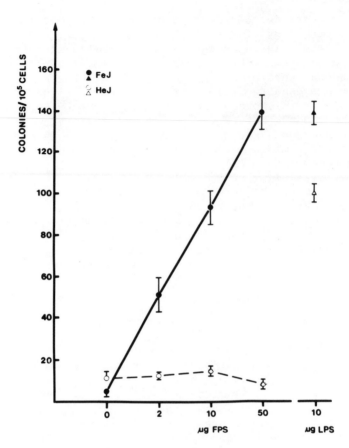

Fig. 7. Serum CSF levels two hr after injection of Freeman-type polysaccharide (FPS) or endotoxin, TCA extract (LPS) in C3H/HeJ mice 0--0,Δ and C3HeB/FeJ mice ●--●,▲ (± SEM).

SUMMARY

    Methylated endotoxin and Freeman-type polysaccharide each stimulate granulopoiesis and the production of CSF in mice. These same preparations also protect pretreated mice from lethal X-irradiation. The role of CSF in stimulating granulopoiesis in vivo was shown by the ability of anti-CSF to reduce the number of CFUc in endotoxin-treated mice. C3H/HeJ low responder mice cannot be protected against lethal X-irradiation by pretreatment with endotoxin and they fail to produce CSF in response to phenol water extracted endotoxin and the Freeman-type polysaccharide, but do respond to trichloroacetic acid endotoxin with elevated serum CSF levels.

ACKNOWLEDGEMENTS

I want to express my gratitude to Dr. Ursula Reincke, from the Brookhaven National Laboratory, Upton, N. Y. (USA), for her essential contributions to the experiments on the stem cell compartments while she was a visiting professor in this Department. I am also grateful to Dr. S. E. Mergenhagen, from the National Institutes of Health, NIDR, Bethesda, MD. (USA), for the helpful discussions and the opportunity to work in his laboratories, where some of these experiments were done. I wish to thank Gertraud Ostwald, Christiane Hoffmann and Rosemarie Hiemesch for their skillful technical assistance.

This investigation was supported by Deutsche Forschungs-gemeinschaft SFB 90, Heidelberg (Germany).

REFERENCES

1. Apte, T. N. and Pluznik, D. H.   J. Cell. Physiol. 89 (1976) 313.
2. Apte, R. N. and Pluznik, D. H., In: N. Müller-Bérat: Progress in Differentiation Research, North-Holland/American Elsevier: (1976) 493.
3. Bona, C., in preparation.
4. Bradley, T. R. and Metcalf, D., Austr. J. Exp. Biol. Med. Sci. 44 (1966) 287.
5. Chervenick, P. A., J. Lab. Clin. Med. 79 (1972) 1014.
6. Chervenick, P. A. and LoBuglio, A. F., Science 118 (1972) 164.
7. Fleming, W. A., McNeill, T. A. and Killen, M., Immunology 23 (1972) 429.
8. Freeman, G. G., Biochem. J. 36 (1942) 340.
9. Golde, D. W. and Cline, M. J., J. Clin. Invest. 51 (1972) 2981.
10. Golde, D. W., Finley, T. N. and Cline, M. J., Lancet 2 (1972) 1397.
11. Hall, B. M., Brit. J. Haemat. 17 (1969) 553.
12. Hanks, G. E. and Ainsworth, E. J., Radiat. Res. 25 (1965) 195.
13. Kurland, J. and Moore, M. A. S., Exp. Hemat. 5 (1977) 357.
14. MacVittie, T. J. and McCarthy, K. F., Exp. Hemat. 2 (1974) 182.
15. McNeill, T. A. and Fleming, W. A., Immunology 21 (1971) 761.
16. Metcalf, D., Immunology 21 (1971) 427.
17. Morley, A., Rickard, K. A., Howard, D. and Stohlman, F., Jr., Blood 37 (1971) 14.
18. Morse, B. S., Rencricca, N. J. and Stohlman, F., Jr., Blood 35 (1970) 761.
19. Nowotny, A., Nature 197 (1963) 721.

20. Nowotny, A., Behling, U. H. and Chang, H. L., J. Immunol. 115 (1975) 199.
21. Pachman, L. M., Schwartz, A. D. and Barron, R., J. Pediat. 87 (1975) 713.
22. Pluznik, D. H. and Sachs, L., J. Cell. Comp. Physiol. 66 (1965) 319.
23. Quesenberry, P., Morley, A., Stohlman, F., Jr., Rickard, K. A. and Howard, D., New Engl. J. Med. 286 (1972) 227.
24. Rytömaa, T., Boll. Ist. Sieroter. Milan 54 (1975) 195.
25. Shadduck, R. K., Carsten, A. L., Chicappa, G., Cronkite, E. P. and Gerard, E., Exp. Hematol. 5, Suppl. 2 (1977) 14.
26. Shadduck, R. K. and Metcalf, D., J. Cell. Physiol. 86 (1975) 247.
27. Shah, R. G., Green, S. and Moore, M. A. S., J. RES 23 (1978) 29.
28. Sinclair, W. K., Science 150 (1965) 1729.
29. Smith, W. W., Brecher, G., Budd, R. A. and Fred, S., Radiat. Res. 27 (1966) 369.
30. Till, J. E. and McCulloch, E. A., Radiat. Res. 14 (1961) 231.
31. Trudgett, A., McNeill, T. A. and Killen, M., Infect. Immun. 8 (1973) 450.
32. Urbaschek, B., Habilitationsschrift, Universität Heidelberg, (1967).
33. Urbaschek, B., In: Kadis, S., Weinbaum, G., Ajl. S. J.: Microbial Toxins, Academic Press, New York/London, Vol. V: (1971) 261.
34. Urbaschek, R., Mergenhagen, S. E. and Urbaschek, B., Infect. Immun. 18 (1977) 860.
35. Urbaschek, R. and Urbaschek, B., Bult 35 (1977) 357.

INTERACTION OF MURINE T-CELL SURFACE ANTIGENS WITH <u>MYCOPLASMA</u>

<u>HYORHINIS</u>

K. S. WISE, P. B. ASA and R. T. ACTON

Department of Microbiology and Diabetes Research and
Training Center, University of Alabama in Birmingham,
Birmingham, Alabama (USA)

Mycoplasms are capable of producing a variety of chronic
diseases in animals and man involving the respiratory tract, joints,
and genitourinary tract (9,20). Recently, Cassell <u>et al</u>. (6) have
discussed the role of the host immune response in determining
characteristic manifestations of chronic mycoplasma disease, which
arise from an extremely complex interplay between these organisms
and the immunological apparatus of the host.

An important feature of many mycoplasmas which may be a central
element in determining the course of chronic disease, is their
striking association with the surface of mammalian cells (2).
This interaction is typified by <u>Mycoplasma hyorhinis</u>, a known
etiological agent for polyarthritis and respiratory disease in
swine (18.22). This report describes a recently developed <u>in</u>
<u>vitro</u> model (26,27) useful in the detailed study of interactions
between <u>M. hyorhinis</u> and mammalian T-lymphoid cells. Observations
are presented which suggest a number of mechanisms by which mycoplasmas may evade, alter, or misdirect the host immune response,
resulting in the onset or protraction of immunopathological disease.
The molecular basis of these interactions may be further examined
using this model system.

MATERIALS AND METHODS

<u>Lymphoid cell cultures and mycoplasma stocks</u>. The propaga-
tion of the BW5147 murine T-lymphoblastoid cell line (17) has been
described previously (32), as has the phenotypic surface expression on these cells of the Thy-1.1 T-cell differentiation alloantigen (30) the H-2K histocompatibility antigens (4) and the

murine leukemia virus (MuLV) related cell surface antigen gp[70] (13).

Identification of M. hyorhinis as a "non-cultivable" contaminant of some BW5147 cultures, (termed "naturally infected") and the detailed methods by which mycoplasmas were purified from the supernatant of these cultures by isopycnic centrifugation on potassium tartrate (KT) gradients have been described elsewhere (27).

Stock cultures of M. hyorhinis (strain GDL) were obtained from Dr. R. F. Ross, Iowa State University, (Ames, Iowa). Maintenance of these cultures and infection of "clean" BW5147 cell cultures with this defined M. hyorhinis stock (referred to as "experimentally infected" cultures) have been described (27). For absorption studies employing broth-grown M. hyorhinis, cultures were centrifuged at 20,000 x g for 30 min at 4 C, suspended in phosphate buffered saline (PBS) and assayed for protein or used in quantitative absorption reactions to assess antigen activity (27).

Cytotoxicity and inhibition assays. Cytotoxicity and quantitative absorption assays were performed with slight modifications of procedures previously described for assessment of Thy-1.1 (30), Thy-1.2 (30), H-2K^k (4) and gp70 (25) antigens. Briefly, the appropriately diluted antisera were incubated with an equal volume of serially diluted absorbing material for 2 hr at 0 C in microtiter plates, and the suspensions centrifuged at 1800 x g for 10 min. An aliquot of the supernatant was transferred to another well, and equal volumes of {^{51}Cr}-labeled target cells and guinea pig complement (C) were then added. The cytotoxic reaction was carried out at 37 C for 90 min with occasional mixing, after which cells were pelleted and the supernatant assayed for released {^{51}Cr}. The dilution of serum added to the absorption reaction and the concentration of target cells added to the subsequent cytotoxicity reaction were as follows: Thy-1.1, (1:100, 1 x 10^7/ml); Thy-1.2 (1:8, 1 x 10^7/ml); H-2K^k (1:50, 1 x 10^7/ml); gp70 (1:70, 5 x 10^6/ml). Antisera and target cells used in these assays have been previously described (4,25,30). The concentration of absorbing material (or the number of cells) added to a reaction resulting in a 50% reduction in specific {^{51}Cr} release (31) was designated the absorption dose$_{50}$ (AD$_{50}$).

C-dependent cytotoxicity of mycoplasma infected BW5147 cells was assessed by identical procedures. Serially diluted mule antiserum to M. hyorhinis or control mule serum which were obtained from the Research Resources Branch, NIH, Bethesda, MD (see ref. 27) were reacted with {^{51}Cr}-labeled BW5147 cells (5 x 10^6/ml), either uninfected or naturally infected with M. hyorhinis in the presence of C as described above.

Immunoprecipitation and SDS - polyacrylamide gel electrophoresis (PAGE) of M. hyorhinis antigens. Purified mycoplasmas from

experimentally infected BW5147 cell cultures were obtained from
KT gradients (27), and labeled with {^{125}I} (sp. activity = 17Ci/mg;
New England Nuclear, Boston, MA) by the choramine-T method (11).
Labeled organisms were disrupted with detergent by incubation in
a buffer containing 0.5% w/v soldium deoxycholate (DOC) and 0.010
M Trishydroxymethylaminomethane (Tris), pH=8.3 (DOC/Tris buffer).
Free iodine was removed by desalting on a Biorad P-2 column
(Biorad Laboratories, Richmond, CA) equilibrated with DOC/Tris
buffer, and the excluded radioactive fractions pooled for use in
precipitation reactions. Immunoprecipitation reactions containing
1 x 10^6 CPM {^{125}I}-labeled M. hyorhinis and 2 μl of the appropriate antiserum in a total volume of 170 μl DOC/Tris buffer were
incubated for 18 hr at 0 C. Antigen-antibody complexes were then
precipitated with formalin-fixed Staphylococcus aureus (Cowan
Strain I) prepared according to the method of Cullen and Schwartz
(7), by adding 100 μl of a 10% v/v suspension in DOC/Tris buffer
and incubating the reaction for an additional 2 hr at 0 C. Precipitates were washed 4 times by centrifugation in DOC/Tris buffer,
and finally placed in a boiling water bath for 5 min in a solution
containing 2% sodium dodecyl sulfate (SDS), 10% v/v glycerol,
0.125 M Tris and 5% 2-mercaptoethanol (pH 6.8). Following electrophoresis, individual channels were removed from the slab gel,
gel strips were sectioned, and each fraction assessed for {^{125}I}
activity. Fluorescent labeled standards of bovine serum albumin
(66,000 daltons), ovalbumin (45,000 daltons), chymotrypsinogen
(25,500 daltons) and myoglobin (17,000 daltons) were electrophoresed simultaneously as molecular weight markers. Sera used in
immunoprecipitation experiments were: a) mule typing serum against
M. hyporhinis and the control serum described above, b) serum from
swine taken six months after experimental infection with M. hyorhinis, and c) serum from swine having chronic respiratory disease,
demonstrating complement fixation titers against M. hyorhinis.
The latter two sera, and their respective control serum from a
caesarian-derived, colostrum-deprived (CDCD) pig, were kindly provided also by Dr. R. F. Ross.

RESULTS

    Selective association of T-lymphoid cell surface antigens
with M. hyorhinis. A number of criteria have been employed to
demonstrate M. hyorhinis in association with the periphery of
BW5147 lymphoblastoid cells in suspension culture (27). In addition to cell-associated organisms, biosynthetic labeling of natu-
rally-infected BW5147 cell cultures resulted in the incorporation
of {^{3}H}-uridine into supernatant material having a buoyant density
on KT gradients of approximately 1.22 g/cm^3, whereas no labeled
material was observed in identically treated supernatants from
labeled, uninfected BW5147 cells (Fig. 1a). This procedure has
been used as a sensitive method of detecting viable mycoplasmas

in cultures infected with these organisms (23,24). Uridine labeling of BW5147 cells experimentally infected with M. hyorhinis
showed the same labeling pattern in supernatant material (Fig. 1b).

Differential and isopycnic sedimentation, yielded a highly
enriched preparation of mycoplasmas from the supernatant of naturally or experimentally infected BW5147 cell cultures (27). A
pronounced, flocculent band (p = 1.20-1.22 g/cm^3) was clearly resolved which revealed a marked predominance of typical mycoplasma
structures by transmission electron microscopy, and contained
large amounts of M. hyorhinis antigenic material (27).

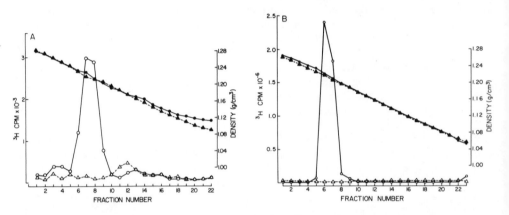

Fig. 1. Isopycnic sedimentation of {5-^{3}H} uridine-containing
material from BW5147 cell culture supernatants. Fractions collected after isopycnic sedimentation of supernatant material
from {5-^{3}H} uridine-labeled BW5147 cultures were analyzed for
the amount of TCA precipitable {^{3}H} (27). Uridine incorporation
into supernatant material from uninfected (Δ----Δ) control BW5147
cultures is compared to that from naturally (A) or experimentally
(B) infected BW5147 cultures (0——0). Densities are indicated
for fractions obtained from infected (●——●) and uninfected
(▲----▲) cultures.

This mycoplasma-containing fraction from BW5147 cells was
further analyzed for associated surface antigens normally present on these T-lymphoblastoid cells, by quantitative absorption
of standard cytotoxic assays specific for the Thy-1.1, H-K^k and
gp70 antigens. Fig. 2 depicts the absorption analysis for the
Thy-1.1 antigen. Mycoplasma isolated from naturally infected
cell cultures demonstrated the presence of the Thy-1.1 alloantigen, showing an AD_{50} of approximately 15 µg protein/ml. This

specific activity was nearly identical to that obtained with mycoplasma derived from experimentally infected cultures. Broth-grown
M. hyorhinis failed to inhibit this reaction significantly at concentrations over 1000 µg/ml. This indicated: a) that the inhibition of cytotoxicity in the Thy-1.1 assay was not due to a component of M. hyorhinis antigenically similar to this T-cell alloantigen, and b) that M. hyorhinis was not anti-complementary in
this assay, since this would appear as an inhibition in the C-
dependent cytotoxic reaction. Furthermore, BW5147 cell-grown M.
hyorhinis isolated from KT gradients did not inhibit the standard,
analogous cytotoxic reaction for the alternate Thy-1.2 allelic
specificity which is not expressed on BW5147 cells (Fig. 2). This
insured that mycoplasma isolated from BW5147 cell supernatants
was not anti-complementary, and that the inhibition observed in the
Thy-1.1 assay was in fact due to the presence of the alloantigen
in the purified mycoplasma material.

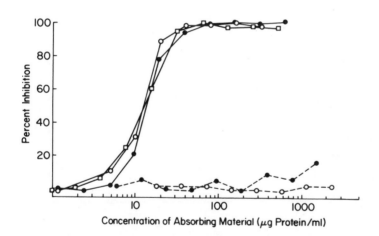

Fig. 2. Quantitative absorption of cytotoxic antiserum against
Thy-1.1 antigen. Absorption of the Thy-1.1 cytotoxic reaction
was carried out with increasing amounts of various absorbing
materials: mycoplasma isolated from naturally infected BW5147
cells (●——●); broth-grown M. hyorhinis (0----0); M hyorhinis
from experimentally infected BW5147 cells (□——□); and BW5147
membranes isolated (21) by isopycnic centrifugation (0——0).
Absorption of the cytotoxic reaction for Thy-1.2 antigen by mycoplasmas isolated from naturally infected BW5147 cells is also
shown (●----●).

The presence of H-2K^k alloantigens in the mycoplasma fraction prepared from BW5147 cell cultures was similarly demonstrated by quantitative absorption procedures (Fig. 3). Broth-grown M. hyorhinis failed to inhibit this reaction, again arguing against an antigenic relationship between M. hyorhinis and H-2K^k allo-antigens, and also against an anti-complementary explanation for this inhibition.

In contrast to H-2K^k and Thy-1.1 surface alloantigens detected in purified M. hyorhinis from lymphoblastoid cell cultures, the MuLV-related gp70 molecule also residing on the surface of BW5147 cells was not detected in the same mycoplasma preparations even at high protein concentrations (4000 µg/ml) of absorbing material (Fig. 4). The inability to detect this surface marker in myco-plasma preparations from BW5147 cell cultures suggested selective association of Thy-1.1 and H-2K^k surface antigens with these or-ganisms. This was confirmed only after showing that the deficiency in gp70 antigen was not due to its inactivation or removal during the KT gradient purification procedures used to prepare mycoplasma, and that the surface expression of antigens was not altered during mycoplasma infection, (a phenomenon known to occur in some myco-plasma-cell interactions in vitro, (19). The first point was established by demonstrating the presence of gp70 a) on purified MuLV virions isolated from the same KT gradient (p = 1.15-1.17

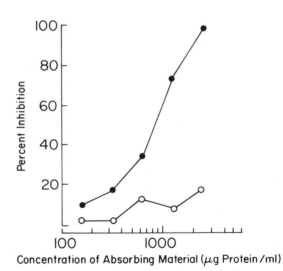

Fig. 3. Quantitative absorption of cytotoxic antiserum against H-2K^k alloantigens. Absorptions were performed as in Fig. 2 to quantitate H-K^k antigens associated with mycoplasma isolated from naturally infected BW5147 cells (●——●) and broth grown M. hyorhinis (0———0).

g/cm^3) used for mycoplasma purification (Fig. 4), and b) on membranes prepared from BW5147 cells and purified on KT gradients
(p = 1.14-1.16 g/cm^3, Fig. 4).   Thus, gp70 was stable to these
procedures, and its absence in the mycoplasma fraction derived
from BW5147 supernatants could not be attributed to its lability
under conditions of purification. Demonstration that mycoplasma-
induced phenotypic change was not a factor in the apparently
selective association of lymphoid surface antigens with M. hyorhinis
is provided in Fig. 5.   Quantitative absorption of Thy-1.1 and
gp 70 cytotoxicity assays showed that even after heavy experimental infection of BW5147 cells with M. hyorhinis (27), the amount
of these antigens exposed on the surface of BW5147 cells was unaltered.

The asymmetry of antigen distribution did not in itself
suggest mechanisms by which antigen acquisition might occur; however, it did argue against a simple contamination by cell membranes during purification as a source of these antigens, since
this would not be expected to result in selective antigen association.   An additional argument against this possibility emerged
from the quantitative measurement of antigens associated with
purified mycoplasma.   The specific Thy-1.1 antigen activity for
mycoplasma obtained from cultures was equal to (or greater than)
that of membranes purified from BW5147 cells (Fig. 2).   Simple

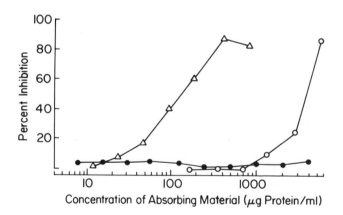

Fig. 4.   Quantitative absorption of cytotoxic antiserum against
gp70 antigen.   Absorptions were performed as in Fig. 2 to quantitate gp70 associated with mycoplasma isolated from naturally
infected BW5147 cells (●———●), BW5147 membranes (0———0) and
MuLV from BW5147 cultures isolated by isopycnic sedimentation
on KT gradients (Δ———Δ).

membrane contamination is difficult to reconcile with thie observation. Interestingly, culture supernatants of BW5147 cells
experimentally infected with M. hyorhinis yielded mycoplasma preparations with Thy-1.1 specific activity was high as that obtained
from naturally infected cultures, even though the quantity of mycoplasma material present in the experimentally infected cultures
was much greater. The high specific activity of Thy-1.1 in these
preparations suggested a selective process capable in some way of
"concentrating" antigens associated with M. hyorhinis.

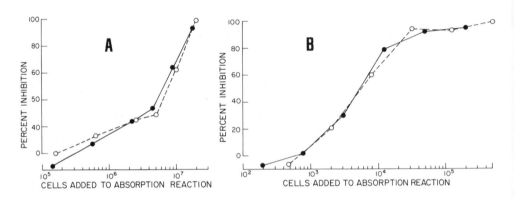

Fig. 5. Phenotypic expression of Thy-1.1 and gp70 antigen on
BW5147 cells. Absorption of gp70 (A) and Thy-1.1 (B) cytotoxic
antiserum was performed using BW5147 cells derived from cultures
either uninfected (●) or experimentally infected (0) with M.
hyorhinis.

        In vitro immunological consequences of mycoplasmas on the
host cell surface. The association between lymphoid cell surface antigens and mycoplasmas on the surface of infected lymphoid
cells was further analysed by studying the C-dependent cytotoxic
properties of antimycoplasma antibodies on infected BW5147 cells
labeled with $\{^{51}Cr\}$. Mule antiserum against M. hyorhinis was
cytotoxic against BW5147 cells infected with this organism, whereas no cytotoxicity was observed with normal control serum (Fig. 6).
When assayed on uninfected BW5147 cells antiserum to M. hyorhinis
showed no cytotoxic activity (Fig. 6). That $\{^{51}Cr\}$ release was
due to cell lysis and not to lysis of surface-associated mycoplasmas (which may have accumulated $\{^{51}Cr\}$) was confirmed by the

observation that infected cells treated with anti-M. hyorhinis
serum were over 95% dead as determined by trypan blue exclusion
(not shown).   This demonstrated that a specific cytolytic reaction
could be mediated by recognition on M. hyorhinis antigens on the
surface of infected BW5147 cells, and suggested a possible mechanism of immunological destruction of lymphoid (or possibly other
host) cells bearing antigens of M. hyorhinis in vivo.

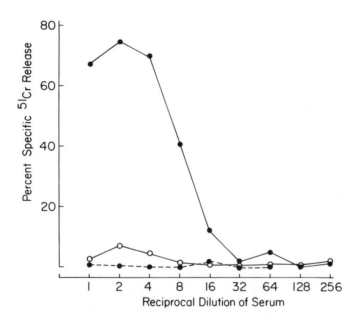

Fig. 6.   Cytotoxic effect of antiserum to M. hyorhinis on mycoplasma-infected BW5147 cells. Varying dilutions of mule antiserum to M. hyorhinis (——·) or preimmune mule serum (-----)
were assessed for C-dependent cytotoxic activity using {^{51}Cr}-
labeled BW5147 cells, either uninfected (0) or naturally infected with M. hyorhinis (●).

Identification of M. hyorhinis antigens recognized in vivo
by chronically infected natural hosts.   In order eventually to
understand the surface interactions between M. hyorhinis and
mammalian cells, and to identify components of these organisms
that may be putative targets in a humoral, immunopathological
response during chronic disease, studies have been initiated to

determine the molecular characteristics of antigenic M. hyorhinis
constituents possibly involved in processes of mycoplasma-cell
interactions. These investigations (1) have aimed at characterizing M. hyorhinis protein antigens by immunoprecipitation of
labeled, detergent-solubilized mycoplasma preparations. SDS-
PAGE analysis of {^{125}I}-labeled mycoplama components precipitated
by standard mule typing serum against M. hyorhinis, revealed a
number of discrete molecular species (ranging in apparent molecular weight from 25,000 to 80,000 daltons) which were not precipitated by control mule serum (Fig. 7a). Serum from experimentally
infected pigs (but not from control, CDCD pigs) showed a similar
pattern of specifically precipitated components (Fig. 7b). With
the exception of an additional 17,000 dalton component, serum from
a pig "naturally" infected with M. hyorhinis also precipitated a
similar pattern of protein antigens (Fig. 7c). None of these sera
precipitated material from {^{125}I}-labeled membranes prepared (33)
from uninfected BW5147 cells, nor from labeled medium used to grow
these cultures. Thus, a number of protein antigens of M. hyorhinis
have been provisionally identified and the IgG class of immunoglobulin measured in this procedure (14) has been demonstrated as a
major component of the humoral response during chronic infection
with M. hyorhinis, a finding in agreement with the results of
others (28).

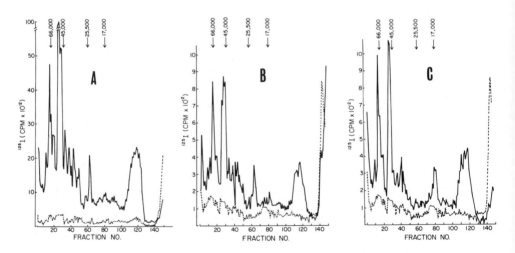

Fig. 7. SDS-PAGE analysis of immunoprecipitated M. hyorhinis antigens. Immunoprecipitates from {^{125}I}-labeled, DOC solubilized M.
hyorhinis obtained with various antisera (——) are compared to
those using respective control sera (----). (A) mule typing serum
against M. hyorhinis; (B) antiserum obtained from swine experimentally infected with M. hyorhinis; and (C) serum from a pig naturally
infected with M. hyorhinis.

DISCUSSION

The results presented here emphasize two major aspects of mycoplasma-host cell interactions: mycoplasmal acquisition of host (lymphoid) cell surface antigens; and possible immunological consequences of a humoral response to mycoplasma antigens, particularly those present on host cell surfaces.

The propensity for mycoplasma to associate _in vitro_ and _in vivo_ with cell surfaces has been extensively documented (2,13,16). A number of reported characteristics of this interaction underscore the close physical and possibly functional relationship between many mycoplasma species and mammalian cells: a) Cell surface adsorption of mycoplasmas may be a very rapid phenomenon _in vitro_ and may lead initially to local clustering of these organisms on the lymphoid cell periphery (29).   b) During the course of "adaptation" of mycoplasmas to cell cultures, the number of organisms capable of associating with the cell surface increases, and has been suggested to reflect alteration in the cellular membrane during progressive mycoplasma colonization of cultured cells (21). c) The ability of mycoplasmas to attach to cells ("cytoadsorption") has also been correlated with their pathogenicity (3). Mycoplasma obtained from animal hosts, as well as the "non-cultivable", cell-adapted forms of M. hyorhinis show particularly striking cytoadsorption (3). The interesting possibility that cell adaptation _in vitro_ by M. hyorhinis may have an _in vivo_ analog has been noted (21).   This interaction may be particularly important in the pathogenesis of mycoplasma disease, and the resulting immunological response.

Within this context, the model system of M. hyorhinis interaction with cultured murine T-lymphoblastoid cells offers further evidence for novel mechanisms of mycoplasma-host cell interactions, and provides for a more precise definition of the cell surface components involved in these processes. The major features described as: a) a selective interaction with lymphoid cell surface components, b) a marked accumulation of host surface antigens by mycoplasmas and c) maintenance of antigen association following mycoplasma detachment from cells. To assess the molecular mechanisms by which these phenomena occur, it is useful to formulate an experimentally testable proposal to explain mycoplasma-cell interactions in a manner consistent with these observations. The five elements of this proposal are briefly outlined as follows:

1. The acquisition of host cell surface components by mycoplasma occurs largely through interactions of these organisms during their physical association with the host cell surface. This is in contrast to alternative, less tenable mechanisms of antigen acquisition, such as binding of cell membrane fragments or "soluble" host antigens to organisms in culture supernatants, which have been discussed elsewhere (27).

2. Host cell constituents interact with surface-associated
mycoplasmas by binding to mycoplasma components expressed on the
surface of these organisms. Both mycoplasma and host cell components are present in multiple copies, thus providing for the
interaction of two multivalent structures. If host cell components are laterally diffusible on the cell membrane, then their
association with mycoplasma may represent the interaction of multiple molecules with a polyvalent "ligand". This would allow for
the accumulation of certain host molecules by surface-associated
mycoplasma. A corollary to this is that mycoplasma may become
mobile on the cell surface following such attachment.

3. The apparent specificity of host component acquisition
by mycoplasma is determined by multiple factors including:
a) the binding affinity of specific or general chemical groups
(e.g., carbohydrate structures) with mycoplasma components, b)
the mobility of host membrane components bearing these groups
(and hence their degree of attachment with the cytoskeletal system) and c) the numerical prevalence of one host surface component (antigen) bearing receptors of equal affinity to those of
other molecules. Thus the Thy-1.1 glycoprotein (31) may selectively associate with mycoplasma due to specific portions of its
protein structure, presence of unique carbohydrage groups, its
high degree of surface mobility (5), or its relatively high concentration on lymphoblastoid cells (30).

4. The association of host membrane components is maintained
during release of mycoplasma from cell surfaces. Little is known
about the mechanisms by which mycoplasma detach from cells.
Mechanisms of "exfoliation" or local fusion of mycoplasma and
cell membranes may be invoked, but with only limited experimental
support for their occurrence in mycoplasma-cell interactions.
The rate and manner of detachment would most likely depend on
the rate of mycoplasma replication, and on the degree of membrane integration and turnover rates of host surface components
interacting with mycoplasma.

This proposal offers one framework, consistent with current
observations, for the experimental evaluation of multiple surface
related processes involved in mycoplasma-cell interactions. Other
factors (such as the ability to utilize cell metabolite pools,
etc.) have been purposely ignored to focus on interactions between
surface molecules. The presence of specific antigenic surface
components in the defined murine T-cell system, and further characterization of M. hyorhinis antigenic constituents identified
in this report, should aid in the evaluation of these phenomena.

A second major consideration relevant to data presented here
concerns possible immunological consequences of mycoplasma-host

cell interactions in vivo. Association of host antigens in general, and particularly of T-lymphoid cell surface antigens with
mycoplasmas residing on cell surfaces, may have profound effects
on the immune response to these organisms during chronic disease.
Possible interactions leading to altered immunological responses
to mycoplasmas can be summarized:

1.   Avoidance of the host immune response may result from
acquisition of host cell antigens, as has been proposed for other
parasitic infections (10,12). This would require fairly complete
masking of mycoplasma antigens, a situation which may not generally
prevail, but which could account for persistence of organisms by
effectively "isolating" a small number of mycoplasma from the
immune apparatus.

2.   As denizens of cell surfaces, mycoplasmas may provide
targets for various immunological effector mechanisms, which
could lead to host-cell damage. One such mechanism is suggested
by the C-dependent lysis of infected BW5147 cells by anti-myco-
plasma antisera. Damage in vivo could result in the production
of antinuclear antibodies, as observed in a number of autoimmune
diseases. An additional similarity to autoimmune phenomena could
result from immune-complex deposition on tissues bearing mycoplasma antigens. This may be particularly relevant to acute
phases of M. hyorhinis-induced polyarthritis in swine (22).

3.   Acquisition of host cell components by mycoplasma may
alter their structure sufficiently to induce an autoimmune
response. Antibodies reacting with normal tissue have been observed in a number of mycoplasma diseases (8). An important
extrapolation of this possibility is the induction of a destructive immunological response to T-lymphoid cells due to acquisition to T-cell antigens by M. hyorhinis, a phenomenon currently
being investigated.

4.   An additional consequence of mycoplasma interaction with
T-lymphoid cells may be the alteration of T-cell function (in
either afferent or efferent immunological processes) due to surface perturbation induced during close contact between lymphoid
cells with mycoplasma-infected tissues. This may cause major,
but presently unpredictable, changes in the immune response to
mycopasmas.

Taken together, these phenomena could lead to a large variety
of mycoplasma-induced modifications of the host immune response.
The final immunological balance between host and persistent pathogenic mycoplasma would obviously be determined by an extremely
complex set of influences. The advantage of the in vitro model
system described herein is that some of these interactions may be
individually dissected to analyze their importance in vivo.

NOTE ADDED IN PROOF

We have obtained evidence for the predicted lateral mobility of mycoplasmas on the surface of BW5147 cells, using immunofluorescent techniques. BW5147 cells chronically infected with M. hyorhinis were obtained from logarithmic phase cultures and fixed with 1% paraformaldehyde. Subsequent immunofluorescent staining of mycoplasmas by a double antibody technique (27), revealed a predominance (80-90%) of lymphoid cells with single aggregates or "caps" of mycoplasmas at one pole. Thus, spontaneous aggregation of mycoplasmas at the cell surface prevailed under these culture conditions. Capping of mycoplasmas in other lymphoid cell systems has been recently reported by others (34). These results further suggest interactions of mycoplasmas with host cell surface components that could be involved both in mycoplasma attachment, and in stabilization of surface aggregates by self agglutination of organisms bearing these host cell constituents.

ACKNOWLEDGEMENT

We thank Dr. G. H. Cassell for continuing support in this work, Ms. Barbara Patterson for expert technical assistance, and Mrs. Candy Gathings for preparation of the manuscript. This work was supported by PHS grants AM-20614, GM-07561, CA-15338, CA-18609 and NSF grant GB-53575X. Ronald T. Acton is an established investigator of the American Heart Association.

REFERENCES

1. Asa, P. B., Acton, R. T., Cassell, G. H. and Wise, K. S. ASM Abstracts (1978) 73.
2. Barile, M. F., In: Cell Culture and Its Applications, (Eds. R. T. Acton and J. D. Lynn), Academic Press, New York (1977) 291.
3. Barile, M. F., Hopps, H. E. and Grabowski, In: Mycoplasma Infection of Cell Cultures, (Eds. G. J. McGarrity, D. G. Murphy and W. W. Nichols), Plenum Press, New York (1978) 35.
4. Barstad, P. A., Henley, S. L., Cox, R. M., Lynn, J. D. and Acton, R. T. Proc Soc. Exp. Biol. Med., 115 (1977) 296.
5. Berlin, R. D., Oliver, J. M., Ukena, T. E. and Yin, H. H. Nature, 247 (1974) 45.
6. Cassell, G. H., Davis, J. K., Wilborn, W. and Wise, K. S. .n Microbiology (Ed. D. Schlessinger), American Society for Microbiology, Washington, D. C. (1978) 399.
7. Cullen, S. E. and Schwartz, B. D. J. Immunol., 117 (1976) 136.

8. DeVay, J. E. and Adler, H. E. Ann. Rev. Microbiol, 30 (1976) 147.
9. Freundt, E. A. Pathol. Microbiol., 40 (1974) 155.
10. Goldring, O. L., Clegg, J. A., Smithers, S. R. and Terry, R. J. Clin Exp. Immunol., 26 (1976) 181.
11. Greenwood, F. C., Hunter, W. M. and Glover, J. S. Biochem. J., 80 (1963) 114.
12. Hall, B. F., Sher, A. and Vadas, M. A. Federation Proceedings, 37 (1978) 1660.
13. Hopps, H. E., Meyer, B. C., Barile, M. F. and Del Guidice, R. A. Ann. N. Y. Acad. Sci., 225 (1973) 267.
14. MacKenzie, M. R., Warner, N. L. and Mitchell, G. F. J., Immunol., 120 (1978) 1493.
15. Old, L. J., Boyse, E. A. and Stockert, E., Canc. Res., 25 (1965) 813.
16. Phillips, D. M., In: Mycoplasma Infection of Cell Cultures (Eds. G. J. McGarrity, D. G. Murphy and W. W. Nichols), Plenum Press, New York, (1978) 105.
17. Ralph, P., J. Immunol., 110 (1973) 1470.
18. Ross, R. F. and Duncan, J. R. J., Amer. Vet. Med. Assoc., 157 (1970) 1515.
19. Shin, S. -Il, and Van Diggelen, O. P., In: Mycoplasma Infection of Cell Cultures, (Eds. G. J. McGarrity, D. G. Murphy and W. W. Nichols), Plenum Press, New York, (1978) 191.
20. Stanbridge, E. J., Ann. Rev. Microbiol., 30 (1976) 169.
21. Stanbridge, E. J. and Katayama, C., In: Mycoplasma Infection of Cell Cultures, (Eds. G. J. McGarrity, D. G. Murphy and W. W. Nichols), Plenum Press, New York, (1978) 71.
22. Switzer, W. P., Amer. J. Vet. Res., 16 (1955) 540.
23. Todoro, G. J., Aaronson, S. A. and Rands, E., Exptl. Cell Res., 65 (1971) 256.
24. Vaguzhinskaya, O. E. J., Hyg. Camb. 77 (1976) 189.
25. Wise, K. and Acton, R., In: Protides of the Biological Fluids, (Ed. H. Peeters), Pergamon Press, Oxford, England, 25 (1977) 707.
26. Wise, K. S., Cassell, G. H. and Acton, R. T., Federation Proceedings, 37 (1978) 1851.
27. Wise, K. S., Cassell, G. H. and Acton, R. T., Proc. Nat. Acad. Sci. (USA), 75 (1978) 4479.
28. Zibb, M., In: Infection and Immunology in the Rheumatic Diseases, (Ed. D. C. Dumond), Blackwell Scientific Publications, Oxford, (1976) 627.
29. Zucker-Franklin, D., Davidson, M. and Thomas, L., J. Exp. Med., 124 (1966) 521.
30. Zwerner, R. K. and Acton, R. T. J., Exp. Med., 142 (1975) 378.
31. Zwerner, R. K., Barstad, P. A. and Acton, R. T., J. Exp. Med., 146 (1977) 986.

32. Zwerner, R. K., Runyan, C., Cox, R. M., Lynn, J. D. and Acton,
     R. T., Biothechnol. Bioeng., 17 (1975) 629.
33. Zwerner, R. K., Wise, K. S. and Acton, R. T., In: Methods
     in Enzymology, (Ed. Jakoby), Academic Press, New York, 58
     (1978) 221.
34. Stanbridge, E. J. and Weiss, R. L. Nature, 276 (1978) 583.

ALVEOLAR MACROPHAGE DYSFUNCTION ASSOCIATED WITH VIRAL PNEUMONITIS

G. J. JAKAB, G. A. WARR and P. L. SANNES

The Johns Hopkins University
School of Hygiene and Public Health, Department of
Environmental Health Sciences, Baltimore, Maryland (USA)

Pulmonary virus infections are known to predispose to bacterial infections in the lung (4). The mechanisms by which acute
viral infections alter normal host resistance to bacterial infection have been studied in a model of murine Sendai virus pneumonia
(6). Quantitative measurements of bactericidal mechanisms during
virus pneumonia have demonstrated that the infection progressively
depresses the in situ phagocytic defenses of the lung reaching
maximal virus-induced suppression of pulmonary anti-bacterial
defenses approximately seven days after viral infection (5).
Thereafter pulmonary phagocytic defenses gradually return to normal. Additional in vivo studies have shown that the virus-induced
suppression of phagocytic defenses is associated with defects in
the alveolar macrophage phagocytic system (7,10). This study
examines the effect of pulmonary virus infection on the ingestion,
phagosome-lysosome fusion, and intracellular killing mechanisms
of alveolar macrophage phagocytosis to relate viral-induced
suppression of pulmonary anti-bacterial defenses to abnormalities
in the subcomponents of the phagocytic process.

MATERIALS AND METHODS

Swiss albino mice were infected by aerosol inhalation with
a sublethal dose of Parainfluenza 1 (Sendai) virus (6). At
various times after infection the lungs of virus infected and
non-infected mice were excised in toto and free pulmonary cells
obtained by lung lavage techniques. The lung cells were suspended
in tissue culture medium 199 (TCM 199) and allowed to form monolayers on coverslips at a cell density of 2 X 10^5.

For the ingestion and intracellular killing experiments lung
macrophages were challenged with freshly grown Candida krusei at
a ratio of 20 yeasts/macrophage. Cultures were maintained at 37 C
in TCM 199 supplemented with 10% heat inactivated fetal calf serum
and 5% guinea pig serum (complement source) (TCM 199 + S). After
the initial challenge period of 30 min, the monolayers were washed
3 times, the culture fluid replenished and incubation continued
for three hr. Macrophage cultures were then treated with a fresh
solution of methylene blue in TCM 199 (0.065 mg/ml). After 5 min
of reincubation the macrophage monolayers were washed 3 times,
the coverslips removed and inverted cell side down on a drop of
the culture fluid to maintain cell viability. By light microscopy intracellular yeasts were counted and the percent dead
yeasts (stained blud) determined (9). The monolayers were then
fixed and stained with Wright-Giemsa to determine phagocytic indices.

Phagosome-lysosome fusion patterns in cells from virus infected and noninfected lungs were visualized by darkfield fluorescent microscopy by a modification of the methods described by
Hart and Young (3). Macrophages from virus infected and non-
infected lungs were monolayered in each of 2 chambers of a 4
chamber Lab-Tek tissue culture chamber slide. To the monolayers
20 μl containing 1 μg of freshly prepared acridine orange solution was added and, after tilting the slides several times to
mix chamber content, the slides reincubated for 20 min. Thereafter, each chamber was washed to remove the non-adherent cells
and excess acridine orange. After washing, the monolayers were
challenged with C. krusei at a yeast to macrophage ratio of 20:1.
After 1 hr incubation the chambers were again washed, the slides
wet mounted with a coverslip and immediately examined with a
Zeiss fluorescent microscope at 1000X. Phagosome-lysosome fusion
patterns were quantitated by randomly selecting and counting 50
macrophages containing intracellular C. krusei and determing
whether the prelabelled lysosomes had fused with the yeast-con-
taining phagosomes as previously described (3). Controls for
the inhibition of phagosome-lysosome fusion were performed with
the lysosomotropic drug suramin previously demonstrated to inhibit the normal fusion process (3). Suramin (250 μg in 20 μl)
was added to the culture chambers containing the lavaged cells
from noninfected mice 10 min after the addition of acridine
orange and removed from the monolayers with the dye. In all
other respects the fusion assay was identical to suramin untreated
cells.

For the ultrastructural cytochemical studies of phagosome-
lysosome fusion the macrophages were suspended in TCM 199 + S
and challenged with viable C. krusei for 1 hr at 37 C. The cells
were then pelleted at 200 x g and fixed with 2% glutaraldehyde,
post-fixed with osmium, and processed for acid phosphatase cyto-

chemistry using a modified Gomorri technique (1) utilizing beta-glycerophosphate as substrate and lead acetate as an electron dense coupler.

RESULTS

Ingestion and intracellular killing of C. krusei by alveolar macrophages during the course of the viral infection is presented in Fig. 1. Under the experimental condition 91.3 ± 1.5% (mean ± S.E.) of the macrophages from noninfected lungs were actively phagocytic ingesting a mean of 6.9 ± 0.3 yeasts. Approximately the same values were observed during the third day of the viral infection. At day 7 the infection induced a reduction in the phagocytic indices so that only 55.0 ± 1.8% of the macrophages were phagocytic each containing 5.1 ± 0.2 yeasts. By day 17 the percentage of the macrophages actively phagocytic was not significantly lower (77.2 ± 5.2%) than the normal values, however, the numbers of yeast ingested was significantly increased to 8.6 ± 0.7 macrophage, a value 25% above normal.

Fig. 1 also shows that in control macrophages 54.5 ± 3.0% of the ingested yeasts were killed within a 3 hr period. Following virus infection the ability of those macrophages which are actively phagocytic to kill microorganisms was progressively reduced. By day 7 only 12.7 ± 2.0% of the yeasts ingested are killed. Those macrophages assayed 17 days following the virus infection were more candidacidal (35.1 ± 2.5%) but were still significantly less active than controls.

Patterns of phagosome-lysosome fusion with normal murine alveolar macrophages were identical to those described with murine peritoneal macrophages (3). Briefly, after ingestion the orange fluorescing lysosomal granules assembled around the unstained yeast cells. Next, these periphagosomal granules disappeared and a bright orange confluent rim of fluorescence appeared around the individual yeasts indicating the discharge of lysosomal content into the phagosomes. Gradually the dye permeated into the yeast cells coloring the whole organism a vivid green. Over the next 30 min the intensity of the green fluorescence faded until sometime later dark holes were seen, suggesting the degradation of the yeast by the lysosomal enzymes. These stages overlapped since after 1 hr of incubation of the yeasts and the alveolar macrophage periphagosomal lysosomes, fluorescent rims and colored yeast were all observed.

Suramin did not appear to interfere with the uptake of the yeasts cells by alveolar macrophages; 1 hr after the start of ingestion, periphagosomal lysosomes were predominant with fluorescent rims and colored yeast being inconspicuous. Concurrent controls showed the normal fusion pattern.

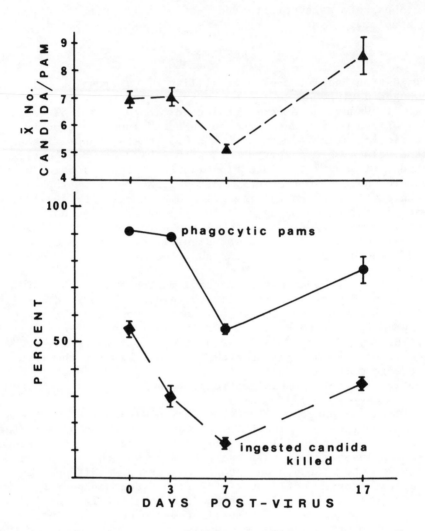

Fig. 1. Ingestion and intracellular killing of C. krusei by
alveolar macrophages during the course of the viral infection.
Each point represents the mean ± S. E. of 10 individual determinations.

Quantitated fusion patterns in free lung cells obtained
during the course of the viral infection is presented in Fig. 2.
In non-infected control macrophages 97 ± 3% of the ingested C.
krusei were fused with the prelabelled lysosomes. Phagosome-
lysosome fusion progressively decreased during the course of the

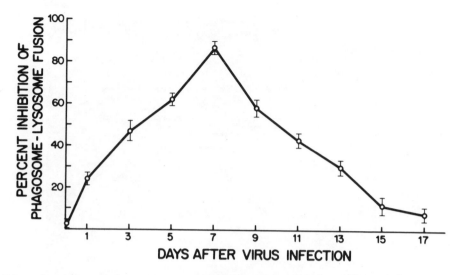

Fig. 2. Phagosome-lysosome fusion patterns in phagocytic cells
during the course of the viral infection. Each point represents
the mean ± S.E. of 10 individual determinations.

viral infection until at day 7 only 13 ± 3% of the intracellular
yeasts showed the normal fusion pattern (Fig. 3). Thereafter,
the fusion patterns gradually returned to normal until at day 17
92 ± 2% of the ingested yeasts containing phagosomes had fused.

The cytochemical studies of the phagosome-lysosome fusion
process are presented in Fig. 4 through 6. In these micrographs
the acid phosphatase reactivity product appear as dark granules
in the lysosomes and within phagolysosomes indicative of phagosome-
lysosome fusion (Fig. 4). Three days after viral infection acid
phosphatase could not be found in the yeast containing phagosomes
of a large number of macrophages (Fig. 5). Those macrophages obtained during the seventh day of the viral infection showed no
evidence of phagosome-lysosome fusion (Fig. 6). However, it
should be noted that acid phosphatase-containing lysosomes within the cytoplasm of these cells is also greatly reduced as compared with control macrophages (Fig. 4) and day 3 macrophages
(Fig. 6).

DISCUSSION

Bacterial multiplication associated with pulmonary virus
infections is related to defects in in situ bactericidal (phagocytic) mechanisms of the lung (4-6). In vivo studies have

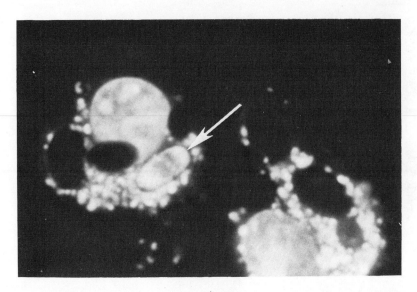

Fig. 3. Acridine orange phagosome-lysosome fusion assay in alveolar macrophages obtained from the lungs during the seventh
day of the viral infection. Note the numerous intracellular
dark oval structures signifying lack of fusion and the fluorescing yeast (arrow) demonstrating successful fusion.

identified that this defect is associated with dysfunctions of the
alveolar macrophage phagocytic system (7,10). In the studies
presented herein we have dissected some of the subcomponents of
the phagocytic process to further define the viral-induced functional lesion.

     The data clearly demonstrate that the phagocytic components
of engulfment, phagososome-lysosome fusion and intracellular
killing are all suppressed by the viral infection. Suppression
of ingestion is evident not only by the reduction of actively
phagocytic macrophages but also by the fewer microorganisms
internalized by each phagocytic cell.

     Virus induced suppression of intracellular killing progres-
sively decreased during the course of the infection reaching a
maximum at day 7 and then gradually returning to normal. The
magnitude and time course of the killing defect paralleled the
defect in phagosome-lysosome fusion. This correlation offers a
possible explanation for the mechanism of the killing defect by
the failure of the potent hydrolytic lysosomal enzymes to reach
the ingested organisms sequestered in the phagosomes. The cyto-

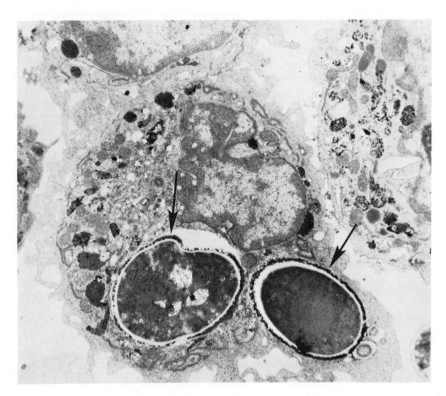

Fig. 4. Electron micrograph of a lung macrophage from a normal
non-infected mouse. The macrophages were challenged in vitro
with Candida krusei for one hr. The macrophage contains two
ingested yeast cells, both of which are surrounded by electron
dense acid phosphatase reaction product (arrows) indicating
lysosomes have fused with the phagosomes.

chemical studies however suggest that the quantity of degradative
enzymes, as determined by the marker enzyme acid phosphatase,
may not be present in sufficient concentration to degrade the ingested cell even if fusion had occurred.

    Following this line of thinking the data suggest another
possible mechanism for failure of macrophages from virus infected
lungs to inactivate ingested organisms. The degradation of ingested organisms by hydrolytic enzymes stands on firm experimental ground (2) and undoubtedly the lysosomal enzymes by sheer
dissolution of the organism also participate in the intracellular
killing of microorganisms. Data, however, suggest that more

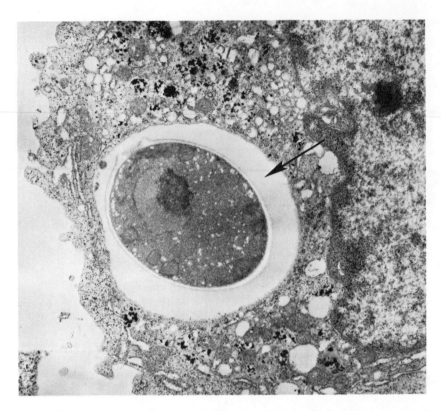

Fig. 5. Lung macrophage from a mouse infected three days earlier
with Sendai virus. The phagosome (arrow) surrounding the ingested yeast cell is devoid of any acid phosphatase reaction
produce indicating the absence of lysosome-phagosome fusion.

rapid and efficient extra-lysosomal (biochemical) killing
mechanisms are the primary participants in the intracellular
inactivation of organisms (8). Thus, an explanation for the
killing dysfunction would also include a defect in the extra-
lysosomal killing mechanisms. Viral infections are known to
predispose to bacterial infections of the lung. Studies on the
virus-induced suppression of pulmonary bactericidal mechanisms
have identified the defect with abnormalities in the alveolar
macrophage phagocytic system. In the investigation presented
herein, we have dissected some of the subcomponents of the phagocytic process and found virus-induced defects in phagocytic ingestion, phagosome-lysosome fusion, and intracellular killing.

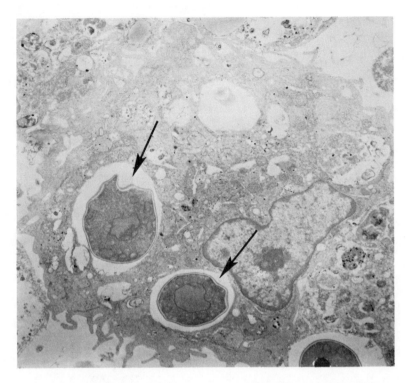

Fig. 6. Lung macrophage from a mouse infected seven days earlier with Sendai virus. The macrophage contains two ingested yeast cells. The phagocytic vacuoles surrounding both yeast cells (arrows) are devoid of acid phosphatase reaction product. The macrophage is devoid of acid phosphatase containing lysosomes normally found within these cells (Fig. 4,5).

SUMMARY

     Viral infections are known to predispose to bacterial in-
fections of the lung. Studies on the virus-induced suppression
of pulmonary bactericidal mechanisms have identified the defect
with abnormalities in the alveolar macrophage phagocytic system.
In the investigation presented herein, we have dissected some
of the subcomponents of the phagocytic process and found virus-
induced defects in phagocytic ingestion, phagosome-lysosome
fusion, and intracellular killing.

ACKNOWLEDGEMENTS

This work was supported by NHLBI grants HL 22029 and HL 14214 (SCOR). Dr. Jakab is the recipient of an NHLBI Research Career Award (HL 00415). Dr. Warr receives support from an NHLBI Research Fellowship Award (HL 05404). Dr. Sannes is supported by NIH postdoctoral fellowship IF 32 GM 05854 from the Institute of General Medical Sciences (USA).

REFERENCES

1. Barka, T., and Anderson, P. J., Histochem. Cytochem. 10 (1962) 740.
2. Goren, M. B., Annual Rev. Microbiol. 31 (1977) 507.
3. Hart, P. D. and Young, M. R., Nature 256 (1975) 47.
4. Jakab, G. J., Bull. Europ. Physiopathol. Resp. 13 (1977) 119.
5. Jakab, G. J. and Dick, E. C., Infect. Immun. 8 (1973) 762.
6. Jakab, G. J. and Green, G. M., J. Clin. Invest. 51 (1972) 1989.
7. Jakab, G. J. and Green, G. M., J. Clin. Invest. 57 (1976) 1533.
8. Klebanoff, S. J. and Hamon, C. B., Antimicrobial systems of mononuclear phagocytes. In: Mononuclear Phagocytes in Immunity, Infection, and Pathology. (Ed. R. van Furth), Blackwell Scientific Publications, Oxford (1975).
9. Schmid, L and Brune, K., Infect. Immun. 10 (1974) 1120.
10. Warschauer, D., Goldstein, E., Akers, T., Lippert W. and Kim, M., Amer. Rev. Resp. Dis. 115 (1977) 269.

B AND T LYMPHOCYTE ACTIVATION BY MURINE LEUKEMIA VIRUS INFECTION

M. BENDINELLI and H. FRIEDMAN

Institute of Microbiology, Pisa (Italy) and University
of South Florida College of Medicine, Tampa, Florida
(USA)

Infection of mice with murine leukemia viruses markedly
affect antibody formation (1,3,6). Both in vivo and in vitro
studies have shown that leukemia virus infection may preferentially
affect antibody forming B cells or their precursors, impairing
their ability to respond normally to antigenic stimulation. Many
studies of this type have suggested that a leukemia virus, when
given before or simultaneously with an antigen such as sheep erythrocytes, depresses subsequent antibody responsiveness. In contrast, studies in this and other laboratories have shown that the
"background" antibody responsiveness to a wide variety of antigens
may be actually stimulated in animals infected with a leukemia virus
alone and not challenged with antigen (4,5). In the present study,
this immunostimulatory effect of Friend leukemia virus (FLV) was
studied in relationship to polyclonal activation of B lymphocytes
or their precursors.

MATERIALS AND METHODS

The FLV was used to infect normal mouse spleen cells in culture. For this purpose, 5×10^6 spleen cells obtained from normal Balb/c mice were cultured in Linbro plates in microtiter wells
(2,7). The antibody responsiveness of the splenocytes was determined by challenge immunization of the cultures with 4×10^6 SRBC.
The number of antibody plaque forming cells (PFC) developing in
the cultures were assessed by the hemolytic plaque assay in agar
gel at various times thereafter (2,7). In order to determine
the effects of FLV, spleen cell extracts were prepared from normal mice injected with 100 ID_{50} virus 7-10 days earlier. Cell-

free extracts were prepared by homogenization of the infected
splenocytes. These extracts were clarified by high speed centrifugation. Graded amounts of the extracts were added to cultures.
The effect of the FLV on the blastogenic responsiveness of the cultures was determined by the standard tritiated thymidine as described elsewhere (2). The stimulation index was assessed by counting triplicate cultures pulsed with thymidine 24-28 hr after treatment with virus as compared to untreated control cultures. The
"background" antibody response was determined in cultures which
were not immunized with SRBC but treated with virus only.

RESULTS

In initial experiments, the effect of FLV infection on the
in vitro antibody response to SRBC was examined. As is evident
in Table I, a rapid increase in total spleen cell number occurred
in infected mice. As the disease progressed there was a concomitant decrease in the ability of the animals to mount an effective

TABLE I

Effect of FLV Infection on SRBC-Induced
and Background PFC Response

Time in Days After In Vivo Infection with FLV[a]	Total no. of Spleen Cells (x 10^8)	PFC per Spleen[b]	
		RBC Immune	Background
None (control)	1.8	47,310 ± 2480	197 ± 46
-1	1.9	51,650 ± 3600	230 ± 32
-3	2.1	31,400 ± 2150	110 ± 18
-5	2.7	10,600 ± 1300	57 ± 14
-8	3.4	5,100 ± 670	40 ± 8
-15	6.5	2,650 ± 530	30 ± 3

[a]Mice injected i.p. with 50-100 ID_{50} FLV on day indicated.
[b]PFC response 5 days after i.p. immunization with 2 x 10^8 SRBC.

immunocyte response to challenge immunization with SRVC. For
example, it is evident that mice infected for only 3-5 days
showed a marked inhibition of the antibody response to SRBC 5
days after challenge immunization. By the end of the first or

second week after infection these animals were markedly immunosuppressed. The "background" antibody response to SRBC in the
animals not challenged with antigen was similarly depressed as
the disease progressed.

When FLV was added to normal spleen cell cultures in vitro,
there was a similar marked depression of immune responsiveness
(Table II). In these experiments FLV was added to spleen cell

TABLE II

Effect of In Vitro Infection of spleen Cell Culture with
FLV on RBC-Induced and Background PFC Response

Time in Days After In Vitro Infection[a]	PFC/10^6 Spleen Cells[b]		Blastogenesis (S.I.)
	Plus SRBC[c]	No RBC	
None (control)	768 ± 82	73 ± 14	1.0
0	206 ± 32	197 ± 36	9.3
+1	240 ± 43	258 ± 28	7.6
+2	478 ± 58	150 ± 30	2.3
+3	610 ± 37	64 ± 21	1.6
+4	689 ± 72	78 ± 13	0.9

[a]Cultures of 5 x 10^6 normal Balb/c spleen cells infected with
100 ID_{50} FLV on day "0".

[b]PFC response 5 days after culture initiation.

[c]Culture immunized with 2 x 10^6 SRBC.

cultures on the day of culture initiation and challenge immunization. Most cultures showed a 70-80% or greater suppression of
antibody responsiveness. When the virus extract was added one
day after culture initiation there was a similar suppression of
antibody responsiveness. However, if virus infection was delayed until the second day or longer after culture initiation,
no significant suppression of the immune response was evident.

In contrast to the above results, when the background antibody response was determined for similar cultures not challenged
in vitro with antigen a dichotomous effect was noted. Those cultures treated with virus on the day of culture initiation or 1
to 2 days later showed a marked increase in background respon-

siveness, as compared to untreated cultures or cultures treated
with virus on days 3 or 4 and then assessed for background PFCs
on day 5 (Table II). Similarly, the blastogenic response of the
splenocytes treated with virus in vitro showed a marked correlation with time of addition of the virus to the cultures. Splenocytes treated with virus on the day of culture initiation had a
nine-fold increase in thymidine uptake as compared to control
cultures (Table II). There was still a significant effect on
the blastogenic response when cultures were treated with virus
one day later and the response determined five days later.
When the virus was added 2-4 days after culture initiation there
was little significant effect on thymidine incorporation.

TABLE III

Effect of FLV Dose on Background PFC Responses

FLV Concentration[a]	Background PFC Response/10^6 Splenocytes[b]				
	day +1	+2	+3	+4	+6
None	18	24	42	96	42
10^0	20	86	142	232	160
10^{-1}	19	58	110	150	105
10^{-2}	28	42	94	106	72
10^{-3}	15	30	49	85	39

[a]Indicated dilution of FLV (undiluted = 1000 ID_{50}) added on
day 0 to 5 x 10^6 normal Balb/c spleen cells.

[b]Average PFC response for cultures on indicated day.

These responses were directly related to the dose of virus
used to stimulate the cultures. The maximum responses occurred
when concentrated virus containing extracts were used (Table III).
Normal spleen extracts had little, if any effect (Table IV).
Furthermore, when the virus containing extracts were heated at
80 C to destroy the infectivity of the virus there was essentially no effect on either antigen induced or background anti-
SRBC responses or the blastogenic response (Table IV).

DISCUSSION

In the present study, the immunostimulatory effects of a murine leukemia virus was studied in terms of effects on antigen induced and background antibody responses to a T-dependent antigen, e.g., sheep erythrocytes, as well as on blastogenesis of the splenocytes. Leukemia virus infection depressed the antigen induced immune response to SRBC, both in vivo and in vitro (1,3,6). However, in vivo there was also a depression of background antibody response, considered an indicator of polyclonal activation of immunocytes, whereas in vitro there was an enhancement of such background responses. This dichotomy appeared related to the possible transformation of lymphocytes in vitro by virus infection. Presumably in vivo there was also a marked transformation and replication of lymphocytes but this could be due to malignant transformation rather than a stimulatory transformation. It is

TABLE IV

Effect of Heating on Background PFC Stimulatory
activity of Friend virus

FLV Preparation[a]	Heating (80 C)	Percent PFC Response of Control Spleen Cells[c] plus SRBC[d]	No RBC	Blastogenesis (S.I.)
Stock FLV	–	4.2%	220.5%	7.3
Infected Spleen	+	83.5%	110.2	2.9
Extract	–	13.6	376.5	9.2
	+	79.8	107.6	2.1
Normal Spleen 1:1		97.6	99.1	1.1

[a]Indicated virus preparation added to cultures of 5 x 10⁶ spleen cells

[b]Heated for 30 min at 80 C

[c]Average PFC response for 3-6 cultures 5 days after culture initiation.

[d]2 x 10⁶ SRBC added to cultures on day 0

possible that in vitro the virus infection occurs at a much slower rate than in vivo because of restrictions induced by the limited growth conditions of the medium, etc. Under such conditions the

leukemia virus appears to cause a moderate proliferative response
which could be reflected not only in thymidine incorporation by
the lymphoid cells but also by increased background PFCs to SRBCs.

The depressed responses of antigen induced PFCs in vitro may
be related to a secondary effect of virus infection in vitro on
antibody forming cells whereas the enhancement of the background
response could be a primary effect related to cell division. Thus
the results of these studies point to a dichotomous effect of
murine leukemia virus infection on lymphoid cell function in vitro
vs. in vivo. It is essential to note that the in vitro responses
may be unrelated to the oncogenic potential of the leukemia virus
infection in vivo. Nevertheless it should be noted that earlier
studies had shown that even in vivo there is a stimulation,
rather than a depression of background antibody responses to a
bacterium such as Vibrio cholerae, which appears to induce a
primary type response in mice rather than the typical responses
noted for SRBC which may reflect a response of animals to an antigen to which they had already been exposed inadvertantly in the
environment. In terms of the response to cholera antigen, immunosuppression did not occur unless mice were infected for a week or
longer with the virus. Those animals given vibrio antigen within
a few days after virus infection showed an enhanced rather than
a suppressed response, suggesting in those studies that the virus
affected primarily antigen stimulated cells rather than "virgin"
immunocompetent cells.

In the present in vitro studies, it is evident that FLV when
added simultaneously to cultures which are not being immunized
with SRBC, an immunostimulatory rather than a suppressive effect
occurs. This, therefore, appears related to the blastogenic
responsiveness of lymphoid cells being infected by the virus.
Active virus replication as a possible mechanism for this effect
is suggested by the finding that heat inactivated virus failed
to cause a similar response. Experiments are warranted to determine the actual cycle or kinetics of virus replication in vitro,
and to relate virus replication to the immunostimulatory and blastogenic responsiveness noted in the present study.

                                    SUMMARY

FLV is suppressive both in vivo and in vitro in terms of the
specific sheep RBC induced antibody response. FLV-containing extracts from infected spleens were found to be markedly immuno-
suppressive. However, these extracts stimulated the background
PFC response to SRBC in vitro, whereas similar background responses
were depressed in infected animals. Furthermore the virus-con-
taining extracts were mitogenic for normal spleen cells in vitro.
Thus, FLV infection may cause immunocyte division (i.e., trans-

formation) as an early event followed later by marked impairment
of the function of the cells as evinced by their failure to
respond normally to challenge immunization.

REFERENCES

1. Dent, P. P., Progr. Med. Virol. 14 (1972) 1.
2. Friedman, H., Ann. N. Y. Acad. Sci. 249 (1975) 264.
3. Friedman, H. and Ceglowski, W. S., Progr. Immunol. 1 (1971)
    815.
4. Hirano, S. and Friedman, H., Nature 224 (1969) 1316.
5. Hirano, S., Friedman, H. and Ceglowski, W. S. J. Immunol.
    107 (1971) 1400.
6. Salaman, M. H., Antibiot. Chemotherap. 15 (1969) 393.
7. Specter, S., Patel, N. and Friedman, H. J. Nat. Canc. Res.
    56 (1976) 143.

ABOLITION OF LYMPHOCYTE BLASTOGENESIS BY ONCORNAVIRAL COMPONENTS

A. HELLMAN[1], A. K. FOWLER[1], D. R. TWARDZIK[1], O. S. WEISLOW[2], and C. D. REED[1]

VOP, NCI, NIH[1] and Litton Bionetics, Inc.[2]
Frederick, Maryland (USA)

Numerous studies have documented immunological alterations associated with a variety of viral infections. These alterations most frequently lead to immune suppression which is observed in both the humoral and cellular compartments of the response, and occur by poorly defined mechanisms. There are at least 20 diseases caused by currently recognized nononcogenic viruses that modify humoral and/or cellular immune function (7). The purpose of this paper is to present data relevant to the retroviruses, a group of RDDP-containing RNA viruses that are transmitted genetically and have been conserved in the genome of most mammals for millions of years.

In those instances where the type C viruses produce a malignancy, it is accompanied by an alteration of immune functions. These modifications are most often early events that may permit tumor progression. Observations by Old (14), a number of years ago, demonstrated a diminished antibody response to an antigen challenge in Friend virus infected mice. Much work has been done since, by other laboratories, to substantiate and expand on these findings. Similarly, abundant data demonstrate suppression of cellular immunity in the host during type C viral induced disease (3). One might still argue which comes first, the suppression leading to disease or the disease leading towards suppression. Our recent data demonstrate that lymphoid cell receptors for the type C virus envelope glycoprotein (gp70) are rapidly saturated in vitro (4) as well as during active viral infection in vivo (unpublished observation) and this may indeed contribute to early events leading to immune modification. In order to focus on the possible generalized immunological modification these viruses may bring about, immune suppression encountered during

99

viral induced leukemia or lymphoma will be of secondary consideration in the context of this paper.

Retroviral genome conservation in the mammal over millions of
years has suggested to us that these agents may serve normal and
necessary physiological functions and only incidentally become
pathogenic under very defined conditions. We would like briefly
to present our evidence and that of others, which support our
contention of the physiological functions of type C viruses. We
will then present our more recent data characterizing and demonstrating an immunological suppressor function for oncornaviral
associated components of murine and nonhuman primate origin and
conclude by suggesting both pathogenic and developmental functions
for these viruses.

We first reported that estrogenic hormones, recognized for
their capacity to modify suppressor genes in target tissue, are
indeed able to derepress type C viral components in the uterus (8).
Viral structural components such as p30 were expressed in ovariec-
tomized mice between 8 and 12 hr after 1 µg of estradiol-17β
administration. Similarly, viral RNA-directed DNA polymerase was
detected within 24-48 hr after estrogen stimulation. More recently,
using cDNA hybridization we have been able to demonstrate the
presence of murine type C viral-specific RNA as early as 4 hr
after estrogen stimulation. When examining the mouse uterine
secretory epithelium during gestation, type C viruses were observed
budding from these cells and mature particles were noted in the
immediate intercellular spaces (5). Interestingly, these particles
were predominately observed shortly after implantation and during
early stages of embryonic development. A component of the placenta
considered to be intricately involved in fetal acceptance, the
syncytiotrophoblast, has also clearly been observed to express
type C viruses in primates, including man (12). Also these
viruses, or their proteins, seem to be sufficiently antigenic
as to bring about in the human female the development of cytotoxic
antibodies directed against cells replicating and expressing on
their cell surface primate type C viral antigens (10). We suggest
that the type C viruses or their components are present at times
in the host when they may have a capacity to exert localized immune
regulation, either in a beneficial or pathogenic mode. We would
like to discuss and characterize such an immune regulator.

We recently described a type C viral associated inhibitor to
cell-mediated immunity in vitro (6). This factor was observed
in various crude viral preparations of murine origin and was found
in the supernatant of multiple freeze-thaw preparations of double
banded type C viral concentrates. These observations have been
confirmed by another laboratory using a FL74 feline leukemia virus
preparation (9) and have since been extended by us to include the
baboon xenotropic type C virus, M-7.

To characterize these suppressor components we utilize an
in vitro CMI assay consisting either of a two-way mixed lymphocyte
reaction between $C_{57}Bl$ and Balb/c spleen cells or phytohemagglutin-P
(Difco) (PHA) mitogen stimulation of Balb/c spleen cells. The
reactions are carried out in microtiter trays containing 1×10^6
cells in 200 μl RPMI 1640 supplemented with either 0.1% BSA or
human serum. The latter was used to rule out a nonspecific polyamine or polyamine interaction product, that could be involved in
suppression resulting from its presence in either the culturing
substrate or the viral concentrate (2). The suppressor fraction
is generally added 30 min prior to mitogen stimulation and the
culture incubated at 37 C. Four to six hr prior to harvest, the
cultures are pulsed with ^{3}H-thymidine, and subsequently harvested
on glass filters, using a Cell-Harvester Model 24V (Biomedical
Research Institute). The radioactivity is then determined in a
Packard scintillation counter (6).

In characterizing the freeze-thaw supernatant we noted that it
is suppressive in the microgram range, as can be seen in Fig. 1.
Based on ^{3}H-thymidine incorporation during mitogen stimulation we
have found that 1 μg of the suppressor reduces the thymidine
incorporation of a CMI response by approximately 50% while 10 μg
of the suppressor totally abrogates the CMI response. As can
be seen in Fig. 2 the suppressive component may be added to the
culture at any time, starting 30 min prior to mitogen addition
and continuing up to 30 hr after mitogen addition, strongly
suggesting that the mechanism of action is not a direct cell
surface competition phenomenon. Also it permits one to deduce
that the phase of sensitization is not altered, but is most
likely influenced by the suppressor during the proliferation
cycle of the cell. The possibility that one is merely observing
an extention of the cell cycle time and that a delay in the DNA
synthesizing cycle is being brought about was ruled out by a
supplementation experiment. As can be seen in Fig. 3, regardless
of the time of ^{3}H-thymidine addition, ranging from 6-92 hr after
mitogen addition to the culture, no increased thymidine incorporation is evident in the suppressed cultures. Therefore, the
suppression does not represent a mere time shift in optimum
thymidine incorporation, at least over the time frame observed.
Direct mitogen competition can also be ruled out since the
addition of mitogen beyond the optimum level does not overcome
the CMI suppression. As can be seen in Fig. 4, 2 ug of the
suppressor, at the optimum level of mitogen 0.075 μl reconstituted
PHA, brings about approximately 85-90% CMI suppression. The
further addition of up to 2.4 μl PHA per culture does not overcome the suppression and, in fact, further depresses thymidine
incorporation, perhaps due to toxicity of the mitogen at these
concentrations.

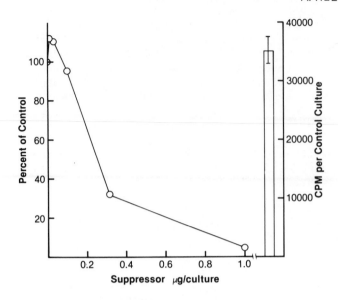

Fig. 1.   Dose response of freeze-thaw R-MuLV supernatant induced
suppression of PHA-P lymphocyte stimulation.

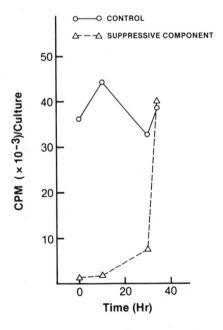

Fig. 2.   Influence of time of R-MuLV suppressor addition of
lymphocyte blastogenic suppression.

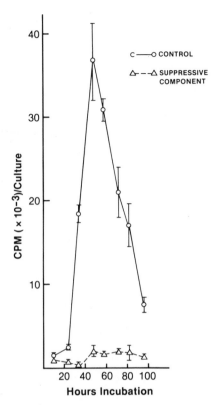

Fig. 3. Comparison of rate of mitogen induced blastogenesis on viral supplemented and control cultures over a 4-day period.

In order to characterize the suppressor more definitevely, double-banded virus (1000 x concentrated) was analyzed. After freeze-thawing three times, the 35K supernatant was chromatogrammed on a Sephacryl 200 gel filtration column. Fractions from this separation were assayed for their capacity to modify either a two-way mixed lymphocyte response or PHA-induced lymphocyte transformation.

A typical elution profile of R–MuLV supernatant is seen in Fig. 5. The CMI responses have provided data indicating that three fractions (A, B, and C) are suppressive; however, the latter is also cytotoxic. Fraction A elutes in the region of the ovalbumin marker, while the other two fractions elute much later, considerably after the 12,000 dalton marker. The molecular weights, of course, are dependent on biophysical properties of the molecule as well as the elution buffer being employed. In most instances our gel filtrations were done in PBS without Ca++ and Mg++. In view of the greater suppression observed with fraction B, and since fraction C

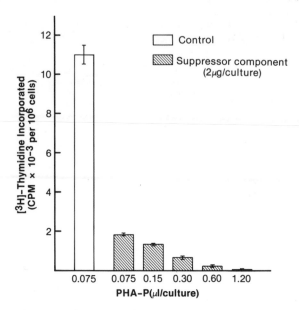

Fig. 4.   The effect of PHA-P level on virus associated suppressor
function.

is cytotoxic and fraction A highly labile, we have concentrated
our efforts on fraction B.   When this fraction is iodinated and run
on SDS-Polyacrylamide gel (SDS-PAGE), Fig. 6 (A), it is found to
consist of at least three components, one with an apparent molecular weight of 70,000 daltons, and two with molecular weights of
10,000 daltons or less.   Fig. 6 (B) denotes an SDS-PAGE of fraction
B stained for protein with Coomassie blue.   A 70,000 molecular
weight peak is readily seen whereas the lower molecular weight
components do not stain.   Similar CMI in vitro responses for fraction B (mitogen competition, time of addition, etc.) as those
mentioned previously for the crude freeze-thaw preparations were
observed.

     The baboon (Papio cynocepholus) retrovirus propagated in
either human or dog cell cultures (concentrated 1000 x) has also
been studied by us to determine if similar suppressive components
could be observed.   Utilizing freeze-thaw supernatant of this virus
preparation, components were separated on a Sephacryl 200 gel
filtration column.   As can be seen in Fig. 7, two major fractions
having suppressive properties were obtained.   One was noted in the
higher molecular weight region of the elution profile and the
other in the lower region.   Significantly, the in vitro CMI suppression brought about by both the baboon and mouse virus components cross species barriers.   That is, the baboon and mouse
components are capable not only of suppressing CMI responses of

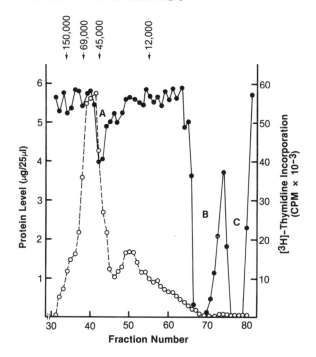

Fig. 5.   Sephacryl gel elution profile of R–MuLV freeze–thaw supernatant preparation (protein O) and (suppressive ●) patterns.

their own cells, but can suppress those of other species, including those of the human.   The feline suppressor component, studied by Olsen (personal communication) shows similar cross species capabilities.

We would like to discuss briefly the possible significance of immune modification brought about by retroviruses, other than those specifically attributed to their etiological neoplastic role.   Most people are aware that a well characterized model for Systemic Lupus Erythematosus is the New New Zealand mouse.   In this particular case, dependent upon the age of the mouse, one notes hyperimmune reactivity in the B cell compartments.   On the other hand, T cell suppression has also been noted (13).   Most intriguing is the role of the murine retrovirus, against which these animals produce abundant antibody, yet in turn show accelerated manifestations to Lymphocytic Choriomeningitis (LCM) or Polyoma.   Perhaps, the hyperimmune activity towards the type C viruses and the abundant presence of such antigens not only are instrumental in the subsequent urological failure, but may also explain accelerated polyoma-associated malignancy brought about by type C virus immunological modification. Other modifying factors permitting retrovirus expression, such as graft-versus-host reactions as well as the age-associated type C

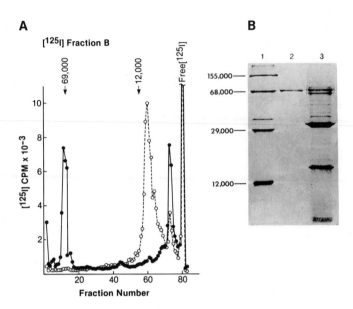

Fig. 6. SDS-PAGE analysis of the major suppressive components:
1) Panel A -- [125]I labeled preparation on disc gel; 2) Panel B --
Coomassie blue on slab gel. (1) Reference standards - 155,000;
69,000; 29,000; 12,000. (2) Sample B. (3) R-MuLV.

virus expression in mice, leading to neoplasia, may be accounted
for by significant contributions of these viruses in their roles
as immune modifiers, rather than, or along with, their direct
role in disease.

An excellent model for studying the immunological ramifica-
tions that retroviruses have on the host is the SPF cat. This
is one of the few models that permits the evaluation of the immune
response to exogenously introduced leukemia virus, since this type
of cat normally does not have leukemia or lymphoma and does not
shed ecotropic virus. In this animal, as well as most mouse
systems it has been extremely difficult to utilize type C viruses
as immunogens and subsequently demonstrate protection against
viral challenge. One reason is, of course, the fact that once
having integrated and tranformed the cell, these viruses do not
require continual proliferation in order to bring about the neoplastic process. Therefore, neutralizing antibody is not
protective for the host. Rather a tumor cell-associated immune
response to FOCMA (feline oncornavirus membrane antigen) is
protective against subsequent viral challenge. Significantly, the
Ohio State Group (personal communication) has demonstrated that
their conventional means of protecting the cat against viral

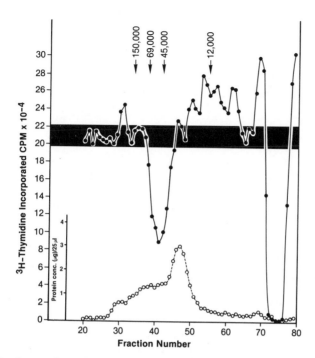

Fig. 7.   Sephacryl gel elution profile of M-7 freeze-thaw supernatant preparation (protein 0) and (suppressive ●) patterns.

challenge, by immunization of the animal with a heat-inactivated
feline lymphoid cell culture (FL74) producing all three types of
feline leukemia virus, can be interfered with by the addition, of
additional high-titered ultraviolet inactivated feline leukemia
virus to this vaccine (15).   This strongly suggests that the
virus preparation has some suppressive component(s) that may
prevent antigen processing, or antibody synthesis.   Similarly,
in both the feline and murine systems, it has been shown that
active immunization with their respective gp70 envelope antigen
is counterproductive for protection to subsequent type C viral
challenge.   Only by passive immunization with anti-gp70 has
protection been achieved (11).   Probably this represents virus
neutralization; however, it may also be that both the envelope
component as well as an immune suppressive component are neutral-
ized by the anti-gp-70 serum.

Other possible functions for immune modifiers can be envision-
ed in the case of chemically induced malignancies.   Let us briefly
consider the situation of tumor promoters in context with the
initiator-promoter hypothesis of carcinogenesis (1).   Tumor

promoters are thought to be agents that increase tumor incidence
when administered after a suboptimal dose of carcinogen, but are
not themselves carcinogens. They appear to function as gene de-
repressors, in a manner analogous to hormonal derepression of
retroviruses and other physiological events. Let us assume the
situation, where promotion of a transformed cell is associated
with the derepression of a retrovirus. This could set the stage
for localized immune suppression brought about by the retroviral
components and the simultaneous replication of the transformed
cell. The latter could escape normal host immune surveillance,
until such time as it has attained sufficient mass to be imper-
vious to host immunological destruction. Of course, these hypo-
thetical viral functions are all physiological in nature and, in
view of the earlier mentioned integrated nature of retrovirus
DNA sequences, would be highly satisfying from a functional point
of view.

One of the more intriguing possibilities for a phsyiological
role for type C viruses is what we have suggested for a number of
years, namely in the maternal-conceptus interaction. Unfortunately,
we still have little if any direct evidence for this hypothesis.
Pregnancy is an interesting paradox involving both immunological
and hormonal controls and modifications. It is recognized that
the pregnant mother, even though immunologically competent, does
not reject the conceptus as she would a typical allograft. Un-
questionably, the fetus and tumor have many similarities, including
a means for escaping immune surveillance. In the past, immunological as well as molecular hybridization data have frequently been
interpreted as suggesting an etiological association between
retroviruses and cancer in many species. Their presence in a
diverse number of animal species without apparent pathology may
suggest, however, other normal physiological functions, such as
cell to cell communication during differentiation and/or immunological regulation.

REFERENCES

1. Berenblum, I. Cancer Res. 14 (1954) 471.
2. Byrd, W. J., Jacobs, D. M. and Amoss, M. S. Nature 267 (1977)
    621.
3. Dent, P. B. Adv. Canc. Res. 22 (1972) 261.
4. Fowler, A. K., Twardzik, D. R., Reed, C. D., Weislow, O. S.
    and Hellman, A. J. Virol. 24 (1977) 729.
5. Fowler, A. K., Strickland, J. E., Kouttab, N. M. and Hellman,
    A. Biol. Reprod. 16 (1977) 344.
6. Fowler, A. K., Twardzik, D. R., Reed, C. D., Weislow, O. S. and
    Hellman, A. Cancer Res. 37 (1977) 4729.
7. Hellman, A. and Weislow, O. S. In: CRC Press, Inc., Cleveland

Ohio (1978) In press.
8. Hellman, A. and Fowler, A. K. Nature New Biol. 233 (1971) 142.
9. Hildebrand, L. C., Mathes, L. and Olsen, R. G. Cancer Res. 37 (1977) 4532.
10. Hirsh, M. S., Kelly, A. P., Chapin, D. S., Fuller, T. C. and Black, P. H. Science 199 (1978) 1337.
11. Hunsmann, G., Moenning, V. and Schaffer, W. Virol. 66 (1975) 327.
12. Kalter, S. S., Heberling, R. L., Helmke, R. J., Panigel, M., Smith, G. C., Kraemer, D. C., Hellman, A., Fowler, A. K. and Strickland, J. E. In: Comparative Leukemia Res. Bibl. Hem. 40 (Eds. Y. Ito and R. M. Dutcher) University of Tokyo Press, Tokyo (1975) 391.
13. Mellors, R. C., Aoki, T. and Heubner, R. J. J. Exp. Med. 129 (1969) 1045.
14. Old, L. J., Clarke, D. A., Benacerraf, B. and Goldsmith, M. N. Y. Acad. Scies. 88 (1960) 264.
15. Olsen, R. G., Hoover, E. A., Schaller, J. P., Mathes, L. E. and Wolf, L. H. Cancer Res. 37 (1977) 2082.

DISTINGUISHABLE BIOLOGICAL EFFECTS OF MURINE LEUKEMIA AND SARCOMA VIRUSES IN LONG TERM BONE MARROW CULTURE

J. S. GREENBERGER, P. B. DAVISSON and P. J. GANS

Joint Center for Radiation Therapy, Sidney Farber Cancer

Institute, Boston, Massachusetts (USA)

Since their discovery, the mechanism of in vitro transformation of fibroblast-lines (14), and rapid induction of erythroleukemia in vivo (18) by murine sarcoma viruses (MSV's) has remained unexplained. In contrast, a comparatively long latent period is required for leukemogenesis following inoculation of murine leukemia viruses (MuLV's), which are also required as "helpers" for replication of the "defective" sarcoma viruses (1). Similar to MSV rapid pathogenicity has been demonstrable with rare other virus isolates. Abelson virus required only 3-4 weeks for either induction of lymphoid leukemia in newborn mice (5) or in vitro transformation of embryo fibroblast or lymphoid cells (19,17). While Friend virus induces erythroleukemia in vivo with a comparably short latent period; no in vitro biologic effect on embryo fibroblasts has been detectable (10).

Recent biochemical evidence indicates that the genomes of murine sarcoma viruses, and perhaps Abelson and Friend virus share the common property of being deletion recombinants (20,24). Viral genetic material of a type-C RNA helper virus has recombined with cellular genetic material from the rat or mouse cells through which the virus was passaged and new gene sequences were acquired with loss of others (20,24). Whether viral genome differences determine the phenotypic differences in the diseases resulting from each virus, or whether cell-specific factors are involved is a subject of controversy.

Attempts to study cell-specific functions in leukemogenesis by both rapid acting and long latent period murine RNA type-C viruses (retroviruses) have been limited by lack of a long-term in vitro culture system for the target organ. Recently, Dr. T. M.

Dexter (7) has developed a method for culture of mouse bone marrow
in vitro, which leads to continued proliferation of granulocyte-
macrophage progenitor cells (CFUc) and pluripotent hemopoietic stem
cells (CFUs) for periods in excess of 14-20 weeks. The biologic
response of these bone marrow cultures to infection with murine
sarcoma or leukemia viruses was evaluated in the present studies.

MATERIALS AND METHODS

Mice. Weanling 6-8 week old NIH/Swiss mice were obtained from
breeding colonies of the National Institutes of Health (Bethesda, MD)

Tissue culture. Continuous cell lines NIH/3T3 (15), Balb/3T3
(2), and NRK (9) and Kirsten murine sarcoma virus transformed non-
producer cell lines of each have previously been described, and are
designated KNIH, KBalb, and KNRK respectively (3). Transformed
non-producer cell lines containing the Moloney and Harvey murine
sarcoma viruses have been reported and are designated H-NRK and M-
Balb (21).

Viruses. A clonal strain of Rauscher murine leukemia virus
has been described (22), and a clonal isolate of the N-tropic
endogenous virus of the Balb/c strain, activated from embryo cells
in vitro following exposure to IUDR, has been reported (4) and is
designated Balb:virus-1. Murine sarcoma virus pseudotypes of each
helper were prepared according to published procedures (3) and are
designated KiMSV (R-MuLV), KiMSV (Balb:virus-1), M-NRK (R-MuLV),
and H-MSV (R-MuLV).

Long term bone marrow culture. The contents of both a mouse
femur and tibia were flushed through a 22 gauge needle into 10.0 ml
Corning plastic flasks in a total volume of 10.0 ml Fisher's medium
supplemented with 25% horse or fetal calf serum (Flow Laboratories,
Rockville, MD) and 10^{-7} M molar hydrocortisone sodium succinate
(Upjohn, Kalamazoo, MI). Previous studies have demonstrated that
corticosteroids will reconstitute the marrow-supportive function
of deficient lots of donor horse serum (11). The cultures were
not recharged with additional marrow at week 4 as in previous
studies (7,11).

Cultures were maintained at 33 C in 7% CO_2 and were de-
populated weekly by removal of 5.0 ml medium containing nonadherent
cell populations generated by the adherent underlayer, and replacement of 5.0 ml fresh medium. Under these conditions marrow cultures
have been demonstrated to generate CFUc, and CFUs for at least 14
weeks (7,11).

Virus infection of marrow. Each 10 ml volume of flushed marrow was centrifuged to a pellet (1000 xg for 3 min) and 1.0 ml Dulbeccos modified Eagle's medium containing 10% fetal calf serum (Colo) and 10^5 Polymerase induction units (PIU) of each virus was added. This 1.0 ml volume was transferred to a 10 ml Corning flask and incubated in shallow monolayer for 2-4 hr at 33 C. Nine ml of medium with 25% serum was then added to each culture. This method allowed both optimal infection and cell adherence.

Colony assays for myeloid and erythroid cells: Cells removed from marrow culture each week were tested for the relative number of granulocyte-macrophage progenitor cells (CFUc) by transferring 1.0×10^5 cells to 1.0 ml cultures containing 0.3% agar (Difco, Detroit, MI) 10% fetal calf serum (Denver, CO) and 10% WEHI-3 colony stimulating factor (CSF) (8). Cultures were incubated at 37 C in 7% CO_2 and the number of $\leq$ 50 cell-containing colonies or 10-49 cell containing clusters were scored at 7 days according to published procedures (16). The presence of erythroid-progenitor cells was assayed by transfer of 1.0×10^5 cells to 0.8% methyl-cellulose-containing medium with 10% fetal calf serum and 0.5 U/ml erythropoietin (sheep source, step III, Connaught Laboratories, Ontario, Canada) (6). Pluripotent hemopoietic stem cells were assayed by transfer of 1.0×10^5 cells to lethally irradiated (1000 rad, total body dose), adult NIH/Swiss mice by tail vein injection. Spleen colonies were scored at day 9 according to published procedures (23).

Hematologic and histochemical staining. Cells removed from long-term marrow culture at weekly intervals, or individual colonies removed from viscous medium after colony assay were prepared as smears on glass coverslips and stained with Wright/Giemsa, or in histochemical methods for myeloperoxidase, esterase-M (ASD-chloroacetate substrate specific), and an immunofluorescence assay for lysozyme (12).

RESULTS

The effect of bone marrow culture conditions on virus replication of leukemia or sarcoma viruses was first evaluated. As shown in Table I, bone marrow cultures infected at time zero with 10^5 polymerase induction units (22) of Rauscher-MuLV, or Balb:virus-1 and grown over a 10-week period in medium containing 25% horse serum and 0.05 ug/ml, (10^{-7}M) hydrocortisone demonstrated persistent reverse transcriptase activity in the culture supernatant measured at weekly intervals. A 5-10 fold higher level of viral reverse transcriptase was detected after week 3 in KiMSV psudotype virus infected cultures. This was associated with simultaneous observation of transformed morphology in the adherent cell layer in culture flasks infected with KiMSV pseudotype viruses but not

TABLE I

Virus Production in Horse Serum Containing Long-Term Marrow Cultures Infected With Balb: Virus-1, Balb:Virus-1 (KiMSV), Rauscher (R)-MuLV, or R-MuLV (KiMSV)[a]

Weeks Culture	Viral Reverse Transcriptase Activity (Polymerase Induction Units) in Cultures Infected With:				
	Nothing	Balb:Virus-1	R-MuLV	Balb:Virus-1 (KiMSV)	R-MuLV (KiMSV)
1	$<10^0$	1.3×10^2	1.2×10^3	3.6×10^2	1.0×10^3
3	$<10^0$	1.5×10^2	1.5×10^2	5.1×10^3	2.1×10^3
5	$<10^0$	1.7×10^2	1.7×10^2	5.5×10^3	3.0×10^3
7	NT	1.3×10^2	1.5×10^2	4.1×10^3	1.5×10^3
8	NT	6.0×10^2	3.2×10^2	5.1×10^3	NT
10	NT	5.0×10^2	1.7×10^2	1.7×10^3	NT
12	NT	NT	NT	5.0×10^3	3.1×10^3
13	NT	NT	5.3×10^2	5.1×10^3	5.1×10^3
15	$<10^0$	3.0×10^2	1.7×10^2	3.5×10^3	NT
16	$<10^0$	5.0×10^2	2.0×10^2	NT	3.5×10^3
20	$<10^0$	1.0×10^2	NT	4.0×10^3	NT

[a] Cultures maintained at 33 C were infected with each virus as described in Materials and Methods and fed weekly by removal of ½ the culture volume (5.0 ml). Serial 10-fold dilutions from 10^{-1} to 10^{-5} were transferred to NIH/3T3 cultures (1.0×10^5 cells per 40 mm petri dish) that had been incubated overnight in 2.0 ug/ml polybrene (22). The polymerase activity in counts per min per ml culture fluid after 7 days at 33 C was plotted (ordinate) against the virus dilutions (abcissa) previously described (22) and an end point titration value extrapolated for undiluted medium. Results are the mean of three cultures at each time given in 25% horse serum and 10^7 M hydrocortisone. NT - not tested.

in helper virus-infected cultures.

Long-term bone marrow cultures established in 25% fetal calf
serum with 0.05 ug/ml hydrocortisone produced higher levels of
virus following infection at time zero compared to cultures grown
in horse serum (Table II). As with horse serum grown cultures transformation of the adherent layer occurred at week 3 in KiMSV infected cultures and virus titer was increased. These data indicated
that virus replication in NIH/Swiss mouse bone marrow·cultures was
more efficient in calf than in horse serum and was higher following
transformation by KiMSV pseudotype viruses.

Effect of serum and corticosteroid on generation of granulocyte-
macrophage progenitor cells and pluripotent hemopoietic stem cells.
As shown in Table III, uninfected long-term marrow cultures growing at 33 C in 7% CO_2 demonstrated continuous generation of between
2×10^5 and 5×10^6 cells in the 5.0 ml volume removed at weekly
intervals. The morphology by differential cell counts was consistent with a gradual decrease in relative numbers of mature myeloid
cells with a shift to more myeloblasts and promyelocytes by week 4.
Recognizable erythroid, megakaryocytic, and lymphoid cells were
markedly decreased by week 3. These data confirm and extend those
of previous reports indicating a "shift to the left" in the hemopoietic cell population produced in long-term marrow cultures (7).

As shown in Fig. 1a, the hemopoietic microenvironment established with cultures growing in horse serum in 10^{-7} M hydrocortisone,
was different from that detected in fetal calf serum in the same
hydrocortisone concentration (Fig. 1b). The difference was in the
generation of islands of lipid-laden fat cells in horse serum
cultures. Previous studies have suggested that adipose-colonies
were absolutely required for long-term in vitro hemopoiesis (7).
Therefore, it was of interest to test whether the large numbers
of non-adherent cells generated in fetal calf serum had lost the
ability to form spleen colonies as well as granulocyte-macrophage
colonies in methylcellulose containing medium in vitro. As shown
in Table IV, calf serum cultures grown for 8 weeks in 10^{-7} M hydrocortisone generated hemopoietic stem cells as measured by CFUs
assay, and CFUc by in vitro assay. In the absence of hydrocortisone, non-adherent cells rapidly decreased in either fetal
calf or horse serum cultures and numbers of detectable CFUs, and
CFUc were markedly decreased by week 4. Transferring calf serum
grown cells to horse serum for 2 hr prior to inoculation into
mice further increased the numbers of detectable spleen colonies
and may present an increase in seeding efficiency to the spleen
stroma (manuscript in preparation).

Thus, the evidence indicated that corticosteroid was required
for generation of hemopoietic cells in long-term marrow culture in
either fetal calf or horse serum. A distinguishable biologic effect

TABLE II

Virus Production in Fetal Calf Serum Containing Long-Term Marrow Cultures Infected with Balb:virus-1, Balb:virus-1 (KiMSV), R-MuLV or R-MuLV (KiMSV)[a]

Weeks Culture	Nothing	Viral Reverse Transcriptase Activity (Polymerase Induction Units) In Cultures Infected With:			
		Balb:Virus-1	R-MuLV	Balb:Virus-1 (KiMSV)	R-MuLV (KiMSV)
1	$<10^0$	1.3×10^3	1.3×10^4	1.5×10^4	2.3×10^4
3	$<10^0$	2.4×10^4	4.1×10^4	4.1×10^4	1.2×10^4
5	$<10^0$	1.3×10^3	5.1×10^3	1.3×10^4	3.1×10^4
7	$<10^0$	4.1×10^3	2.1×10^3	4.3×10^4	3.0×10^3
10	$<10^0$	5.0×10^3	6.5×10^3	5.1×10^4	2.1×10^4
15	$<10^0$	1.0×10^3	3.0×10^3	1.4×10^4	3.1×10^4

[a]Results are as described in the legend to Table I and are the mean of 3 cultures at each time grown in 25% fetal calf serum (Flow) and 10^{-7} M hydrocortisone.

TABLE III

Proliferation of NIH/Swiss Mouse Marrow in Long-Term Tissue Culture

Weeks Culture	Total Cells Removed (x 10^5)[a]	Colony Forming (Progenitor Cells) /10^5 Cells[b]		Differential Cell Count (%)[c]					
		CFUc (CSA)	CFUe (EP)	Immature Myeloid	Mature Myeloid	Ery	Lymph	Mega	Mac
1	42.0	103 ± 7.1	67 ± 3.1	8	30	25	8	1	3
2	31.0	117 ± 3.2	15 ± 1.7	NT	--	--	--	--	--
3	38.3	115 ± 1.7	1	21	55	4	2	3	20
4	45.6	68 ± 2.1	1	41	27	0	0	1	31
5	57.3	217 ± 8.1	38 ± 0.8	NT	--	--	--	--	--
7	33.3	331 ± 9.1	8 ± 1.7	NT	--	--	--	--	--
9	28.1	373 ± 6.1	1	37	28	0	0	0	35
11	37.1	279 ± 3.1	1	NT	--	--	--	--	--
13	18.1	371 ± 8.7	1	NT	--	--	--	--	--
15	17.1	193 ± 10.3	1	46	18	0	0	0	36
17	8.3	117 ± 3.1	1	33	31	0	0	0	36
19	9.1	86 ± 4.1	1	NT	--	--	--	--	--
21	2.3	23 ± 3.1	1	17	21	0	0	0	61

[a]Results are expressed as the mean of total nucleated cells counted in weekly 5.0 volumes re-moved from at least 3 flasks at each time point.

[b]Results are expressed as the mean ± SEM of at least (2) 1.0×10^5 - cell containing 1.0 ml cultures from 3 experiments (total 6).

[c]The differential cell counts are presented as the average of 3 at each time point. NT = not tested. *Mega = metakaryocyte; Mac = macrophage; Immature myeloid = myeloblast, promyelocyte, myelocyte; Mature myeloid = metamyelocyte, band form, polymorphonuclear leukocytes.

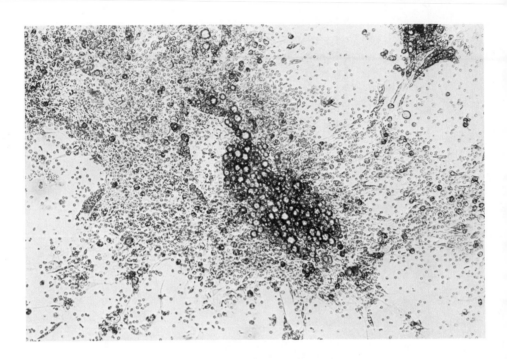

Fig. 1. Morphologic appearance of 5 week cultures of NIH/Swiss
mouse marrow infected with: a) R–MuLV in 25% horse serum + 10^{-7} M
hydrocortisone (OHC); b) R–MuLV in 25% FCS + 10^{-7} M (OHC) (x200);
c) R–MuLV (KiMSV) in 25% horse serum + 10^{7} M OHC (x400).

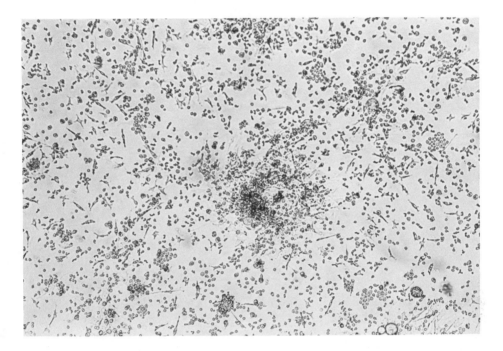

Fig. 1b

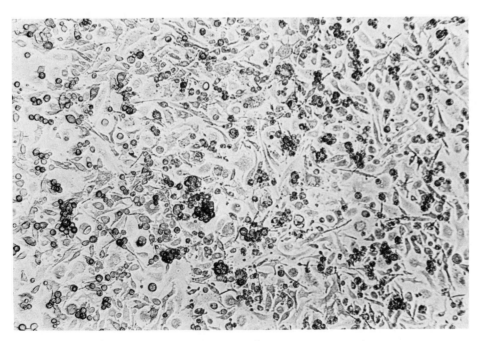

Fig. 1c

TABLE IV

Comparison of CFUs and CFUc Generated in Uninfected Marrow
Cultures Grown in Steroid-Enriched Horse or Fetal
Calf Serum[a]

	CFUc/CFUs In Cultures Grown In Fisher's Medium With:			
Weeks Culture	25% FCS Alone	25% FCS + 10^{-7}M OHC	25% Horse Serum Alone	25% Horse Serum + 10^{-7}M OHC
1	7000/30	21,000/.240	18,000/120	33,000/420
3	3000/0	18,000/170	7,000/30	12,000/330
5	200/0	20,000/75	140/0	21,000/200
7	0/0	7,000/43	35/0	9,700/120
8	0/0	11,000/117	20/0	13,000/70
10	0/0	4,000/50	0/0	8,100/52
15	0/0	5,200/30	0/0	3,500/20

[a]Results are the mean of total numbers of CFUc and CFUs in 5.0 ml
removed volumes from 3 cultures at each time grown in horse or
fetal calf serum (FCS) with or without hydrocortisone (OHC).

was noted in horse serum with a generation of large numbers of
adipose-rich colonies formed in the adherent underlayer between
weeks 1 and 4. Thus, 2 effects of hydrocortisone in long-term
marrow culture are separable: increased hemopoiesis as measured
by numbers of hemopoietic cells generated, and an effect on fibro-
blast-derived cells in the adherent layer which can accumulate
lipid in the presence of some other substance concentrated in horse
serum.

Effect of leukemia and sarcoma viruses on hemopoiesis in vitro.
As shown in Table V, infection of cultures at time zero with R-Mulv,
Balb:virus-1, or KiMSV psudotype viruses of each helper virus,
produced strikingly different biologic effects on the numbers and
biologic activity of cells removed. The number of non-adherent
cells and CFUc removed per week was increased 2-5 fold in each
helper leukemia virus infected culture between weeks 2 and 8
compared to uninfected cultures (Table III) CFUs were not detect-
ably different from uninfected cultures (data not shown).

In contrast, cultures infected with KiMSV-pseudotype viruses
of each helper virus demonstrated a rapid decrease in the total
number of cells removed at weekly intervals and a decrease in
the number of functionally detectable CFUc and CFUs (Table V).

TABLE V

Effect of In Vitro RNA Type-C Leukemia or Sarcoma Virus Infection on NIH/Swiss Mouse Marrow Cultures

Weeks in vitro culture	Balb:virus-1		R-MuLV		KiMSV (Balb:virus-1)		KiMSV (R-MuLV)	
	Tot. cells[a]	CFUc[b]	Tot. Cells	CFUc	Tot. Cells	CFUc	Tot. Cells	CFUc
1	56.0 ± 7.1	107	49.3 ± 6.1	117	59.0 ± 6.1	118	48.0 ± 3.1	107
2	51.1 ± 7.9	116	37.0 ± 9.1	86	83.1 ± 10.7	103	45.8 ± 3.2	96
3	33.6 ± 5.1	87	37.7 ± 1.6	76	51.3 ± 7.3	83	61.7 ± 2.7	87
4	27.6 ± 6.3	79	18.6 ± 3.7	58	18.4 ± 6.1	63	13.8 ± 3.3	57
5	61.3 ± 7.1	291	91.6 ± 7.1	287	73.7 ± 3.7	107	87.0 ± 16.0	108
7	51.7 ± 3.1	837	196.0 ± 8.7	1070	36.3 ± 7.1	51	38.1 ± 9.3	53
9	73.6 ± 1.9	1073	126.0 ± 3.7	1107	1.6 ± 0.7	27	18.3 ± 1.7	14
13	108 ± 9.7	1173	108.0 ± 6.7	1191	0.6 ± 0.01	73	0.3 ± 1.8	67

Virus - Added

[a]Total cells removed (5.0 ml)[1] x 10^5 (Cell counts are as described in the legend to Table III).
[b]Colonies/10^5 cells(CFUc).

A striking observation was the increased number of macrophage
clusters formed in KiMSV-infected marrow in methylcellulose containing medium or 0.3% agar in the absence of added colony stimulating
activity. These data extend our previous observations that murine
sarcoma viruses can stimulate proliferation of granulocyte-macrophage progenitor cells in the absence of added CSF (13). As shown
in Fig. 1C, the morphologic appearance of cells in the adherent
layer was markedly altered by 5 weeks after sarcoma virus infection.
An increased number of transformed macrophages overgrew the adherent
layer and was associated with destruction of adipose-cell colonies
in horse serum grown cultures, and a loss of hemopoietic cells in
calf or horse serum grown cultures. Similar results were observed
with H-MSV (R-MuLV) and M-MSV (R-MuLV). Leukemia virus infected
cultures were morphologically similar to controls at week 5
(Fig. 1a-b). Thus distinguishable morphological and biological
effects were detectable in cultures infected with leukemia
compared to sarcoma virus.

                              DISCUSSION

     The present studies demonstrate distinguishable biological ef-
fects of murine leukemia and sarcoma viruses in a unique long-term
bone marrow culture system. The Dexter-system (7) is based upon
the establishment of a microenvironment in vitro on a plastic
surface by whole marrow. The microenvironment contains several
populations of cells including adipose-laden fibroblasts, normal
fibroblasts, macrophages, and endothelial cells (7). On this
adherent microenvironment a population of round hemopoietic cells
proliferate in sheets and releases clusters and single cells into
the supernatant. The initial studies of Dexter et al. (7) suggested
a requirement for certain lots of donor horse serum which induced
both adipose adherent colonies and maintained hemopoiesis. It has
been assumed that these 2 phenomenon were associated with the
presence of a factor(s) in the horse serum.

     Due to the shortage of special lots of horse serum, it was
necessary to reconstitute the horse serum available in the USA.
Studies from this laboratory have demonstrated that addition of
corticosteroid at 10^{-7}M will reconstitute most lots of horse serum
to the potency of Manchester horse serum, in both ability to
induce adipose-colonies and sustain hemopoiesis for periods of
at least 14 weeks (11).

     The present data demonstrate that calf serum can also be
reconstituted to a condition associated with prolonged hemopoiesis
by addition of 10^{-7}M corticosteroid; however, visible adipose cells
in the adherent cell layer are not detected. The presence of
detectable CFUs (pluripotent stem cells), and CFUs (granulocyte-
macrophage progenitor cells), during a 15 week culture period in

the absence of visible adipose colonies indicates that the effect of hydrocortisone in reconstituting hemopoiesis is separable from its effect on stimulating lipid uptake in horse serum by preadipocytes.

The effects of a murine leukemia virus of known in vivo oncogenicity, Rauscher-MuLV and an endogenous virus on the Balb/c mouse strain which is not leukemogenic in its strain of origin, (Balb:virus-1) were compared in long-term marrow culture. Leukemia virus infected cultures generated larger numbers of non-adherent cells in weekly removed fractions, and produced larger numbers of cells capable of forming colonies in viscous medium in the presence of CSF. These data suggest that murine leukemia viruses may stimulate proliferation of a cell which is destined to proliferate in response to specific stimulatory macromolecules.

In contrast, infection of long-term marrow cultures with murine sarcoma virus pseudotypes of each leukemia helper virus was associated with destruction of the hemopoietic microenvironment by 4 weeks, including loss of adipocyte colonies, proliferation of macrophages and decreased numbers of non-adherent cells detectable as CFUs and CFUc. These results confirm and extend those of Dexter, et al. (8). The fact that murine sarcoma virus pseudotypes of each leukemia virus induce erythroleukemia in vitro suggests that a mechanism to bypass the marrow destructive effect is operative in the animal. Further studies with the Dexter in vitro culture system should aid in defining the mechanism of leukemogenesis by these 2 classes of murine RNA tumor viruses.

REFERENCES

1. Aaronson, S. A. and Rowe, W. P. Virol. 42 (1970) 9.
2. Aaronson, S. A. and Todaro, G. J. Science 164 (1968) 1024.
3. Aaronson, S. A. and Weaver, C. A. J. Gen. Virol. 13 (1971) 1133.
4. Aaronson, S. A. and Stephenson, J. R. Proc. Natl. Acad. Sci., USA, 70 (1973) 2055.
5. Abelson, H. T. and Rabstein, L. S. Cancer Res. 30 (1970) 2213.
6. Cooper, M. C., Levy, J., Cantor, L. N., Marks, P. A. and Rifkind, A. A. Proc. Natl. Acad. Sci. USA. 71 (1974) 1677.
7. Dexter, T. M. and Testa, N. C. In: Methods in Cell Biology, XIV, Chap. 34 (1976) 387.
8. Dexter, T. M., Scott, D. and Teich, N. M. Cell 12 (1977) 355.
9. Duc-Nguyen, H., Rosenbaum, E. N. and Ziegel, R. F. J. Bacteriol. 92 (1966) 1133.
10. Friend, C. J. Exp. Med. 105 (1957) 307.
11. Greenberger, J. S. Nature (1978) in press.
12. Greenberger, J. S., Aaronson, S. A., Rosenthal, D. S. and

Moloney, W. C.   Nature 257 (1975) 143.

13. Greenberger, J. S., Davisson, P. B. and Gans, P. J.   Clin. Res. (Abstr.) 26 (1978) 347A.

14. Harvey, J. J. and East, J.   In: The Murine Sarcoma Viruses (MSV), Academic Press, New York, (1971) 265.

15. Jainchill, J. C., Aaronson, S. A. and Todaro, G. J.   J. Virol. 4 (1969) 549.

16. Moore, M. A. S., Williams, N. and Metcalf, P.   J. Natl. Canc. Inst. 50 (1973) 603.

17. Rosenberg, N., Baltimore, D. and Scher, C. D.   Proc. Natl. Acad. Sci. USA, 72 (1976) 1932.

18. Scher, C. D., Scolnick, E. M. and Siegler, R.   Nature (Lond.) 256 (1975) 225.

19. Scher, C. D. and Siegler, R.   Nature (Lond.) 253 (1975) 729.

20. Scolnick, E. M., Goldberg, R. J. and Williams, D.   J. Virol. 18 (1976) 559.

21. Scolnick, E. M. and Parks, W. P.   J. Virol. 13 (1974) 1211.

22. Stephenson, J. R. and Aaronson, S. A.   Virol. 48 (1972) 749.

23. Till, J. E. and McCulloch, E. A.   Radiat. Res. 14 (1961) 213.

24. Troxler, D. H., Boyars, J. K., Parks, W. P. and Scolnick, E. M.   J. Virol. 22 (1977) 361.

Part II

Nature, Activation and Interactions of the Reticuloendothelial System

During the last decade it has become apparent that a complex interaction occurs among cells constituting the RE System. The first paper in this section is based on a major address given by Dr. Yoffey at the Congress. He reviews the interaction of lymphocytes and macrophages in the lymphomyeloid complex. In this section the genetic control of lymphocyte and macrophage interaction in regard to immune responsiveness is also described. The effects of various agents, including BCG, in activating "macrophages" is also included, especially in terms of tumor cells, cytotoxicity and antibody formation. It is apparent that a wide variety of soluble factors may also be involved in the interaction as well as activation of many diverse cell types in the immune response system. Furthermore, the recognition phase considered an important aspect of immune competence may also be intimately involved with specific receptors and factors. Thus, the activation and interaction of cells within the RE System constitute a complex issue in need of greater understanding through further work and careful interpretation of current data.

LYMPHOCYTES AND MACROPHAGES IN THE LYMPHOMYELOID COMPLEX

J. M. YOFFEY

Department of Anatomy and Embryology, The Hebrew
University-Hadassah Medical School
Jerusalem (ISRAEL)

It was in 1926 when I started to work on what I later termed
the Lymphomyeloid Complex. In some ways life then was very simple.
The prevailing view was that all lymphocytes were identical, and
that they were mature cells without any capacity for growth or
development. This sounds very strange to us now, but such in fact
was the case until what one may aptly describe as the Great Lymphocyte Revolution began about 1960, following the introduction of
PHA. Now we have of course made very great advances since then.
But despite the enormous amount of work performed on the lymphomyeloid complex since 1960, including the wide variety of immunological studies on its lymphocytes and macrophages, there are
still many striking gaps in our knowledge, and I shall draw particular attention to some of these in the course of my address.

As far as macrophages are concerned, the interest in recent
years seems to have been directed almost entirely to their immunological role. Since there are special sessions on immunological interactions between lymphocytes and macrophages, I shall
deal in the main with the more general and non-immunological
aspects of their activity.

THE LYMPHOMYELOID COMPLEX

Fig. 1 is a general scheme of the lymphomyeloid complex as
we now know it, with its six major contitutents: bone marrow,
thymus, spleen, lympho-epithelial tissues, lymph nodes, and connective tissues, CT in the diagram (Fig. 1). The term connective
tissue includes the serous cavities, notably the peritoneum,
which contains cell populations very like those of the connective

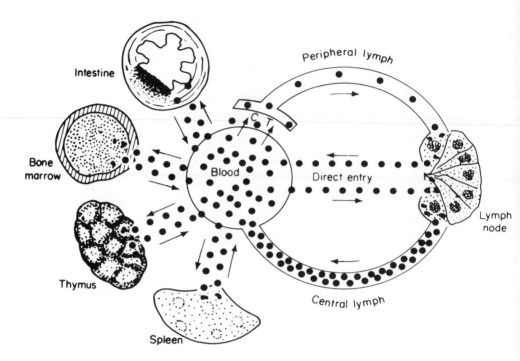

Fig. 1. A scheme of the lymphomyeloid complex, and the integration
of its constituent parts by cellular migration streams, comprising
both a variety of lymphocytes, and of macrophages or macrophage
precursors.   Cells reach the blood stream either by first obtaining access to the lymph stream (indirect entry) or by passing
through walls of blood capillaries directly. Lymphocytes from bone
marrow and spleen reach the blood by direct entry. Lymphocytes
from lymph nodes and thymus are of both the direct and the indirect entry type, in varying proportions. The connective tissue
migration streams (CT) include the serous cavities, such as the
peritoneum (61).

tissues in general, but with a fluid matrix. When I began my own
work in 1926, the lymphomyeloid complex was largely terra incognita
and its constituent elements were regarded as discrete entities,
functionally unrelated to one another. Not knowing quite where to
start, I began by trying to obtain some idea of the magnitude of
the problem, by means of quantitative data on the number of lymphocytes produced.

     The initial working hypothesis was that most lymphocytes en-
tered the blood via the thoracic duct, and that these were mainly
newly formed cells, arising in lymph nodes and alimentary lymphoid
tissue (58). From this starting point I argued that since the

number of lymphocytes in the blood remained fairly constant, and
since there was no evidence of lymphocytes being destroyed in the
blood, the only way in which the blood lymphocytes could remain
constant was by cells leaving the blood at the same rate as they
were entering. This of course raised the obvious question: Where
did they leave the blood? In answer to this question I speculated
that lymphocytes left the blood to enter the bone marrow and act
as stem cells, to replace those stem cells which were constantly
undergoing differentiation. It all sounded very plausible at
the time, though unfortunately it later turned out not to be true.
One of the early arguments against this concept was the idea that
lymphocytes entering the blood were not newly formed, but were undergoing recirculation, as suggested by a Swedish worker, Sjövall,
in 1936 (47).

    I thought of this recirculation in terms of lymphocytes pas-
sing out of the blood into the connective tissues, then into the
lymph, in which they returned to the blood after traversing one or
more lymph nodes. Now we did find a small number of cells in lymph
when it was first formed, peripheral lymph as we termed it (62),
but there were about thirty times as many cells in the efferent
lymph leaving the node, so we concluded that there was indeed a
small amount of recirculation, but that most of the lymphocytes
leaving the lymph node were newly formed. This was about 25 yr
before the discovery of the more massive recirculation from blood
into lymph node and lymph via the post-capillary veins, marked in
Fig. 1 "direct entry" (16). In dealing with the problem of lymphocyte migration we had to introduce a number of new terms: peripheral
lymph, which had not yet passed through any nodes; intermediate
lymph, which had passed through one or more nodes but had yet to
traverse others; and central lymph, which had no more nodes to
traverse before entering the blood. At a later date, to cope with
our expanding knowledge of lymphocyte kinetics, additional terms
were introduced. Direct entry lymphocytes entered the blood stream
by passing directly through the walls of the blood capillaries in
the tissue in which they were formed. Indirect entry lymphocytes
first entered the lymph stream, through which they then reached
the blood (61).

                QUANTITATIVE DATA ON LYMPHOCYTE PRODUCTION

    My initial working hypothesis was that the indirect entry
lymphocytes, mainly thoracic duct cells, were the most numerous
of all the lymphocytes entering the blood, but it later became
evident that the direct entry lymphocytes were far more numerous
than the indirect. Quantitative data collected over many years,
mainly on dogs, guinea pigs and rats, with the help of several
colleagues at the University of Bristol, bring this point out very
clearly. For every lymphocyte present in the blood of the young

adult guinea pig three are daily entering via the thoracic
duct, while 20 are present in the bone marrow, with a turnover
time of 2-3 days. The number of direct entry lymphocytes entering
the blood from the bone marrow was enough to replace those in the
blood about 6 times daily, while in addition there is substantial
lymphocyte production in the thymus (12). While these are the
major sources of lymphocyte production, a fair number of cells are
formed in the remainder of the lymphomyeloid complex, so it follows
that the blood lymphocytes are a rapidly changing population. It
is here that we encounter one of the most striking gaps in our
knowledge. We do not have the faintest idea how the level of the
blood lymphocytes is normally kept so constant, and a balance
maintained between those entering and those leaving the blood.
Reviews of the various possible factors which may control lymphocyte production (1, 61) seem to throw little light on the control
of the blood lymphocyte level.

     The direct entry lymphocytes of the bone marrow, predominantly
B lymphocytes, have been repeatedly observed in passage through
the sinusoidal endothelium (4, 6, 23), but we do not know what
causes them to migrate in this manner. Possible control mechanisms
for marrow lymphocyte production have recently been discussed by
Rosse (45). Some of the factors which influence the output of
thoracic duct lymphocytes have been discussed by Reinhardt (39),
who noted inter alia an inverse relationship between the size of
the animal and the number of thoracic duct lymphocytes.

     The changing blood lymphocyte population is not only a ques-
tion of the numbers of cells entering and leaving the blood.
There are also important qualitative changes. Throughout foetal
life and up to the time of birth the blood lymphocytes are a rather
different population from those in the adult, for one finds among
them a number of more primitive cells, with leptochromatic nuclei
and high N:C ratio, which in their morphology are very like the
primitive transitional cells in bone marrow (15, 66).

                        CELLULAR MIGRATION STREAMS

     My initial mistaken hypothesis about the thoracic duct lympho-
cytes passing through the blood to the bone marrow did have one
valuable result. It led us at an early stage to the idea of
streams of migrating cells passing through the blood from one
constituent of the lymphomyeloid complex to another, thus making
possible the integration of the complex into a functional whole.
The existence of these cellular migration streams is something
we now take for granted. But I can still recall how at a conference in Salt Lake City in 1959, when together with Dr. W. O.
Reinhardt and the late Dr. Everett (63), we first put forward
the general concept of cellular migration streams, it came in for

a good deal of criticism. There are several such migration streams
of which we now have some knowledge, and no doubt there are some
of whose existence we have yet to learn. But here, too, there is
a major gap in our knowledge. We have yet to obtain really convincing evidence - in the normal animal - of biotactic stimuli
which can cause lymphocytes to leave the blood in any particular
situation. One of the outstanding examples is the migration of B
and T cells to more or less specific zones in lymph nodes. The
mechanism controlling this migration is far from clear.

Using parabiotic rats, in which one parabiont was labelled
in vivo with thymidine, Tyler and Everett (51, 52) obtained
interesting data on lymphocytic migration in rats, as did Rosee
(43) in guinea pigs.

The efferent stream of lymphocytes from the bone marrow consists mainly of B lymphocytes, but there is also a small but
important number of primitive cells such as those proceeding to
the thymus to act as T cell precursors. The bone marrow is the
major source of the primitive pluripotent immunohemopoietic stem
cells which may occur in small numbers throughout the lymphomyeloid complex, but whose major and primary habitat is the bone
marrow - with the exception of the very small laboratory animals
such as the mouse, where the spleen plays a very similar role.
The marrow also contains monocyte and macrophage precursors, so it
must be regarded as the great cellular power house of the lymphomyeloid complex.

CELL MIGRATION THROUGH CONNECTIVE TISSUE

The central problem of the lymphomyeloid complex is the
extent and control of the various cellular migration streams which
serve to integrate the scattered elements of the complex. One of
the major blind spots in our understanding of the complex is in
the connective tissues of the body - CT in Fig. 1. The connective
tissues, here shown as a narrow strip, are in fact a vast area,
possibly the largest part of the lymphomyeloid complex in terms
of size, though we have no way of measuring its lymphocyte content.
Under normal circumstances there is a slow but steady drift of
lymphocytes from the blood through the connective tissues, then into the peripheral lymph to the regional node. About 20% of the
cells in peripheral lymph are monocytes or macrophages. The slow
stream of lymphocytes from blood through the connective tissues into peripheral lymph seems, under normal conditions, to be largely
independent of the level of the blood lymphocytes, which can show
quite wide variations with relatively minor changes in the cell
content of peripheral lymph (62). According to Engeset et al.(10)
peripheral lymph contains more T than B cells.

The cells in peripheral lymph presumably reflect their state in the connective tissues from which they have just emerged, and it is interesting therefore to note that one finds not infrequently in peripheral lymph what one might almost regard as the "exploring" lymphocyte, which puts out numerous long fine processes, 30-40 μ in length, or even longer, which wave about for a time and then retract. This is a different type of movement from that generally seen, for the cell is not now moving from place to place, but is greatly increasing its surface area, presumably thereby giving itself a much better chance of contacting any substance which might influence its further development (61). Another interesting finding in peripheral lymph is the very close association often seen between lymphocytes and macrophages (61). The fate of the monocytes and macrophages constantly reaching the node via peripheral lymph is not known.

In response to stimulation, the lymphocyte and macrophage content both of the connective tissues and of peripheral lymph may undergo marked changes. In the sheep, Hall (19) found that peripheral lymph draining a skin homograft contained a higher percentage of macrophages than normal peripheral lymph, around 75% as opposed to 25%, though there was no significant increase in the total cell content. On the other hand, Smith et al.(48) produced granulomata in the legs of sheep by the subcutaneous injection of incomplete Freund's adjuvant + influenza virus, and found over a 9 wk period that there was a great increase in the cell content of peripheral lymph, attributable in part to the active proliferation of cells in the granuloma and in part to accelerated movement of lymphocytes from blood into peripheral lymph by the development of post-capillary veins in the granulomata.

Another problem which has been with us since the start of the century concerns the origin of the connective tissue macrophages. Rebuck and Crowley (38), observing connective tissue changes by the skin window technique, concluded that tissue macrophages could develop from blood-borne lymphocytes, while others have suggested their origin from monocytes (27). These two origins are not mutually exclusive, while one must also allow for the local proliferation of pre-existing macrophages, though this appears to be a somewhat variable phenomenon. But whatever the origin of the macrophage precursors in connective tissue, they appear to be largely hematogenous, and to arise in the bone marrow. Volkman and Gowans (56, 57) applied the skin window technique in rats, and showed that the macrophages which appeared were hematogenous, as Rebuck and Crowley (38) had maintained, since they failed to appear in rats given 750R, but appeared as usual if the marrow was shielded. Everett and Tyler (13) also investigated the source of the macrophages which appear in skin window preparations in rats, and they considered the precursors to be "monocytoid" in type.

Spector and Willoughby (49) found in rats that local inflammatory
reactions could be abolished after the destruction of bone marrow
and lymphoid tissue by irradiation, but restored by transfusion of
marrow cells, though not of suspensions of lymph node or thymus.
Detailed histological study of some of the inflammatory foci
showed a perivascular infiltration by mononuclear cells, many of
which looked like lymphocytes.

From a technical point of view, the peritoneum is simpler
to deal with than the other connective tissues, and one can
readily inject carbon particles and identify the phagocytic cells.
It contains in fact a wide variety of mononuclear cells in which
one can see various sizes, ranging from an occasional pachychromatic
small lymphocyte to a large macrophage. While one may now and
again see a typical small lymphocyte which has been phagocytic
(46), most of them are not. That cells with typical small lymphocyte structure may occasionally be phagocytic has also been noted
by other observers (5, 71), the former with CLL lymphocytes.
However, these are few in number, in comparison with the somewhat
larger and more frequently seen phagocytic cells, sometimes termed
"lymphocyte-like", with a high N:C ratio and a more leptochromatic
nucleus than the small lymphocyte. These larger cells are in fact
not unlike the transitional cells of bone marrow, and between
them and the typical large macrophage one may see numerous intermediate stages. Typical monocytes are not too common, though in
this respect there are species differences.

A consideration of the varied morphology of the mononuclear
cells of the peritoneal cavity suggests that one may have to consider the possibility of macrophage formation through several different lines of development: (1) from monocytes, (2) from a special
subgroup of phagocytic small lymphocytes, (3) from larger "lymphocyte-like" cells resembling the smaller transitional cells of bone
marrow, (4) from the division of pre-existing macrophages, occurring only to a small extent under normal conditions.

On the whole, it seems now to have become generally accepted
that peritoneal macrophages are of bone marrow origin, as shown
by Virolainen (54) in mice, using chromosome markers, and Volkmann
(55) in rats. Volkmann transfused rats with a suspension of
thymidine-labelled marrow cells, and found labelled "lymphocyte-
like" cells in the peritoneum. He considered it "paradoxical that
more lymphocyte-like cells in the exudates could be derived from
transfused marrow than from thoracic duct lymphocytes." But it
is not paradoxical if the peritoneal macrophages are derived from
transitional cells, which are present in the marrow in appreciable
numbers, but are not found in thoracic duct lymph. Furthermore,
the data both of Volkmann (55) and of Van Furth and Dulk (53)
indicate that the macrophage precursors are rapidly proliferating

cells which the latter authors termed "promonocytes", carrying
with it the implicit assumption that all macrophage production
passed through a monocyte stage. This may not always be the case.

MACROPHAGES IN BONE MARROW

Although the kinetic data point to the bone marrow as the
major center for the production of macrophages from rapidly-
growing precursors, the marrow itself contains very few free and
readily mobilizable macrophages. The endothelium of the blood
sinusoid is actively phagocytic, but its cells are fixed, an
integral part of the wall of the sinusoid (22, 24). Another extremely active macrophage is the cell in the center of the erythroblastic island - a very remarkable cell, with no obvious immunological role, though the possibility cannot be entirely ruled out.
This central macrophage is surrounded by developing erythroblasts,
and is very actively phagocytic (2). The view now generaly held
is that as the erythroblasts mature, their extruded nuclei are
rapidly ingested and digested by this macrophage, which we sometimes refer to as the central reticular cell. If the generally
accepted view is correct, it seems to be essential for normal
erythropoiesis, probably for a number of reasons. But one of its
more obvious roles is to remove extruded nuclei as quickly as
possible, to prevent the marrow being cluttered up by their accumulation. Youse (70) endeavored to quantitate the reticuloendothelial cells in rat marrow, and concluded that about 1 cell
out of every 1,000 was phagocytic. The endothelium of the sinus-
oids, in addition to being actively phagocytic, also readily allows the passage of large molecules, including particulate matter,
from the blood stream into the marrow parenchyma. Since the endothelium also allows the free passage of blood plasma, the trans-
parenchymal flow of this plasma quickly brings the particles into
the neighborhood of the erythorblastic islands. Hence, intravenously injected carbon particles can be found ingested by the
central reticular cells within a quite short time (22).

THE TRANSITIONAL CELL COMPARTMENT

Neither the phagocytic endothelium, nor the central reticular
cells of the erythroblastic islands, which are fixed cells, can
be regarded as migrating macrophage precursors, which must therefore be sought elsewhere in the marrow. In the concluding section
of this address I would like to discuss the cell group which I now
believe to contain the fundamental primitive stem cells in the
lymphomyeloid complex, the cells on which ultimately all the rest
of the complex depends, and this means all the different cell
groups in the marrow, including macrophage precursors.

TRANSITIONAL CELLS

As already noted, the initial working hypothesis was that
thoracic duct lymphocytes were newly formed cells, which were
continually migrating through the blood stream to the bone marrow
to act as stem cells. Once in the marrow, it was assumed that the
small lymphocyte would enlarge, and that as it did so the typically pachychromatic nucleus would gradually become leptochromatic.
After a time, the cytoplasm would increase in amount, and become
basophilic, at which stage the cell would have become a typical
blast cell, in the main either proerythroblast or myeloblast.
When, after obtaining quantitative data on the thoracic duct lymphocyte output, we turned our attention to the bone marrow, the
appearance at first seemed to fit in with this view. One could
see a whole spectrum of cells, ranging in size from the pachychromatic small lymphocyte, passing apparently through progressively enlarging cells with leptochromatic nuclei, and reaching
finally the blast cell stage. All these intermediate stages between small lymphocytes and blast cells were termed transitional
cells. Transitional cells have a high N:C ratio like small
lymphocytes, from which however they are readily distinguished by
their larger overall size and leptochromatic nuclei. When PHA
was introduced, and one could see small lymphocytes enlarging in
just this way, passing through a typical transitional cell stage
before becoming a typical PHA blast cell, it seemed to clinch the
matter.

However, kinetic studies with tritiated thymidine (34) showed
that, far from small lymphocytes enlarging in the bone marrow to
form transitional cells, the reverse was the case since transitional cells were dividing to give rise to small lymphocytes,
as shown by the sequential labelling pattern in the marrow after
tritiated thymidine in vivo. The transitional cells label first,
to be followed by the labelled small lymphocytes resulting from
their division. Rosse (42) observed the phenomenon in vivo, and
noted that a few hr elapsed after the division of the transitional
cells before the nuclear chromatin became condensed and fully
pachychromatic. Rosse (44) was also able to show that transitional cells could differentiate either into the erythroid or the
lymphocytic cell line in the experimental conditions with which
he was dealing.

These and many other experimental findings led us to formulate a stem cell scheme presented in Fig. 2. The transitional
cell compartment contains a spectrum of cells, ranging from large
to small, and these have frequently been illustrated (64). This
compartment needs a high proliferative capacity, since in addition
to the production of small lymphocytes, it also provides stem cells
for the formation of large numbers of red cells and granulocytes,
as well as for the smaller numbers of other cells, including mono-

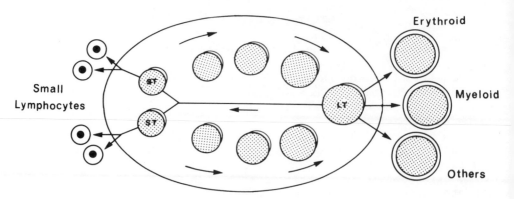

Fig. 2.   A scheme of the transitional cell (stem cell) compartment
in bone marrow.   The compartment has two essential functions,
namely: (a) self-maintenance , (b) differentiation into the various
blood cells which leave the marrow.   In the process of self-
maintenance, large transitionals (LT) divide into small ones (ST)
which then enlarge.   The growth of small into large transitionals
gives rise to a spectrum of cells of all sizes.   In addition,
there is probably an intermediate group of transitionals, not
shown in the diagram, so that there may be two self-maintenance
cycles, between small and medium, and medium and large transitionals.   The differentiation of transitional gives rise to the
various groups of blood cells, of which the most numerous are small
lymphocytes, erythrocytes and granulocytes.   The size of the
compartment is the result of a dynamic equilibrium between the
two processes of self-maintenance and differentiation.

cytes.   Osmond et al.(35) in a careful kinetic analysis of transitional cells (which they term lymphoid) have shown that the proliferative capacity is sufficient to cope with self-maintenance
as well as differentiation into the various cell groups required.
For the purposes of self-maintenance, small transitional cells enlarge, and the large cells then divide to give rise to small ones.
The result of this is a continuous size spectrum between the small
and large transitionals.

Lymphocyte production in the marrow continues throughout life,
though it appears to slow down with age (30).   While most of the
marrow lymphocytes are destined to become B cells, one must still
keep an open mind on the possibility that there may be a small
number which are unspecialized and are capable of enlarging and
re-entering the transitional cell compartment.   If this were to
turn out to be the case, it would to some extent accord with our
original concept, and with the experimental findings of Fliedner
and his co-workers (17, 50).

The transitional cells are a very rapidly proliferating population, and have a remarkably high labelling index with tritiated thymidine, higher in the larger transitionals than in the smaller. In some recent studies on rat marrow, the transitional cell compartment as a whole has been found to have a labelling index of around 50%, ranging from 32-69% in different functional states (68). An analysis of the compartment is complicated by the varying proportions of committed and uncommitted stem cells. This aspect of the problem has recently been reviewed by Rosse (45). In their morphology, the smaller transitional cells resemble the phagocytic "lymphocyte-like" cells which one finds in the peritoneum. Histochemical studies may help to decide whether these latter are in fact derived from migrating transitional cells which do not pass through a typical monocyte stage.

TRANSITIONAL CELLS AND CFU

There seems now to be little doubt that the various colony-forming units have transitional cell morphology. Although it has become somewhat of a fetish for many workers to assert dogmatically that the colony-forming cells cannot be identified morphologically, and in consequence to refrain from ever looking at the cells concerned, a number of workers have done so, and the results seem quite clear. Observations such as those of Moore et al. (32), Rosse (44), De Gowin and Gibson (7), Dicke et al. (8) and Riches et al. (40) have shown that the CFU possess both the morphology and the kinetic properties of transitional cells. Furthermore, the high thymidine suicide rate of the various colony-forming units is explicable only on the basis of their identity with transitional cells. There is no group of undifferentiated cells other than the transitionals which has the high proliferative capacity required to give rise to a thymidine suicide rate in the neighborhood of 50%. The identity of CFU and transitional cells explains why marrow suspensions with increased numbers of transitional cells confer protection more effectively than normal marrow (21, 33, 35).

THE SIZE SPECTRUM IN THE TRANSITIONAL CELL COMPARTMENT

The rapid turnover of marrow lymphocytes demonstrated by Osmond and Everett (54) suggested that there could only be two or three mitoses in the course of the lymphocyte production pathway for B lymphocytes, as compared with an estimated eight mitoses in the course of the production of T lymphocytes in the thymus. The former was therefore designated the short production pathway, in contrast to the long production pathway in the thymus (61). Since for several reasons the distinction between the two pathways appeared to be a fundamental one, a study was undertaken to ascertain whether more accurate measurement of the size spectrum of the cells

in the short production pathway would throw further light not only
on the kinetics of lymphocyte production, but also on the stem
cell compartment as a whole (65). Highly enriched populations,
consisting mainly of transitional cells of all sizes and pachychromatic small lymphocytes were measured in an improved Coulter
counter, and four peaks were obtained, corresponding to four
distinct cell types, on the basis of volume and density. There
was one peak for the small lymphocytes, and three peaks for the
transitional cells: small, medium, and large. These findings
therefore provide additional evidence that marrow lymphocytes –
for the most part presumably B lymphocytes – are formed via a
short production pathway involving only two or three mitoses.
The shortness of the pathway explains the observation of Everett
and Caffrey (11) that in radioautographs after the administration
of tritiated thymidine, there is markedly denser labelling in
marrow lymphocytes than in those of the thymus. In a short pathway there is bound to be much less label dilution.

Apart from lymphocyte production, the size spectrum of the
transitional cell compartment carries with it the necessary corollary that hemopoietic stem cells should exist in different sizes.
It is interesting therefore to note that a number of investigators
have recently shown this to be the case, by the application of cell
fractionation techniques (25, 29). The first-named authors noted
that in the main it was large CFUs which were in cycle, whereas
the smaller ones were not. This observation is an additional
pointer to the identify of CFU and transitional cells, since the
differential labelling pattern of large and small transitional
cells has been noted repeatedly (35, 45, 60).

TERMINOLOGY

In view of the fundamental importance one must now attach to
the transitional cell, a brief comment on the question of terminology is necessary. A full discussion will be found elsewhere (45,
60). The term transitional is not now fully applicable in the
sense in which it was originally intended. But it has been retained for several reasons. Within the compartment itself, one does in
fact find a continuous series of transitions between the small and
the large transitionals. In addition, there is the possibility
that, as already mentioned, there may be a special group of small
lymphocytes which is capable of enlarging and re-entering the
transitional cell compartment, in which case the original use of
the term would be entirely valid. Furthermore, other names which
have been suggested are unsatisfactory. "Lymphocyte-like" and
"Lymphoid" are not satisfactory, since these names hold good for
many cells throughout the lymphomyeloid complex, whereas, subject
to the provisos already made, transitional cells are first and foremost cells of the bone marrow.

CONTROL OF THE TRANSITIONAL CELL COMPARTMENT

From a kinetic point of view, the size of the transitional cell compartment at any time is the result of a dynamic equilibrium between very active self-maintenance, and the demand for differentiation. In the steady state the compartment can cope adequately with all demands, and it even has some margin of reserve for increased demands, but beyond a certain point the compartment cannot meet all the stem cell requirements, and then something has to give.

One of our main experimental tools has been hypoxia, since in erythropoietic stimulation additional stem cells, i.e., transitional cells, are directed into erythropoietic channels. For these studies a quantitative technique was developed, giving absolute counts of marrow cells. A full account of this work has been given elsewhere (60), so only a brief reference will be made here to some salient features. One of the early experiments was to compare the effect of weak erythropoietic stimulation, at a simulated altitude of 10,000 ft, with stronger stimulation at 20,000 ft (67). The working hypothesis was that with strong stimulation, as many more stem cells differentiated into the erythroid series, not enough would be left for granulocyte and lymphocyte production, which might therefore be impaired. This in fact was found to be the case, but the granulocytes seem to be affected before the lymphocytes. There is a significant fall in the granulocytes at 10,000 ft, and an even more marked fall at 20,000 ft. Lymphocytes, on the other hand, are not affected at 10,000 ft, but fall quite sharply at 20,000 ft. The transitional cells show a slight increase on day 1 at 10,000 ft, but remain unchanged for the subsequent 4 days. At 20,000 ft, the transitional cells fall steadily during the 5 days of hypoxia. If these results can be confirmed, they imply that lymphocytes have priority over granulocytes, at least under the conditions of these experiments.

The standard experimental animal selected for the study of the transitional cell compartment was one subjected to hypoxia for 7 days at 17,000 ft, and subsequently kept in ambient air for times ranging from 7-14 days. During the period of hypoxia, red cell production rises sharply for a few days, then levels off, while both lymphocyte and granulocyte production fall sharply. It should be emphasized that in a quantitative analysis of bone marrow changes, these are the three major cell groups constituting the bulk of the nucleated cells of the marrow, and making the biggest demand on the stem cells. At 17,000 ft there is a demand for greatly increased numbers of transitional cells to feed into the red cell compartment, with the result that not enough are left to meet granulocyte and lymphocyte production, so that these undergo a marked fall. During the hypoxic period polycythaemia develops. When the animal is taken out of the decompression chamber, since it

now has excess oxygen-carrying capacity red cell production falls
sharply, and there are now once again sufficient transitional cells
to give rise to granulocytes and lymphocytes. During this post-
hypoxic period, therefore, granulocyte and lymphocyte production
rebound, granulocytes return to their control level and lymphocytes
to well above. For this reason we refer to the state of the marrow during this post-hypoxic period as <u>rebound</u>. For several days
during rebound we have a marrow with hardly any erythroid cells,
normal numbers of myeloid cells, and greatly increased numbers of
transitional cells and lymphocytes. Full details of these changes
have been given elsewhere (60).

During hypoxia, while lymphocytes and granulocytes are falling,
the transitional cells are nevertheless proliferating very actively,
since increased numbers of them are required for the increased
erythropoiesis. Studies now in progress on rat bone marrow show
that during hypoxia there is a rise in the thymidine labelling index of the transitionals (68). When rebound begins, and erythropoiesis falls abruptly, the increased proliferation of the transitionals seems unable to slow down immediately, but goes on for
some days, so that more are formed than are needed for lymphocyte
and granulocyte production, and their numbers rise sharply. So for
several days during rebound we have a marrow with hardly any erythroid cells, normal myeloid cells and greatly increased numbers of
transitional cells and lymphocytes. These latter seem to be increasing steadily, so that one would expect, in the course of a few
days, to have a marrow consisting almost entirely of transitional
cells and lymphocytes. But this does not happen, for suddenly some
sort of brake mechanism comes into play, the transitionals cease to
proliferate for the most part, and the majority divide to produce
small lymphocytes, which for a day or two constitute 60-70% of the
marrow cells. It was this enriched rebound marrow which formed
the starting point for our study of the size spectrum of lymphocytes
and transitional cells (65).

We do not know what factor or factors control the activity of
the transitional cell compartment, but we are hoping that the
changes occurring in hypoxia and rebound will provide a useful approach to this fundamental problem.

HISTORICAL REFLECTIONS

The lymphocyte has been the object of intense study and violent
controversy for the greater part of a century. It has generated a
vast literature, containing hypothesis after hypothesis which has
been propounded and then discarded. Once thought to be useless,
the lymphocyte now seems to be ushering in what one might almost
term a Lymphocytic Era in biology and medicine. "The stone which
the builders rejected" has become the cornerstone of a vast new

edifice. Yet our ignorance of many fundamentals seems to be as
profound as ever, and even the most recent literature abounds in
the same confessions of ignorance as one encountered almost a
century ago.

In 1898, Virchow, the founder of modern pathology, was at-
tending the annual meeting of the German Pathological Association,
where he saw some preparations by a young pathologist, Felix
Marchand. Marchand (28) reports how Virchow threw up his hands in
dismay and said, "Now I know I shall never live to see the leukocyte problem solved". This had a profound effect on Marchand, who
worked for the next fifteen years on the lymphocyte and what appeared to be related cells, and in 1913 (28) he gave a lengthy
paper on the lymphocyte - again to an annual meeting of the German
Pathological Association. At the end of his paper he recalled
Virchow's words in 1898, and concluded rather sadly, "We too shall
not live to see the solution of this problem, though we can affirm
that the investigations of the last two decades have greatly clarified our knowledge of these matters. But as new results are obtained, new questions arise."

The years 1959-60 saw the start of the Great Lymphocyte
Revolution, with the introduction of PHA, and it looked as though
a new era was about to dawn. Immunology was rapidly expanding.
In 1967, when I was retiring from the Chair of Anatomy at Bristol,
we had a symposium on "The Lymphocyte in Immunology and Hemopoiesis"
and when writing the preface (59) I took Galen's famous description
of the spleen "Organon Plenum Mysterii" (an Organ Full of Mystery)
and applied it to the lymphocyte, which I described as "Cellulax
Plena Mysterii" (a Cell Full of Mystery). I then commented rather
hopefully, "The full extent of the Mysterium is now beginning to
unfold." Since then a vast army of immunologists have been at
work, and we have all had high hopes that they would solve the
Mysterium. But this is apparently not to be - not yet, at any rate.
In a book published last year by Katz (26), entitled Lymphocyte
Differentiation, Recognition and Regulation, he writes at the out-
set: "It will be apparent that a considerable number of uncertainties exist in all of the various areas of cellular immunology; indeed, it is perhaps more accurate to state that very few certainties
can be cited with any comfortable degree of assurance that a given
one will not be perceived as something different in a matter of
time."

In view of sentiments such as these, we may perhaps be excused
for feeling, like Marchand in 1913 (28), that "we too may not live
to see the solution of this problem." But I hope you will have an
interesting and enjoyable time trying to solve it and that this
Congress will provide the answers to at least some of the outstanding questions.

REFERENCES

1. Astaldi, G. and Lisiewicz, J. Lymphocytes. Structure, Production, Functions. Edelson, Naples. 1971.
2. Ben-Ishay, Z. and Yoffey, J. M. Irs. J. Med. Sci. 7 (1971) 948.
3. Balckett, N. M. J. Natl. Canc. Inst. 41 (1968) 908.
4. Campbell, F. R. Am. J. Anat. 135 (1972) 521.
5. Catavsky, D. Scand. J. Haemat. 19 (1977) 211.
6. De Bruyn, P. P. H., Michelson, S. and Thomas, T. B. J. Morphol. 133 (1971) 417.
7. De Gowin, R. L. and Gibson, D. P. Blood 47 (1976) 315.
8. Dicke, K. A., van Noord, M. J., Maat, B., Schaefer, U. W. and van Bekkum, D. W. In: Haemopoietic Stem Cells. (Eds. G. E. W. Wolstenholme and M. O'Connor) Ciba Foundation Symposium, p. 47 (1973).
9. Drinker, C. K. and Yoffey, J. M. In: Lymphatics, Lymph and Lymphoid Tissue. Harvard University Press. (1941).
10. Engeset, A., Froland, S. S. and Bremer, K. Scand. J. Haemat. 13 (1974) 93.
11. Everett, N. B. and Caffrey, R. W. In: The Lymphocyte in Immunology and Haemopoiesis. (Ed: J. M. Yoffey) Edward Arnold, London. p. 108 (1967).
12. Everett, N. B. and Tyler, R. W. Int. Rev. Cytol. 22 (1967) 205.
13. Everett, N. B. and Tyler, R. W. Biochem. Pharmac. Suppl. (1968) 185.
14. Everett, N. B. and Tyler, R. W. Cell Tiss. Kinet. 2 (1969) 347.
15. Faulk, W. P., Goodman, J. R., Maloney, M. A., Fudenberg, H. H. and Yoffey, J. M. Cellular Immunol. 8 (1973) 166.
16. Gowans, J. L. and Knight, E. J. Proc. Roy. Soc. Biol. 159 (1964) 257.
17. Haas, R. J., Bohne, F. and Fliedner, T. M. Proc. Monaco Symp. International Atomic Energy Agency 205 (1968).
18. Haas, R. J., Hans-Dieter, F., Fliedner, T. M. and Fahe, I. Blood 42 (1973) 209.
19. Hall, J. G. J. Exp. Med. 125 (1967) 737.
20. Harris, P. F. Acta Haematol (Basel) 23 (1960) 293.
21. Harris, P. F. and Kugler, J. H. Acta Haematol. (Basel) 32 (1964) 146.
22. Hudson, G. and Yoffey, J. M. Proc. Roy. Soc. Lond. (Biol.) 165 (1966) 486.
23. Hudson, G. and Yoffey, J. M. J. Anat. (Lond.) 97 (1963) 409.
24. Hudson, G. and Yoffey, J. M. J. Anat. (Lond.) 103 (1968) 515.
25. Inoue, S. and Ottenbreit, M. J. Blood 51 (1977) 195.
26. Katz, D. Lymphocyte Differentiation, Academic Press. (1977).
27. Lennert, K. and Leder, L. D. Proc. IV Internat. Symp. RES 25 (1964).
28. Marchand, F. Verhandlungen der Deutsch. Pathologis. Gesellsch. 16 (1913) 5.
29. Metcalf, D. and MacDonald, H. R. Cell. Tiss. Kinet. 8 (1975) 97.

30. Miller, S. C. and Osmond, D. G. Cell. Tiss. Kinet. 8 (1975) 97.
31. Monette, F. C., Gilio, J. and Chalifoux, P. Cell. Tiss. Kinet. 7 (1974) 443.
32. Moore, M. A. S., Williams, N. and Metcalf, D. J. Cell. Physiol. 79 (1972) 283.
33. Morrison, J. H. and Toepffer, J. F. Am. J. Physiol. 213 (1967) 923.
34. Osmond, D. G. and Everett, N. B. Blood 23 (1964) 1.
35. Osmond, D. G., Miller, S. C. and Yoshida, Y. In: Haemopoietic Stem Cells. (Eds. Wolstenholme, G. E. W. and O'Connor, M.) Associated Scientific Publishers, p. 131. (1973).
36. Pedersen, N. C. and Morris, B. J. Exp. Med. 131 (1970) 936.
37. Prindull, G., Prindull, B. and Yoffey, J. M. Acta Anat. 100 (1977) 95.
38. Rebuck, J. W. and Crowley, J. H. Ann. N. Y. Acad. Sci. 73 (1955) 8.
39. Reinhardt, W. O. Ann. N. Y. Acad. Sci. 113 (1964) 844.
40. Riches, A. C., Sharp, J. C., Littlewood, V., Briscoe, C. V. and Thomas, D. B. Proc. Anat. Soc., J. Anat. Lond. 122 (1976) 717.
41. Rosse, C. Blood 38 (1971) 372.
42. Rosse, C. In: Proceedings of the 6th Leucocyte Culture Conference (Ed. M. R. Schwarz) Academic Press, p. 55 (1972).
43. Rosse, C. Blood 40 (1972) 90.
44. Rosse, C. In: Ciba Foundation Symposium on Haemopoietic Stem Cells. (Eds. G. W. E. Wolstenyolme and M. O'Connor) Associated Scientific Publishers p. 105. (1973).
45. Rosse, C. Internal. Rev. Cytol. 45 (1976) 155.
46. Shipman, J., Hunt, C. and Yoffey, J. M. J. Anat. (Lond.) 102 (1967) 140.
47. Sjovall, H. Experimentelle Untersuchungen uber des Blut und die blutbildenden Organe - besonders das Lymphatische Gewebe - des Kaninchens bei widerholten Anderlassen. Hakan Ohlssons Boktrycheri, Lund. (1936).
48. Smith, J. B., McIntosh, G. H. and Morris, B. J. Anat. (Lond.) 108 (1971) 87.
49. Spector, W. G. and Willoughby, D. A. J. Path. Bact. 96 (1969) 389.
50. Thomas, E. D., Fliedner, T. M., Thomas, D. and Cronkite, E. P. J. Lab. Clin. Med. 66 (1965) 64.
51. Tyler, R. W. C. and Everett, N. B. Blood 28 (1966) 873.
52. Tyler, R. W. and Everett, N. B. Blood 39 (1972) 249.
53. Van Furth, R. and Dulk, M. M. C. J. Exp. Med. 132 (1970) 813.
54. Virolainen, M. J. Exp. Med. 127 (1968) 943.
55. Volkmann, M. J. Exp. Med. 124 (1966) 241.
56. Volkmann, A. and Gowans, J. L. Brit. J. Exp. Path. 46 (1965) 62.
57. Volkmann, A. and Gowans, J. L. Brit. J. Exp. Path. 46 (1965) 50.
58. Yoffey, J. M. J. Anat. (Lond.) 67 (1932) 250.

59. Yoffey, J. M.   In: The lymphocyte in immunology and haemo-
    poiesis. (Ed. Edward Arnold) London (1967).
60. Yoffey, J. M.   In: Bone marrow in hypoxia and rebound.
    (Ed. Chac. C. Thomas) Springfield (1974).
61. Yoffey, J. M. and Courtice, F. C.   In: Lymphatics, lymph
    and the lymphomyeloid complex. Academic Press (1970).
62. Yoffey, J. M. and Drinker, C. K.   Anat. Rec. 73 (1939) 417.
63. Yoffey, J. M., Everett, N. B. and Reinhardt, W. O.   In:
    Cellular migration streams in the haemopoietic system.   (Ed.
    F. Stohlman) Grune and Stratton, New York, p. 69 (1959).
64. Yoffey, J. M., Hudson, G. and Osmond, D. G.   J. Anat. (Lond.)
    99 (1965) 841.
65. Yoffey, J. M., Patinkin, D. and Grover, N. B.   The short
    production pathway for marrow lymphocytes. The significance
    of the size spectrum of the lymphocyte-transitional cell com-
    partment.   In press.
66. Yoffey, J. M., Ron, A., Prindull, G. and Yaffe, P.   Clin.
    Immunol. Immunopathol. 9 (1978) 491.
67. Yoffey, J. M., Smith, N. C. W. and Wilson, R. S. E.   Scand. J.
    Haemat. 4 (1967) 145.
68. Yoffey, J. M. and Yaffe, P.   The thymidine labelling index of
    transitional cells in rat bone marrow in different functional
    states.   (1978) Unpublished data.
69. Yoshida, Y. and Osmond, D. G.   Blood 37 (1971) 73.
70. Youse, J. H. and Barry, W. E.   J. Reticuloendoth. Soc. (1973)
    258.
71. Zucker-Franklin, D., Davidson, M. and Thomas, L.   J. Exp. Med.
    124 (1966) 533.

ULTRASTRUCTURAL STUDIES ON BRONCHIAL-ASSOCIATED LYMPHOID TISSUE
(BALT) AND LYMPHOEPITHELIUM IN PULMONARY CELL-MEDIATED REACTIONS
IN THE RABBIT

Q. N. MYRVIK, P. RACZ, and K. T. RACZ

Department of Microbiology and Immunology
Bowman Gray School of Medicine of Wake Forest University
Winston-Salem, North Carolina (USA)

The BALT represents a highly organized lymphoid tissue which
occurs in and around the walls of the large and medium-sized
bronchi, particularly at points of branching. The BALT-associated
epithelim (BALT-AE) differs from that over the rest of the bronchial mucosa in being flattened instead of columnar and ciliated;
furthermore, it is often heavily infiltrated by lymphocytes and
contains no goblet cells. Although the study of this tissue has a
long history, Bienenstock and his colleagues (1,2) recently have
drawn the attention of the immunologists to the morphologic and
functional similarities between BALT and gut associated lymphoid
tissue (GALT).

With the 1000 R irradiated allogeneic rabbit cell transfer
model of Craig and Cebra (9), Rudzik et al. have demonstrated (22)
that BALT lymphocytes repopulate the bronchial and gut lamina propria with predominantly IgA-containing cells. On the basis of
these and other recent data it has been suggested that IgA precursors sensitized in the Peyer's patches (9) or BALT (3) migrate from
here through the lymphatics, regional lymph nodes, thoracic duct,
into the blood circulation and then preferentially home in the
lamina propria of the different mucosal layers. According to this
concept, lymphocytes sensitized at one mucosal membrane can provide
protection for another.

We (19) found that morphologic similarities between BALT of
BCG-immunized rabbits and the Peyer's patches of normal animals
are even more impressive than that between normal BALT and GALT.
The lack of continuous or comparable antigenic stimulation of the
BALT in normal lungs could be an explanation for this.

145

In the present paper, we report on the morphology of the BALT-AE, horseradish peroxidase (HRP) transport in normal and BCG-immunized animals, the capability of lymphoepithelial (LE) cells for transporting bacterial antigens (Ag) and the changes of different areas of the BALT in animals undergoing a pulmonary granulomatous reaction.

MATERIALS AND METHODS

White New Zealand outbred rabbits of either sex were used. The animals were sensitized s.c. with 200 µg of head-killed BCG-suspended in 0.2 ml of mineral oil (11). Three weeks later all rabbits showed a positive skin reaction when tested with 25 µg of PPD (24 hr). Two days after skin testing, the animals were challenged intratracheally (i.t.) with 3 mg of heat-killed BCG suspended in phosphate buffered saline (pH 7.4). Groups of animals were sacrificed at 9, 16 and 24 hr, 2 days, 1, 2 and 3 weeks after the challenge dose. Control groups consisted of 14 non-treated animals. These rabbits were sacrificed at time points corresponding to those in the experimental groups. Sample pieces from lung tissue and BALT were fixed and processed for light and electron microscopy (19). The sections for light microscopy were stained with hematoxylin and eosin, Giemsa's stain, Alcian-blue-PAS and Ziehl-Neelsen's stain.

Infection with living BCG. The 8 day-old cultures of BCG in Dubos medium were washed several times with sterile medium according to Hsu (13). The pellet was resuspended in sterile saline and adjusted so that each rabbit received approximately 1×10^9 organisms suspended in 10 ml of saline via a plastic catheter. The animals were sacrificed 12, 24, 48 and 72 hr after the infection.

Horseradish peroxidase reaction. Untreated, normal as well as sensitized and challenged (S-C) rabbits were anesthetized i.v. with Napental 2 days after the challenge. Following tracheostomy, 10 mg of HRP (Sigma, Type VI) in 1 ml of saline were instilled through a premature infant feeding tube into the trachea. At 3, 10, 30 and 60 min groups of animals (3 rabbits per group) were sacrificed by an overdose of Napental. Specimens containing the BALT were handled as previously described (19). The histochemical demonstration of HRP was performed according to Graham and Karnovsky (12).

Ruthenium red (RR) staining. Lungs of 3 untreated and 3 sensitized and challenged rabbits were removed. Tissue pieces containing the BALT were fixed in RR-containing fixatives according to Luft (15). For the electron microscopic analysis of the presence of HRP as well as for the demonstration of the surface coat unstained sections were used. In specified instances uranyl acetate and lead citrate stained preparations were used.

RESULTS AND DISCUSSION

The BALT-AE consists of an epithelial reticulum. This reticulum is formed mainly by LE cells. In addition, we observed several interspersed ciliated cells, intermediate cells and basal cells participating in the reticulum. The tight junctions between the cells were closed. The LE cells were flattened and their apical surface showed irregular microvilli with prominent axial filaments. Between the microvilli deep invaginations were observed. The apical cytoplasm contained numerous vesicles and vacuoles, well developed mitochondria, and scanty endoplasmic reticulum. The number of lysosome-like bodies was very limited showing that these cells are more involved in the transport of antigen than in its digestion. The LE cells revealed several characteristics similar to those of intestinal tuft cells (14, 16) and of the brush cells (6) of the airways.

Owen (17) emphasized that the M cells of the Peyer's patches did not have a glycocalyx over their surfaces. Thiery (23) raised the hypothesis that in the appendix of the rabbit the enterocytes differentiate into LE cells under the influence of the interepithelial lymphocytes. He felt that during this process enterocytes pinocytosed their surface coat. Using RR staining, we could demonstrate the presence of an extraneous coat on the apical surface of LE cells of the BALT-AE. This layer stained by RR was continuous down to the outer cell membrane (Fig. 1). Our results are in agreement with Rao's et al. (21) postulation, that cells require a glycocalyx in order to effect endocytosis. Bockman and Cooper (5) studied the epithelium covering the bursa of Fabricius and rabbit, mouse and human Peyer's patches. They proposed to name these epithelia follicle-associated epithelium (FAE). They reported that FAE was capable of transporting ferritin or India ink from the gut lumen to the underlying lymphoid tissue. To clarify the interaction between the LE cells and the interepithelial lymphocytes, they examined the embryonal development of the Peyer's patches. Lymphoid cells were seen earlier than LE cells in the area corresponding to what later became the Peyer's patches. Similarly, Bienenstock et al. (2) observed the development of BALT in mouse fetal lungs implanted s.c. in adult recipients without antigenic stimuli. After birth, however, the antigen transported by the LE cells still had an influence on the underlying lymphoid tissue. It enhanced the accumulation of lymphocytes since in germ-free animals the Peyer's patches were only poorly developed (18). Similar to the Peyers' patch associated epithelium, the epithelium covering the BALT could also interiorize ferritin. This was reported in rabbit (4) and rats (10).

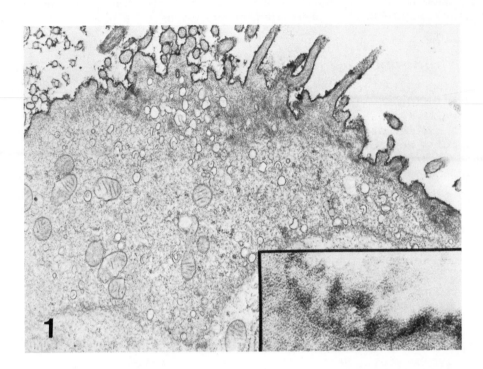

Fig. 1. Lymphoepithelial cell of a sensitized rabbit 2 days after
the challenge. A surface coat stained by RR is present on the
apical surface of the LE cell. This layer is incorporated into
the outer leaflet of the cell membrane (insert). Note the presence of numerous vesicles and mitochondria in the apical cytoplasm 4600 X; insert 110,000 X.

        In the present experiments, following i.t. infection with
living BCG we observed the presence of mycobacteria within the
LE cells at all time intervals. The bacteria were transported to
the underlying BALT. Using HRP as a marker, we found the antigen-
transporting capability of the LE cells greatly exceeded that of
the adjacent ciliated cells. At the first examined time interval,
3 min following instillation of HRP, the tracer was adsorbed to
surface of the LE cells both in normal and in S-C animals (Fig.
2a,b). In contrast, none or very limited amounts of HRP was
demonstrated on the surface of the surrounding ciliated epithelial cells. These findings showed that the surface properties of
the LE cells were more suitable for antigen adsorption than those
of the ciliated cells. The LE cells in non-immunized animals

contained only a few HRP positive vesicles and the tracer protein
was found mainly in the deep surface invaginations. In the LE
cells of S-C rabbits the number of HRP-containing structures was
significantly higher and they were evenly distributed in the cytoplasm.

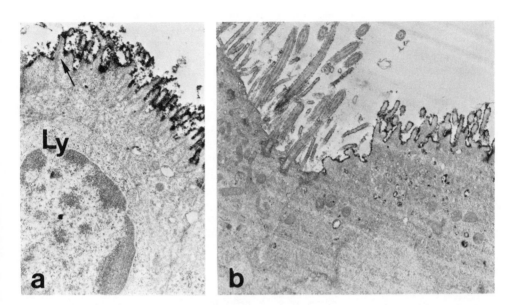

Fig. 2. Part of the BALT-AE 3 min after i.t. instillation of HRP.
a. The tracer protein is located mainly on the apical surface of
the LE cell. Note the axial filaments in the microvilli (arrows).
Normal rabbit: Ly = lymphocyte 1800 X.   b. S-C animal. The
HRP-containing structures are evenly distributed in the cytoplasm
of the LE cell. There is none or minimal amounts of HRP adhering
to the surface of the adjacent ciliated cell.   1800 X.

     Ten min following the instillation of the tracer, the distri-
bution and the amount of HRP containing vesicles in control animals, corresponded to those seen in S-C rabbits at the previous
time interval. There was a marked increase in the amount of HRP
in the LE cells of S-C animals.

     At the 30 min interval of the apical surface of LE cells
showed only limited amounts of adsorbed HRP both in normal and
S-C rabbits. We assume that the cells have interiorized the

majority of the original cell membrane and that the capability of
the remaining membrane for antigen adsorption was less than that of
the original membrane.

At one hr after instillation, the LE cells in the S-C animals
have already transported the majority of the tracer to the interepithelial lymphocyte clusters and the BALT (Fig. 3a,c). In contrast, in control animals the LE cells contained a significant
amount of HRP and the amount of HRP in the interepithelial lymphocyte clusters was significantly less than in S-C rabbits.

Our findings suggest that BCG S-C increases the intensity of
the transport of an unrelated Ag by the BALT-AE. It has been
demonstrated that the GALT represents one of the most important
portals of entry of antigen from the gut lumen (7,8). Our results
confirm our earlier data (19) and the data found in literature
(2,10) that the BALT, like Peyer's patches, has a major role in
the antigen uptake.

On the basis of morphologic characteristics and similarities
to the analogous areas of the Peyer's patches, we (19) proposed to
divide the BALT into 3 contiguous areas. These areas are: a. the
dome area (DA) which is a band of lymphoid tissue adjacent to the
lymphoepithelium, b. the follicular area (FA), and c. the para-
follicular area (PFA) containing a thymus dependent zone. This
division has proved to be useful for analyzing the reaction of BALT
in the present study.

The DA basically corresponds to the interfollicular and
superfollicular areas of the lymph node, which are located beneath the subcapsular sinus. The DA is that area which first
comes in contact with antigen transported by the LE cells. Following the i.t. challenge of sensitized animals there was an increase in the number of macrophages and lymphoblasts in the DA.
The number of plasma cells remained limited. In contrast, an
increased number of plasma cells were seen in the adjacent BALT-
AE. This observation supports the concept (3,9) that plasma cells
do not directly migrate from the BALT into the epithelial layer
but migrate out of the capillary network lying beneath the epithelial layer. The possibility of a bacterial transport by the LE
cells was demonstrated by the findings that following the i.t.
injection of living BCG, macrophages containing acid-fast bacteria
were found in the DA.

Following i.t. challenge, the FA showed a marked activation.
The number of mitoses was especially high one and two weeks following the challenge. It is likely that the production of the precursors of IgA-producing plasma cells took place in the FA.

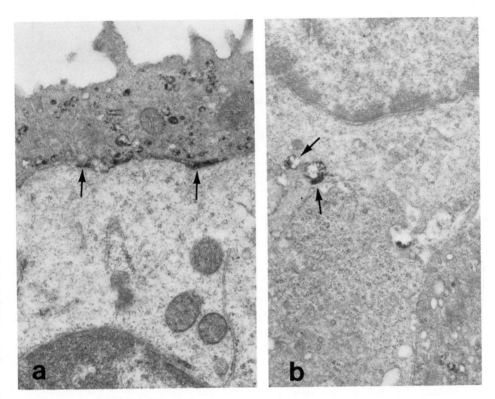

Fig. 3.   Sixty min after instillation of HRP.   a. S-C rabbit.
Minimal amounts of HRP are seen on the apical surface of a LE
cell.   Note the presence of the tracer between the LE cell and
the lymphocyte (arrows) 9500 X.   b. S-C rabbit.   HRP-positive
vesicles (arrows) in an interepithelial lymphocyte 9500 X.

An increased number of lymphoblasts and a proliferation of
high endothelial venules were seen in the thymus-dependent areas.
These changes were especially intensive two days following the
i.t. challenge.   A similar reaction was found in the paracortical
area of the hilar lymph nodes (20).   In the non-thymus dependent
part of the PFA epithelioid granulomas were seen two and three
weeks after the i.t. challenge.   This observation is compatible
with antigen being transported to the PFA.

The data presented in this paper underline the important
role of BALT-AE and BALT in the immunology of the lung.

ACKNOWLEDGMENT

The work for this project was done through a grant from the National Institutes of Health, HL 16769.

REFERENCES

1. Bienenstock, J., Johnston, J. and Perey, D. Y. E., Lab. Invest. 28 (1973) 686.
2. Bienenstock, J., Johnston, N. and Perey, D. Y. E., Lab. Invest. 28 (1973) 693.
3. Bienenstock, J., Clancy, R. L. and Perey, D. Y. E., In: Immunological and Infectious Reactions in the Lung. (Eds. C. H. Kirkpatrick and H. Y. Reynolds) Marcel Dekker, Inc., New York and Basel (1976) 29.
4. Bienenstock, J. and Johnston, N., Lab. Invest., 35 (1976) 343.
5. Bockman, D. E. and Cooper, M. D., Am. J. Anat. 136 (1973) 455.
6. Breeze, R. G. and Wheeldon, E. B., Am. Rev. Resp. Dis. 116 (1977) 705.
7. Cebra, J. J., Gearhart, P. J., Kamat, R., Robertson, S. M. and Tseng, J., In: Cold Spring Harbor Symposia on Quantitative Biology, 41 (1977) 201.
8. Cebra, J., J., Kamat, R., Gearhart, P. J., Robertson, S. M. and Tseng, J., In: Immunology of the Gut, Ciba Foundation Symposium 46 (new series) (1977) 5.
9. Craig, S. W. and Cebra, J. J., J. Exp. Med. 134 (1971) 188.
10. Fournier, M., Vai, F., Derenne, J. P. and Pariente, R., Am. Rev. Resp. Dis. 116 (1977) 685.
11. Galindo, B., Myrvik, Q. N. and Love, S. H., J. Reticuloendothel. Soc. 18 (1975) 295.
12. Graham, R. C., Jr. and Karnovsky, M. J., J. Histochem. Cytochem. 14 (1966) 291.
13. Hsu, H. S., Am. J. Resp. Dis. 100 (1969) 677.
14. Isomaki, A. M., Acta Pathol. Microbiol. Scand. 240 (Suppl.), (1973) 1.
15. Luft, J. H., Anat. Rec. 171 (1971) 369.
16. Nabeyama, A. and Leblond, C. P., Am. J. Anat. 140 (1974) 147.
17. Owen, R. L., Gastroenterology, 72 (1977) 440.
18. Pollard, M., Sharon, M. and Sharon, N., Infect. Immun. 2 (1970) 96.
19. Racz, P., Tenner-Racz, K., Myrvik, Q. N. and Fainter, L. K., J. Reticuloendothel. Soc. 22 (1977) 59.
20. Racz, P., Tenner-Racz, K., Myrvik, Q. N., Shannon, B. T. and Love, S. H., J. Reticuloendothel. Soc. (1978) in press.

21. Rao, S. N., Mukherjee, T. M. and Williams, A. W., Gut, 13 (1972) 33.
22. Rudzik, R., Clancy, R. L., Perey, D. Y. E., Day, R. P. and Bienenstock, J., J. Immunol. 114 (1975) 1599.
23. Thiery, G., C. R. Acad. Sci. Paris Serie D. 277 (1973) 413.

ULTRASTRUCTURAL AND CYTOCHEMICAL STUDIES OF MOUSE NATURAL KILLER (NK) CELLS

R. KIESSLING, J. C. RODER and P. BIBERFELD

The Department of Tumor Biology, Karolinska Institute
and the Department of Pathology, Karolinska Sjukhuset
Stockholm (SWEDEN)

There is a growing list of non-thymus dependent cytostatic and cytolytic effects which can be active against growing tumor cells. Activated macrophages, as well as antibody dependent cell mediated cytotoxicity (ADCC) by a variety of different cell types are two such alternatives to T-cell dependent mechanisms. Yet, another example is the natural killer (NK) cell, the subject to be dealt with in this paper. Similar to activated macrophages, NK cells preexist in unimmunized mice at high levels and, therefore, might be expected to provide the organism with a first line of defense against growing tumor cells. A number of experiments indeed seem to indicate that NK cells play a major role in rejecting transplantable tumor cells in vivo (7).

NK cells seem to arise in the bone marrow (2) and develop without the influence of a functional thymus (8,4). Efforts to classify this killer cell within the known groups of lymphocytes or monocytes - macrophages have so far been fruitless (8,4), and it was proposed that this cell type might constitute a "new" cell type, distinguishable from mature T or B cells (8). According to recent reports, however, the active population has low amounts of Thy. 1 antigen (5) and receptor for the hemagglutinin Helix pomatia (3). All available data so far support the notion that NK cells are small lymphocytes; they are low-adherent and non-phagocytic (8,4), have a size and density distribution corresponding to that of small and medium sized lymphocytes (6) and can be readily distinguished from activated macrophages by their range of specificity and genetic regulation (10). Moreover, in spleen cell populations which have been strongly enriched for NK cells by various cell fractionation procedures, the majority of cells (> 95%) morphologically seem to consist of small lymphocytes (8).

It is noteworthy, however, that all efforts to characterize NK
cells so far have been at the population level. For a more
precise characterization of this cell type an assay was, therefore, required to identify the NK cell at the single cell level,
as has previously been done with CTL (9,14) effector cells. In
the present report we will present such an assay system allowing
us to identify the NK cells which bind to sensitive tumor targets.
Evidence will be summarized suggesting that the majority of nylon
column-passed mouse spleen cells which bind to NK sensitive targets
are cytolytic NK cells. A partial characterization of this target
binding cell (NK cell) by cytochemistry and ultrastructural studies
will be presented.

RESULTS AND DISCUSSION

In order to identify the NK cell morphologically, we have
devised an assay system in which NK cells were studied when
binding to sensitive tumor targets. For this purpose a rosetting
assay of the same type as used by others for studying binding of
CTL was used. As summarized in Table I, we have found two types
of target binding cells (TBC) in the various lymphoid organs of
normal, non-immunized mice. The first cell type is not adherent
to nylon wool columns and binds in a selective fashion to a large
number of tumor cell targets which are susceptible to lysis (11).
The rise and fall in the frequency of these TBC, with age, closely
parallels the NK cell activity in these mice and TBC were specific
since they could be inhibited by cell surface glycoproteins of
sensitive but not insensitive targets (12). The genes controlling
the frequency of these TBC are inherited in a dominant fashion
and are linked to the H-2 region of chromosome 17 (11).

The strong correlation (r = .95) between the frequency of TBC
in various populations and the level of lysis provides strong
indirect evidence that the TBC may be related to the NK cell (11).
This suggestion was supported by the observation that the majority
of single target-effector conjugates contained lysed targets when
isolated in droplets under oil and incubated for several hours at
37 C (13).

In contrast, the second cell type, a nylon adherent population,
was not subject to any genetic control and bound to targets in a
nonspecific manner (Table I). Furthermore, these nylon adherent
cells differed from nylon non-adherent TBC in their lack of
correlation with lysis, age variations, organ distribution and
kinetics of formation (11). In conclusion, the data listed in
Table I would then strongly support the notion that the majority
of TBC from nylon non-adherent mouse spleen cells are actively
cytolytic NK cells. This system provided us with a unique possibil-

TABLE I

A Comparison of Target Cell Binding by Nylon Adherent and Non-
Adherent Spleen Cells

Characteristics	Nylon non-Adherent TBC	Nylon Adherent TBC	Reference
Follows NK genotype pattern	Yes	No	11
Shows H-2 linkage in backcross	Yes	No	11
Follows age pattern of NK cell	Yes	No	11
Organ distribution follows NK cell	Yes	No	11
Correlates well with NK lysis in kinetics experiments (r = 0.86)	Yes	No	13
Blocking by target cell sonicates	Yes	No	11,12
Time requirement for max. target cell binding	30 min	1 min	13
Mean number of targets bound per affector	1.3	3.27	11
TBC disrupted by EDTA	Yes	Yes	13
Binding of 0 C	Yes	Yes	13
Kills attached target	Yes	No	13
Frequency in whole spleen population	0.6 - 2.4%	15%	11

ity to more directly study the nature of the NK cell when binding
to a tumor target. For that purpose, direct staining of TBC with
cytochemical methods as well as electronmicroscopical studies of
the ultrastructure of TBC have been performed.

In order to have a high proportion of NK cells in the spleen
cells used for these studies, enrichment of NK cells was performed
prior to formation of target/effector conjugates. Thus, spleen
cells from homozygous nude mice were passed over nylon wool
followed by another passage over anti-Ig columns, a procedure
known to yield highly active NK cells (8). After fractionation,
TBC were formed at 4 C or 20 C, and the morphology, ultrastructure
and cytochemistry of these target/effector conjugates was then
examined.

The results of the cytochemical studies are summarized in Table II. In fixed cells, positive reactions were usually weaker but more distinct, otherwise no significant difference was observed in fixed and unfixed cells. The lymphocytes attached to YAC-cells were completely negative for peroxidase and ANAE and only faintly positive for acid phosphatase, usually localized within the cytoplasm corresponding to the Golgi area. No major difference was observed in TBC versus non-binding lymphocytes in these pre-selected populations. In contrast, YAC-cells were clearly positive for acid phosphatase and ANAE and in additional preparations, normal T lymphocytes were also ANAE positive.

Morphologically, the lymphocytes "rosetting" around the target YAC-cells were readily distinguishable from the target cells both in TEM and SEM due to their small size, characteristic mode of contact (cf. below) and the fact that virtually all YAC-cells contained abundant virus particles in the cytoplasm (Fig. 1-3). The general ultrastructural appearance of the rosetting NK-cells was consistent with that of "resting" lymphocytes, with high N/C ratio, scanty cytoplasm, relatively numerous large mitochonria, inconspicuous Golgi zones, a lack of endoplasmic reticulum and polyribosomes, and a predominantly heterochromatic nucleus with a "crescent" nucleolus (Fig. 1-3). The surface was mostly rather villous both in TEM and SEM preparations particularly in prepara-tions incubated at 20 C (Fig. 2).

TABLE II

Cytochemistry of Mouse-NK-Target Cell (YAC) Conjugates

Reaction	NK[a]	YAC[a]
Acid phosphatase	weak[b]	+ to ++
Peroxidase	−	weak to +
ANAE	−	+ to +++

[a]The results were similar irrespective of incubation temperature (4 C or 20 C) used for conjugate formation.

[b]The reactions were scored as negative (−), weak or clearly positive (+).

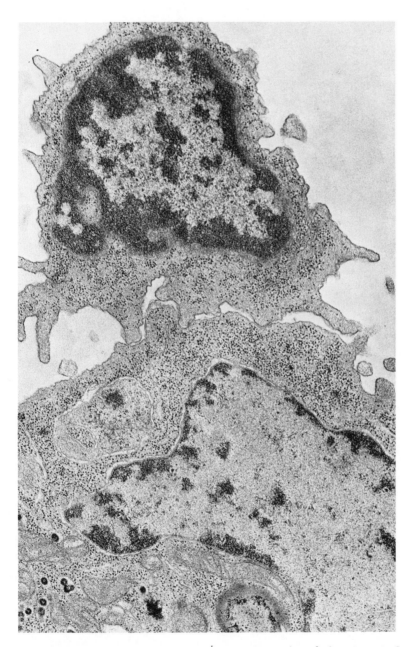

Fig. 1. Transmission electron micrographs (TEM's) of TBC from
nylon non-adherent, anti-Ig passed Balb/c nude spleen cells (For
details of electron microscopy see Ref. 13). TBC were formed
with YAC tumor cells at 4 C. (Mag. 17,000 and 34,000 X, respectively).

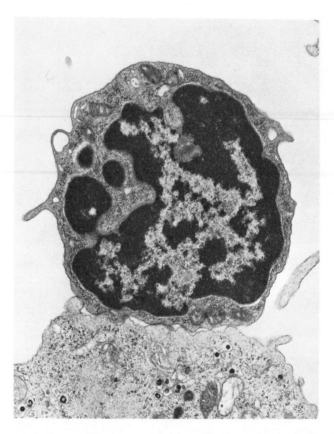

Fig. 2. Transmission electron micrographs (TEM's) of TBC from
nylon non-adherent, anti-Ig passed Balb/c nude spleen cells (For
details of electron microscopy see Ref. 13). TBC were formed
with YAC tumor cells at 20 C. (Mag. 17,000 and 34,000 X, respective
ly).

TBC and non-binding lymphocytes were similar in morphology with
the exception that TBC were usually somewhat more villous than the
nonrosetting cells especially in the 20 C preparations. The contact
between lymphocytes and target cells usually involved broad
irregular or villous surface areas of the effector cells (Fig. 3).
The physical interaction was always established by point contact
of interdigitating villi or processes extending between the cells.
Rather often, the lymphocytes appeared to be in the process of
"engulfing" small villi of the target cells (12). No local cyto-
pathogenic membrane or cytoplasmic changes were observed in contact
areas. However, in the 20 C preparations, YAC cells were frequently
observed in various stages of lytic-osmotic degeneration and
lymphocytes were only occasionally seen still attached to these
degenerating or dead cells (13).

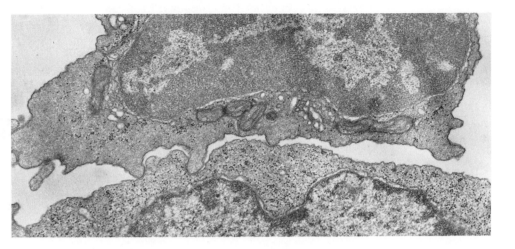

Fig. 3.   TEM of the contact areas between spleen cells (upper)
and YAC target cells (lower).   (Mag. 32,000 X).

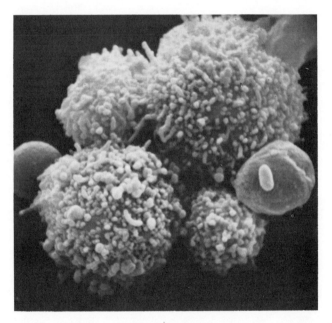

Fig. 4.   Scanning electron micrograph showing two large YAC cells
with two small spleen cells attached by numerous villi.   The smooth
cells are erythrocytes.   (Mag. 8,500 X).

The morphological and cytochemical observation on the effector cells attached to YAC cells are consistent with the characteristics of small, metabolically inactive lymphocytes. It was also clear that TBC were not significantly different from non-attached lymphocytes by the tests applied on these preselected populations. Since most of the spleen cells attached under these conditions were shown to be functionally active NK cells, as already discussed, it can be concluded that NK cells are not distinguishable from normal lymphocytes by morphology or the investigated cytochemical reactions.

The association of some lymphocytes with dead or degenerating YAC cells further suggests that they function as effective NK cells This also indicates that the killing event is definite in time and probably of short duration since no localized or progressive degenerative changes of the target cells were observed. In this respect, the NK effect is similar to other forms of lymphocyte mediated cytotoxicity (1). The often elaborate interdigitations of effector and target cell surfaces seem to indicate that the contact phase triggers major membrane and membrane associated cytoplasmic changes within the contact areas. These changes may be necessary for lysis to occur since colchicine, a disrupter of cell architecture, inhibits lysis but not cell contact. These membrane specializations probably represent a dynamic but relatively strong association between effector and target cells comparable to that observed in the CTL system (14).

Studies of surface markers on TBC are still in progress but several lines of evidence suggest that TBC are not mature B or T cells. The frequency of TBC was not lower in nude mice (11) or in nylon non-adherent spleen cell populations which were almost completely depleted of surface Ig-bearing cells on anti-Ig columns (13). It still remains to be established, however, whether the TBC express low amounts of Thy. 1 antigen, as has been suggested for the mouse NK cell (5).

In conclusion, these studies of the cytochemistry and ultra-structure of TBC strongly support the notion that NK cells are lymphocytes. Further work is necessary to delineate whether they belong to any of the already defined lymphocyte lineages, or to a separate class of lymphocyte differentiation.

ACKNOWLEDGEMENTS

This work was supported by the Killam Program of the Canada Council, The Swedish Cancer Society and the National Cancer Institute (USA) Contracts. During the study, Dr. R. Kiessling was a Fellow of the Cancer Research Institute, New York (USA) and Dr. J. C. Roder was a Research Scholar of the Canada Council, Ottawa.

REFERENCES

1. Cerottini, J. C. and Brunner, K. T. In: B and T Cells in Immune Recognition (Eds. F. Loor and G. E. Roelants) London (1977).
2. Haller, O., Kiessling, R., Örn, A. and Wigzell, H. J. Exp. Med. 145 (1977) 1411.
3. Haller, O., Gidlund, M., Hellström, U., Hammarström, S. and Wigzell, H. (1978) Submitted for publication.
4. Herberman, R. B., Nunn, M. E. and Lavrin, D. H. Int. J. Cancer (16 (1975) 230.
5. Herberman, R. B. and Holden, H. T. In: Adv. Cancer Res. (Eds. G. Klein and S. Weinhouse) Academic Press, New York (1977).
6. Kärre, K., Becker, S., Haller, O., Örn, A., Anderson, L. C., Ranki, A., Kiessling, R. and Hayry, P. (1978) Submitted for publication.
7. Kiessling, R. and Haller, O. In: Contemporary Topics in Immunobiology (Eds. N. Warner and M. Cooper) (1978) In press.
8. Kiessling, R., Klein, E., Pross, H. and Wigzell, H. Europ. J. Immunol. 5 (1975) 117.
9. Martz, E. J. Immunol. 115 (1975) 261.
10. Roder, J., Lohmann-Matthes, M. L., Kiessling, R. and Haller, O. (1978) Submitted for publication.
11. Roder, J. C. and Kiessling, R. Scand. J. Immunol. 38 (1978) In press.
12. Roder, J. C., Rosen, A., Fenyö, E. M. and Troy, F. A. (1978) Submitted for publication.
13. Roder, J. C., Kiessling, R., Andersson, B. and Biberfeld, P. (1978) Submitted for publication.
14. Sanderson, C. J. and Glauert, A. M. Proc. R. Soc. London, (B) 198 (1977) 315.

MACROPHAGE-LYMPHOCYTE INTERACTION AND GENETIC CONTROL OF IMMUNE RESPONSIVENESS

J. W. THOMAS, J. SCHROER, K. YOKOMURO, J. T. BLAKE
and A. S. ROSENTHAL
Laboratory of Clinical Investigation, National Institute
of Allergy and Infectious Diseases, National Institutes
of Health, Bethesda, Maryland (USA)

PHYSICAL INTERACTIONS BETWEEN MACROPHAGES AND LYMPHOCYTES

The physical interaction between lymphocytes and macrophages has been established as a biological event serving a number of functions such as the maintenance of viability (4) and the promotion of functional maturation and differentiation of thymocytes (25). The binding of macrophages presumably bearing an antigenic signal is seen in vivo (23) and in vitro in several species including the mouse (24), rabbit (14, 22), guinea pig (37) and man (14, 22). The functional nature of these interactions is not clear. However, detailed investigation has indicated the importance of macrophages for the in vitro induction of primary (24) and secondary (16) antibody responses as well as antigen mediated lymphocyte proliferation in vitro (5). Macrophage-lymphocyte interactions could well provide an efficient mechanism for presentation of specific and non-specific signals to immune lymphocytes.

Quantitation and characterization of these physical interactions have been carried out in the guinea pig by Lipsky and Rosenthal (19, 20). Glass adherent macrophages from various sources, including peritoneal exudate, resident peritoneal, splenic and alveolar macrophages were observed to bind thymocytes to a greater extent that either polymorphonuclear leukocytes or fibroblasts. Thymocytes and lymph node lymphocytes were bound by macrophages in numbers significantly greater than L_2C guinea pig leukemia cell line, erythrocytes or mouse thymocytes. These interactions were present when no antigen was involved and suggest the existence of a cellular recognition mechanism. However, no selectivity for T or B lymphocytes was observed - each being bound to macrophages in proportion to their frequency in the population.

165

Such interaction requires viable macrophages while the role of the
lymphocyte is passive, so that binding is not decreased by metabolic poisons or heat killing of the lymphocytes.

    Further studies on antigen independent macrophage-lymphocyte
interaction have demonstrated its dynamic character. Upon addition to macrophage monolayers, lymphocyte binding increases until
a maximum is reached after 30-60 min of incubation. Experiments
using radiolabeled thymocytes confirm this plateau to represent
an equilibrium between cellular-associated and dissociated lymphocytes (34). The microcinematographic studies of Salvin et al.(37)
also support the dynamic character of these interactions. The in
vitro characteristics of the antigen-independent binding of thymocytes or lymphocytes by macrophages are summarized in Table I.

    To examine the effects of specific antigen on macrophage-
lymphocyte interaction, established macrophage monolayers are exposed to antigen prior to the addition of lymphocytes. After 60
min at 37 C the excess antigen is washed away and nylon wool passed lymph node lymphocytes from guinea pig previously immunized
with antigen in complete Freund's adjuvant are added. During the
first hr of observation, no difference could be noted between lymphocyte interactions with antigen bearing macrophages or control
macrophages. After 1 hr, a difference could be noted and this
difference became statistically significant after 6 hr, was maximal by 20 hr and extended for at least 72 hr. The specificity of
the binding depended upon the immune status of the lymphocyte. The
immune status of the animal from which the macrophages were obtained was found to be irrelevant. Similar exposure of lymphocytes
to antigen did not result in antigen mediated interaction when

                              TABLE I

              Characteristics of Antigen-Independent Binding
                       of Lymphocytes by Macrophages

Dependent on active macrophage but not lymphocyte metabolism
Abolished by trypsinization of macrophage but not lymphocyte
Temperature dependent
Dependent on divalent cations
Cannot distinguish T from B cells
Binding is not inhibited by excess immunoglobulin
"Reversible"

---

added to macrophages, nor did it block the development of antigen
dependent interactions when these cells were added to antigen
pulsed macrophages. When hapten protein conjugates were used,
the antigen dependent binding was found to be carrier rather than
hapten specific. To the declining phase of antigen specific interactions (24-72 hr) the re-addition of antigen has been shown
to restore optimal binding (2). Thus, dissociation appears to be
dependent upon antigen degradation and subsequent lack of macrophage related changes.

The functional significance of antigen specific binding has
been assessed by autoradiographic studies of bound and unbound
lymphocytes using tritiated thymidine incorporation. ^{3}H-thymidine
incorporation of macrophage bound lymphocytes is seen after 48 hr
in culture whereas unbound lymphocytes are not found to be undergoing synthesis until 72 hr of culture - a time when maximal
dissociation is occurring. These data suggest that DNA synthesis
is initiated while lymphocytes are macrophage bound.

Other evidence indicates that the antigen mediated binding
precedes lymphocyte activation and is not dependent on initiation
of DNA synthesis. Immune lymphocytes which have been treated
with Mitomycin C, an inhibitor of DNA synthesis in response to
antigen, will participate in antigen-dependent macrophage-lymphocyte interaction as well as untreated control lymphocytes. In
addition, when immune lymphocytes are exposed to both antigen-
bearing and control macrophages simultaneously, antigen mediated
binding involves only those macrophages actually bearing antigen.
This lack of enhancement of co-culture suggests that antigen-
mediated binding is a primary event developing between an immune
lymphocyte and an antigen-bearing macrophage and does not represent a non-specific event resulting from lymphocyte activation.

The role of histocompatibility linked determinants in the
development of both antigen-independent and antigen mediated
macrophage lymphocyte interaction has recently been examined. In
the absence of antigen no significant differences were noted in
the ability of either strain 2 or strain 13 macrophages[1] to bind
syngeneic or allogeneic lymphocytes. However, antigen mediated
macrophage-lymphocyte interactions were found to require that
lymphocytes and macrophages share histocompatibility linked
identities. This restriction has been shown to exist for the
central lymphocyte of the cluster but not for the peripheral
lymphocytes in the cluster. Experiments were also performed with
F_1 (2 x 13) lymphocytes immunized with DNP-GL (an antigen towards
which only strain 2 guinea pigs respond). It was found that only
strain 2 macrophages were able to support clusters with F_1 lympho-
----
[1]Strain 2 and strain 13 are inbred guinea pigs which differ at
the region of their major histocompatibility loci.

TABLE II

Genetic Restriction of Macrophage-Lymphocyte
Antigen Dependent Interaction

		Mϕ-LNL Clusters (#/culture)	
Lymphocyte	Macrophage	PPD	DNP-GL
F_1 (2 x 13)	F_1 (2 x 13)	442 $\neq$ 25	103 $\neq$ 9
F_1 (2 x 13)	2	256 $\neq$ 37	153 $\neq$ 11
F_1 (2 x 13)	13	212 $\neq$ 63	34 $\neq$ 8

cytes. Table II demonstrates the genetic restrictions in both
strain 2 and strain 13 guinea pigs. Thus, it appears that the
antigen specific clusters require MHC similarity before physical
interactions can take place. In addition, these interactions can
be blocked by antisera directed at the alloantigen of the
macrophage involved.

THE ROLE OF THE MACROPHAGES IN ANTIGEN PROCESSING

The role of macrophages in lymphocyte activation entails not
only physical interaction between these 2 cells but also the uptake
and degradation of antigen and subsequent presentation of T
lymphocytes. Maximum DNA synthesis in T lymphocytes can be induced by macrophages exposed to antigen for as short as 30 min at
either 4 C or 37 C. However, a combination of metabolic inhibitors
such as sodium azide and 2-deoxyglucose will inhibit activation at
37 C but these are not effective at 4 C. In addition, cytochalasin
B, an agent which blocks classical pinocytosis does not reduce
antigen uptake. These results appear to indicate that uptake of
immunologically relevant antigen proceeds by at least two steps.
The initial step, though sensitive to early trypsination, is not
affected by temperature or metabolic inhibitors and would appear
to be represented by antigen interaction with a site on the macrophage surface. The later step during antigen which is internalized,
requires metabolically derived high energy intermediates and is not
related to simple fluid phase pinocytosis.

The intracellular fate of numerous antigenic proteins has
been studied. Most iodinated proteins, including mouse serum
albumin (38), bovine gamma globulin (7), bovine serum albumin
(18), keyhole-limpet hemocyanin (47) and DNP-GPA (9) undergo

extensive catabolic release of 75-90% of the initially cell-bound
radiolabel within the first 24 hr of culture. Thereafter, residual
macrophage-bound protein remains stable both qualitatively and
quantitatively (9). However, there are some antigens which undergo continued catabolism, although slow, following the initial
catabolic burst as with human serum albumin and hemoglobin (7, 8).
Of the retained antigen, 20-30% can be localized in a stable
macromolecular surface associated pool and 70-80% is intracellular -
also stable in macromolecular form (9). Removal of the membrane
bound antigen by trypsination does not reduce activation of in
vitro T cell proliferation in the guinea pig, nor does it affect
MIF production or the formation of antigen specific clusters.
However, macrophage surface-associated antigen may have major
relevance in the in vivo antibody response in the mouse (46).
These differences may indicate the surface pool is important for
macrophage-B cell interaction and the intracellular pool necessary
for macrophage related T cell activation.

     Other data have added support to the concept that a stable
surface pool was neither the sole nor the critical site of antigen
retention for T lymphocyte activation. Ellner and Rosenthal (9)
have demonstrated that antibody against antigen (DNP-OVA or horseradish peroxidase) was unable to inhibit activation of immune
lymphocyte proliferation by macrophage-associated antigen. Moreover, in studies of Lipsky such antibody was unable to inhibit
antigen dependent cluster formation. Recent data of Thomas et
al.(45) using TNP conjugated macrophages, indicated that anti-TNP
antibody inhibited the antigen induced lymphocyte proliferation
by such macrophages immediately after conjugation but such
inhibition was lost if macrophages were cultured prior to mixture
with T cells. Such results are likely the result of internalization
or redistribution of antigen upon the presenting cell surface.
These results seem to indicate that a nonspecific display of antigen is unlikely to be important in T cell activation. Rather, a
local display of macrophage associated antigen to specific receptors
might be critical for T cell activation.

     The use of fragments of whole molecules such as cytochrome (44)
and insulin (Thomas and Rosenthal, unpublished observations) may
give insight into the metabolic fate of antigen. In the case of
insulin, a 16 amino acid peptide is fully cross-reactive at the T
cell level with the whole molecule. Animals immunized with the fragment do not produce antibodies against the insulin molecule. Further
studies are underway to determine if this fragment cross-reacts with
anti-insulin antibodies. In the absence of macrophages the fragments fail to activate primed T cells, indicating the role of the
macrophage is not simply antigen degradation. Consonant with the
observation that T cell triggering can be blocked by antisera
against MCH-linked Ia antigens (43), one can construct a model
in which a degradative product or antigen fragment will combine

with such surface antigen to create a new structure for antigen
recognition and subsequent T cell activation. Failure of antibodies directed against the native molecule to block such activation may be explained by the inability of such antibodies to
bind the important fragment.

MACROPHAGE FUNCTION IN THE PROLIFERATION RESPONSE TO PROTEIN
ANTIGEN, MITOGENS, HISTOCOMPATIBILITY ANTIGENS
AND CHEMICAL MODIFICATION OF CELL SURFACE

The result of the previously outlined studies have documented
that macrophages process antigen and interact physically with
lymphocytes. The functional significance of these observations
are demonstrated in studies of the T cell response in vitro and
in vivo. The simplest of these techniques is to restore the
proliferative capacity of populations of lymphoid cells depleted
of macrophages. Such restoration is not supplied by lymphocytes,
granulocytes, or fibroblasts (29, 33, 48). In addition, the
antigen presenting cell must share histocompatibility linked
determinants with the responding T cells (34). Studies in the
mouse using peritoneal exudate T lymphocytes (PETELS) (4) and lymph
node T cells (35) have examined the interactions between the antigen presenting cell and the T cell. In PETELS system, the interaction requirement could be mapped to a more precise region of the
MHC - the IA subregion. Rossenwasser (35), using lymph node lymphocytes obtained by nylon wool purification, produced a population
of T cells which had an absolute requirement for an adherent cell
population, even in the presence of continuous antigen. The requirement for macrophages was found to differ with the nature of
the antigen to which the T cells were sensitized. Complex multideterminant soluble protein antigens such as DNP-OVA are dependent
on the production of a soluble factor which is not antigen specific
nor related to the haplotype origin of the adherent cell. However,
when an antigen such as syngeneic terpolymer L-glutamic acid, L-
lysine, L-tyrosine (GLT) which is under IR control is used,
the interaction requires identity in the MCH between macrophage and
primed lymphocytes. Table III demonstrates the difference in
macrophage requirement for T cell response for the antigen GLT and
DNP-OVA.

T cell proliferation depends upon the macrophage not just for
antigen induced proliferation but also for less specific mitogen
induced responses. Using guinea pig lymph node derived T lymphocytes, Lipsky et al.(21) were able to sufficiently deplete macrophages to abolish the proliferation response to phytohemagglutinin
(PHA). However, unlike the antigen response, restoration was not
restricted to syngeneic macrophages as both allogeneic macrophages
and fibroblasts restored PHA responsiveness. Thymocytes or polymorphonuclear leukocytes were ineffective in restoring the response.

TABLE III

Supernatants of Cultured PEC Enhance the Response of Immune
T Cells to DNP-OVA, but Have Little Effect on Response to
GLT[15]. Response of BALB/c LNL Primed In Vivo
with 100 μg GLT[15] and 10 μg DNP-OVA Per Mouse

PEC/Supe	[a] Δcpm + S. E. ^{3}H-Tdr Incorporation	
	GLT[15] 200 μg/ml	DNP-OVA 200 μg/ml
0	0.04 + 0.01	1.21 + 0.3
BABL PEC	11.11 + 2.84	31.92 + 1.55
B6 PEC	0.24 + 0.14	24.23 + 4.31
BALB Supe	0.03 + 0.02	10.57 + 1.19
B6 Supe	0.10 + 0.04	12.79 + 5.17

[a]mean Δ cpm + S. E. for three experiments; Δ cpm is (Expt'1-
Control) for each experiment

The accessory cell function is unlikely to be that of maintenance
of viability since 2-ME did not permit an effective PHA-induced
lymphocyte response. One must conclude, therefore, that accessory
cells have an additional function. This could include effects
upon cell density or even contamination of re-added cells with
macrophages. Using the in vitro plaque forming system, different
results have been reported (4, 30).

The mixed leukocyte reaction (MLR) in both man and the guinea
pig are much more efficiently stimulated by macrophages (11, 12, 32).
The role of the macrophage has not been studied in the mouse MLR.
However, unlike the guinea pig, both B and T lymphocytes have been
reported to have considerable stimulating activity (10, 15). Com -
paring the presentation of antigen in the guinea pig proliferation
assay to that of MHC antigens in the MLR, the obvious notation is
that the histoincompatible macrophage is the stimulator. The difference may well reside on cell surface alloantigen display as con-
trasted with soluble protein antigen bound by macrophages. Alter-
nately, an analogy can be drawn from the MLR and the previously
mentioned model in which antigen is theorized to combine with "self"
surface proteins to create a modified self determinant which can
activate T cells.

Alteration of cell surface molecules can be studied via
chemical modification vida infra. The generation of aldehyde
moieties on lymphocytes either by gentle treatment with sodium

metaperiodate ($NaIO_4$) or sequential neuraminidase and galactose oxidase (NG) treatment will induce extensive blastogenesis in lymphocytes from several species (26, 27, 28). In the guinea pig studies have shown that macrophages are required for lymphocyte transformation regardless of how or where the aldehyde is generated (11, 12). If lymphocytes are treated in the absence of macrophages, the latter are still required for interaction before blastogenesis can occur. In addition, if macrophages are treated, they can themselves stimulate a lymphocyte proliferative response. These two mechanisms for activation are not totally identical for macrophage aldehyde "presentation" function, which is resistant to proteolytic treatment and persists in culture up to 48 hr, whereas aldehyde modified lymphocytes are sensitive to proteolytic enzymes and aging. The kinetics of such chemically induced proliferation resembles that of soluble antigen and other cell types such as thymocytes, fibroblasts and PMNs and cannot reconstitute the responses. However, it does differ in that both syngeneic or allogeneic macrophages may stimulate. Such a chemically altered surface could act as a final common pathway for the "activation" phase of macrophage lymphocyte interaction. The initial phase of such an interaction could involve either binding of antigen specific T cells, induction of MLR or mitogen responsiveness.

FUNCTION OF THE MACROPHAGE IN THE GENETICS OF THE IMMUNE RESPONSE

The immune response to many antigens has been noted to be linked by dominant inheritance to the major histocompatability complex (MHC). These immune response genes (Ir) have been studied most extensively in the guinea pig and mouse and have been shown to control various T cell dependent responses, such as delayed hypersensitivity, T cell proliferation, and induction of antibody production. One interpretation is that Ir genes function via the production of a cell surface product which plays a role in the mechanism of antigen recognition by the T lymphocyte. The extension of studies which demonstrated the critical role of macrophages in an antigen induced T cell proliferation showed that efficient interaction was only observed when the macrophage and T lymphocyte were syngeneic (34). Still more important was the observation that F_1 T cells, which are normally activated by macrophage from either parent, can only be stimulated by the Mø of the responder haplotype when the immunizing antigen is under Ir gene control (43). To explain histocompatability restrictions in macrophage T interaction, a "cellular interaction structure" model was proposed. Since I region differences appeared responsible for the restriction in the guinea pig, Ia antigens seemed a likely candidate for this structure. In addition, I region alloantisera directed against such differences can block the MLR between the two strains when directed against the stimulating macrophage but has no effect on the responding lymphocyte (13).

In a similar fashion, when T lymphocytes are treated with sodium periodate and mixed with untreated macrophages, the resultant stimulation is markedly inhibited by an alloantisera directed against the macrophage, but not the proliferating T cells. Recent observations in our laboratory also indicate that alloantisera can specifically inhibit the antigen dependent physical interactions between responding macrophages and F_1 T cells (Braendstrup, Werdlin and Rosenthal, submitted for publication). Attempts to define the site of action of the alloantisera using combinations of antige-pulsed macrophages and T cells are difficult because of the pre-viously noted MLR which is stimulated by allogenic macrophages. However, in an in vivo system which eliminates alloreactivity with bromodeoxyuridine (BUdR) and light, T cells can be specifically primed with allogeneic macrophage bound antibody or TNBS modified macrophages (45). In the same in vitro system using F_1 T cells, the genetic restrictions in a secondary response could be imposed by the macrophage type used for priming.

One possible explanation for the failure of the non-responder macrophage to activate the (non-responder x responder) F_1 T cell is an intrinsic defect of the Ir gene product in the non-responder macrophage. The most direct approach to the analysis of the deter-minants mediating macrophages and/or T cells would be from an ani-mal which bears a recombinant chromosome in which genes coding for alloantigens and Ir gene products are separated. Unfortunately in the offspring of (2 x 13) F_1 x parental animals, no animals pos-sessing recombinant chromosomes have been found.

Though I region differences appear to play no role in T cell cytotoxicity, the mechanism proposed by Shearer et al. (42) and Doherty et al. (6) does have relevance for an understanding anti-gen specific induction of T cell proliferation. They proposed that immune recognition took place, an "alteration of self", as in TNBS modification or virus infection. Thus, strain 13 macro-phages pulsed with PPD failed to activate immune strain 2 T cells not because strain 2 T cells have never previously seen PPD but rather in the primary immunization they were sensitized to "PPD-altered self" (Table IV). This hypothesis does not explain why antigen pulsed non-responder macrophages fail to activate (re-sponder x non-responder) F_1 T cells. In order to explain the defect one must postulate that the macrophages of non-responders lack an I region determinant which can be suitably altered to be recognized as "altered self". Another explanation has been ap-plied to an antibody forming cell assay to the terpolymer GAT (31). In this system F_1 mice (responder x non-responder) can be primed with either parental macrophages pulsed with antigen and subse-quent restriction to the immunizing macrophage strain ensues. However, when the F_1 is immunized with soluble antigen, the secon-dary response is restricted to the responder strain macrophage. The alterante hypothesis suggests that helper T cells are primed

TABLE IV

Activation of (2 x 13) F_1 PELs
by Antigen-Pulsed Macrophages[a]

Antigen	F_1 Macrophages	Strain 2 Macrophages	Strain 13 Macrophages
		NGPS	
DNP-GL	14,539	23,402	2,992
PPD	28,117	21,919	28,048
PHA	34,710	55,021	67,538
		13 anti-2 serum	
DNP-GL	0	1,840	69
PPD	19,333	2,167	31,648
PHA	50,208	61,249	75,052
		2 anti-13 serum	
DNP-GL	16,517	29,363	0
PPD	18,538	26,113	119
PHA	60,098	18,963	77,449

[a](2 x 13) F_1 strain 2, or strain 13 macrophages were pulsed with
either 100 µg/ml of DNP-GL and 10 µg/ml PHA. Macrophages were
washed, and then mixed with immune (2 x 13) F_1 PELs. Results
are expressed a Δ cpm/culture; each value is the mean of 3 determinations.

preferentially to soluble antigen responder macrophages and that
non-responder macrophages are not capable of stimulating this subpopulation.

A simple hypothesis has been developed in our laboratory which
states that a given macrophage's repertoire of Ir gene products
function to select specific antigenic determinants. Most complex
antigens such as tuberculin (PPD) or the random copolymers do not
have defined structure and thus do not permit precise intramolecular mapping of those areas responsible for immunogenicity. By
contrast, polypeptides of known structure such as insulin, offer
a unique opportunity to characterize those regions of the molecule
regocnized by the T cell receptor or antibody.

The immune response to insulin, in both mouse (17) and guinea
pig (1) is under MHC-linked Ir gene control. When immunized with

either pork or beef insulin CFA, both strain 2 and 13 guinea pigs
respond by antigen specific lymphocyte proliferation and synthesis
of specific activity. Even though the specificity of antibodies
is undistinguishable between these inbred strains, the T cell's
response is directed at distinct regions of the molecule – alpha
loop of A chain in strain 2 and B chain in strain 13.

If Ir gene function operates in the lymphocyte, both of these
determinants should be simultaneously recognized by F_1 T cells
independently of the macrophage presenting the antigen. If, however, determinant recognition depends on the genetic profile of
the macrophage, the Ir gene function must also be operating at this
cell level. A strong proliferative response is observed when pork
insulin pulsed macrophages from either strain are added to primed
F_1 (2 x 13) guinea pig T cells. However, when different species
variants of intact insulin are presented to these same F_1 pork
insulin immune T cells, 2 different patterns of response are seen.
When strain 2 macrophages are used to present beef, sheep or pork
insulin, the amount of T cell activation varies with the degree of
identity within the alpha loop region of the A chain. On the other
hand, when strain 13 macrophages are used, no difference in T cell
reactivity can be detected. This suggests that the strain 13 macrophage is providing the B chain determinant which is identical in
all these species. In order to corroborate these findings, we
studied the response of oxidized insulin B chain immune F_1 T cells
to parental macrophages pulsed with either natural insulin or B
chain. As shown in Table V, only strain 13 macrophages can present
B chain to the F_1 T cells. Despite the capacity of strain 2 macrophages to present insulin to insulin immune T cells, they cannot
initiate DNA synthesis on B chain immune F_1 T cells.

From these experiments it appeared that 2 distinct clones of
T cells are generated in the F_1 – 1 responsive to amino acid dif-
fuse with the A chain alpha loop and the other responsive to the
B chain determinant. Using BUdR and light to eliminate responsive
clones, F_1 T cells initially stimulated with strain 2 macrophages
lost on subsequent stimulation with strain 2 but not with strain
13 macrophages (Table VI). Conversely, exposure F_1 T cells strain
13 macrophages bearing pork insulin eliminates 97% of responsiveness on repeat culture to pork insulin on strain 13 macrophages but
does not affect the response of F_1 T cells to strain 2 macrophages
bearing insulin. Such data showed that at least 2 distinct clones
of insulin reactive T cells exist in F_1 animals and that the macrophage plays a critical role in selecting the moieties of complex
antigens recognized by immune T cells. In order to further examine
the possibility that the genetic restriction in the macrophage
might result from the priming process as indicated by the previously mentioned studies of Pierce et al. (30, 31), guinea pigs were
immunized with antigen pulsed macrophages in vivo. The results
indicate that F_1 (2 x 13) guinea pigs can be primed with oval-

TABLE V

DNA Synthetic Response of T Cells from Oxidized Insulin B Chain
Immunized F_1 (2 x 13) Guinea Pigs to Parental
Macrophage Pulsed with Native Insulin and Isolated B Chain[a]

Macrophages Pulsed with	Macrophage Genetic Background	
	Strain 2	Strain 13
	^{3}H-TdR incorporation (Δ cpm x 10^{-3})	
PPD	145,810	98,010
Pork insulin	100	13,160
Oxidized B chain	6,840	66,900

[a]F_1 (2 x 13) guinea pigs were immunized with 10 µg of B chain in
CFA, 2-3 weeks prior to use. Oil induced, macrophage-rich peritoneal exudate cells were pulsed with 100 µg/ml of antigen and
40 µg/ml of mitomycin-C at 37 C for 60 min. After 4 washes, 1.2
x 10^5 of these cells were added to 2.4 x 10^5 responding peritoneal
exudate lymphocytes depleted of adherent cells (PELs) in 200 1
of 5% heat inactivated male guinea pig serum in RPMI-1640 + 2.5
x 10^{-5} M of 2-mercaptoethanol in round bottom microtiter plates.
After 48 hr of culture, 1 µc of ^{3}H-methyl-thymidine (New England
Nuclear, sp. act. 6.7 µc/mM) was added to each well for an additional 24 hr of culture. At this time cells were harvested on
glass fiber filters with a semi-automated microharvester from
Adaps Corporation (Boston, Massachusetts) and ^{3}H-thymidine incorporation determined by liquid scintillation spectrometry.

bumin on either of their parental macrophages and that in vitro
secondary DNA synthetic responses can be recalled only with the
macrophages used for priming. However, in contrast to the results of Pierce et al.with GAT, F_1 guinea pigs can be immunized
with the B chain of insulin only when pulsed on macrophages of
responder genetic background (strain 13) (Yokomuro and Rosenthal,
submitted for publication).

These results add support to the possibility that the responses to multideterminant antigens in F_1 guinea pigs is the
result of a macrophage dependent process of determinant selection.
Our studies in insulin further indicate that a selected amino acid
sequence and/or conformation of the antigen is seen by the responding cell and that these determinants are made available
through immune response genes functioning at the level of the

TABLE VI

BUdR and Light Elimination of Antigen Specific F_1 T Cell
Proliferation: Intramolecular Determinant
Selection by Pork Insulin–Bearing Parental Macrophages[a]

Macrophages used in First Culture	% Elimination of F_1 T Cell DNA Synthetic Response on 2nd Culture Macrophage Used:	
	Strain 2	Strain 13
Strain 2	96	12
Strain 13	0	97

[a] Immune PELs at a concentration of 1 x 10^6/ml were cultured first
with 3 x 10^5 mitomycin–C treated insulin pulsed macrophages for
48 hr in 12 x 75 mm capped plastic tubes. At the end of this time
2 μg/ml of freshly prepared 5-bromodeoxyuridine (BUdR) was added
to the cultures. 24 hr later, the cell pellets were exposed to
light by placing the culture tubes directly on an array of 3
fluorescent light bulbs for 90 min. After 4 washes of the cell
pellet with Hanks BSS, the BUdR and light treated cells were
cultured a second time in microtiter plates (as described in
Table V) in the presence of added pork insulin-pulsed macrophages.
Data are expressed as % inhibition of DNA synthesis remaining
after BUDr and light treatment. BUdR is a thymidine analog which
if present during the S phase of the cell cycle is incorporated
into newly synthesized DNA and cross-links DNA strands upon light
activation. Treatment of activated lymphocytes with BUdR and
light leads to an irreversible block in cell replication.

antigen presenting cell.

Two general mechanisms by which gene products on macrophages
might function can be suggested. One possibility is that immune
response genes define a class of receptors on broad specificity
which recognizes molecular shape and thus have the unique ability
to focus or orient distinct regions of the antigen for presentation to the T cells. A second possibility is that immune response
gene products are/or regulate the ability of enzymes which modify
or metabolize polypeptide antigens. These would be able to define
restricted areas of the molecule for display to the T cell receptor.

SUMMARY

We have reviewed briefly some of the diverse functions of
macrophages in the immune response. Clearly, this population of
cells interact physically with lymphoid cells, are required for
activation of T cells, and process various protein antigens.
Finally, we have studied the immune response to insulin in order
to unify these previous data in such a way to demonstrate the
active role of macrophages in the regulation of the immune response. The function of the Ir gene in the guinea pigs appears to
be an intramolecular selection of discrete regions within the
antigen for recognition by the T cell. The data presented suggest
that this function operates at the level of the macrophage.

REFERENCES

1. Barcinski, M. A. and Rosenthal, A. S. J. Exp. Med. 145 (1977)
    726.
2. Ben-Sasson. J. Immunol. 120 (1978) 1902.
3. Boehmer, H. J. Immunol. 112 (1974) 70.
4. Chen, C. and Hirsch, J. G. J. Exp. Med. 136 (1972) 604.
5. Cline, M. J. and Swet, V. C. J. Exp. Med. 128 (1968) 1309.
6. Doherty, P. C., Bladen, R. V. and Zinkernagel, R. M.   Trans-
    plant. Rev. 29 (1976) 89.
7. Ehrenreich, B. A. and Cohn, Z. A. J. Exp. Med. 126 (1967)
    941.
8. Ehrenreich, B. A. and Cohn, Z. A. J. Cell. Biol. 38 (1968)
    244.
9. Ellner, J. J. and Rosenthal, A. S. J. Immunol. 114 (1975)
    1563.
10. Fathman, C. G., Handwergie, B. S. and Sachs, D. H. J. Exp.
    Med. 140 (1974) 853.
11. Greineder, D. K. and Rosenthal, A. S. J. Immunol. 114 (1975)
    1541.
12. Greineder, D. K. and Rosenthal, A. S. J. Immunol. 115 (1975)
    932.
13. Greineder, D. K., Shevach, E. M. and Rosenthal, A. S. J.
    Immunol. 117 (1976) 1261.
14. Hamfin, J. M. and Cline, M. J. J. Cell. Biol. 46 (1970) 97.
15. Harrison, M. R. J. Immunol 111 (1973) 1270.
16. Katz, D. H. and Unanue, E. R. J. Exp. Med. 137 (1973) 967.
17. Keck, K.   Eur. J. Immunol. 5 (1975) 801.
18. Kolsch, E. and Mitchison, N. A. J. Exp. Med. 128 (1968) 1059.
19. Lipsky, P. E. and Rosenthal, A. S. J. Exp. Med. 138 (1973)
    138.
20. Lipsky, P. E. and Rosenthal, A. S. J. Exp. Med. 141 (1975)
    138.
21. Lipsky, P. E., Ellner, J. J. and Rosenthal, A. S.   J. Immunol.
    116 (1976) 876.

22. MaFarland, W., Heilman, D. H. and Moorehead, J. F. J. Exp. Med. 124 (1966) 851.
23. McGregor, D. D. and Logie, P. S. Cell. Immunol. 18 (1975) 454.
24. Mosier, D. E. Science 151 (1967) 1573.
25. Mosier, D. E. and Pierce, C. W. J. Exp. Med. 136 (1972) 1484.
26. Novogrodsky, A. and Kathchalski, E. Fed. Eur. Biol. Sci. 12 (1971) 297.
27. Novogrodsky, A. and Kathchalski, E. Proc. Nat. Acad. Sci. USA 69 (1972) 3207.
28. Novogrodsky, A. and Kathchalski, E. Proc. Nat. Acad. Sci. USA 70 (1973) 1824.
29. Oppenheim, J. J., Levinthal, B. G. and Hersch, E. M. J. Immunol. 111 (1968) 58.
30. Pierce, C. W., Kapp, J. A., Wood, D. D. and Benaceraff, B. J. Immunol. 112 (1974) 1181.
31. Pierce, C. W., Germain, R. M., Kapp, J. A. and Benacerraf, B. J. Exp. Med. 146 (1977) 1827.
32. Rode, H. N. and Gordon, J. Cell. Immunol. 13 (1974) 87.
33. Rosenstreich, D. L. and Rosenthal, A. S. J. Immunol. 112 (1974) 1085.
34. Rosenthal. A. S, and Shevach, E. M. J. Exp. Med. 138 (1973) 1194.
35. Rosenwasser, L. J. and Rosenthal, A. S. J. Immunol. 120 (1978) 1991.
36. Rosenwasser, L. J., Schwartz, R. H. and Rosenthal, A. S. (1978) In preparation.
37. Salvin, S. B., Sell, S. and Nichio, J. J. Immunol. 107 (1971) 655.
38. Schmidtke, J. R. and Unanue, E. R. J. Immunol. 107 (1971) 331.
39. Schwartz, R. J., Jackson, L. and Paul, W. E. J. Immunol. 115 (1975) 1330.
40. Schwartz, R. H. and Paul, W. E. J. Exp. Med. 143 (1976) 529.
41. Sharp, J. A. and Burwell, R. G. Nature 188 (1960) 474.
42. Shearer, G. M., Rehn, T. G. and Schmitt-Verhulst, A. M. Transplant. Rev. 29 (1976) 89.
43. Shevach, E. M. and Rosenthal, A. S. J. Exp. Med. 138 (1973) 1213.
44. Sollinger, A., Schwartz, R. W. and Paul, W. E. (1978) Presented at the 4th Ir Gene Workshop.
45. Thomas, D. W., Yamashita, U. and Shevach, E. M. Immunol. Rev. 35 (1977) 97.
46. Unanue, E. R. and Cerottini, J. C. J. Exp. Med. 131 (1970) 711.
47. Unanue, E. R., Cerottini, J. C. and Bedford, M. Nature (London) New Biol. 272 (1969) 1193.
48. Waldron, J. A., Horn, R. G. and Rosenthal, A. S. J. Immunol. 111 (1973) 58.

ENHANCEMENT OF SPREADING, PHAGOCYTOSIS AND CHEMOTAXIS BY MACROPHAGE STIMULATING PROTEIN (MSP)

E. J. LEONARD and A. H. SKEEL

Immunopathology Section, Laboratory of Immunology
National Cancer Institute
Bethesda, Maryland (USA)

It is now generally believed that the macrophage originates from a bone marrow precursor, has a developmental period as a circulating blood monocyte, and resides as a mature cell in tissues, where its function is determined in part by the organ in which it settles (6). Infectious and other stimuli alter profoundly the metabolic and functional state of macrophages recovered from the tissues (Fig. 1). Inflammatory stimuli increase the flow of macrophages into the tissue site. The recently arrived macrophages can be distinguished functionally and cytochemically from normal tissue macrophages. Furthermore, they can be activated to become cytotoxic in a series of steps initiated by a product of antigen-stimulated lymphocytes (Macrophage Activation Factor). Recent developments in the elucidation of this pathway will be discussed by Dr. M. S. Meltzer from our laboratory elsewhere in this book and have been reported earlier (2, 3, 4). In this presentation, we will describe a serum protein, Macrophage Stimulating Protein (MSP), that affects several functions of the normal tissue macrophage. The exquisite specificity of MSP is shown by the fact that it has no effect on the activated macrophage; the activated macrophage, however, is affected by macromolecules other than MSP in normal serum.

MSP was discovered during a study of the chemotactic response of resident peritoneal macrophages, obtained by washing out the normal mouse peritoneal cavity with tissue culture medium. Chemotaxis chambers were filled with complement or lymphocyte derived chemotactic factor. A polycarbonate membrane with 5 μm diameter pores separated the bottom well from the top where the cell suspension was added. After a 3 hr incubation at 37 C, the cells were removed and the membrane was inverted onto a glass slide,

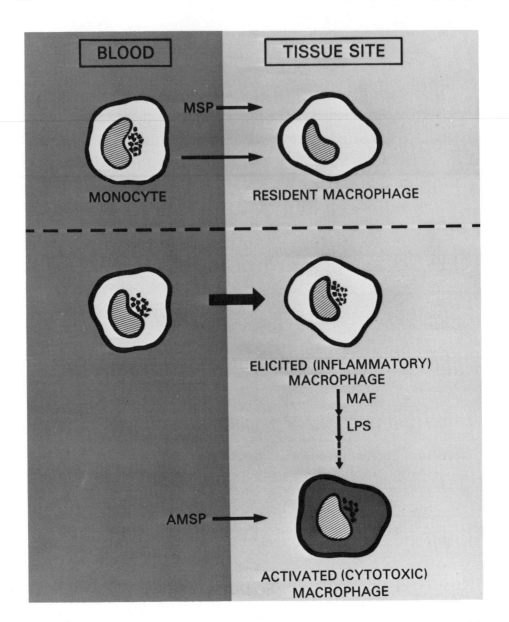

Fig. 1. Top: peroxidase-positive blood monocytes become peroxidase
negative tissue macrophages. MSP affects chemotactic and phagocytic responses of resident macrophages. Bottom: flow of macrophage precursors into tissue is increased by inflammation. A
series of steps converts them into activated macrophages. Chemotactic responses of activated macrophages are affected by serum
macromolecules (ASMP), but not by MSP.

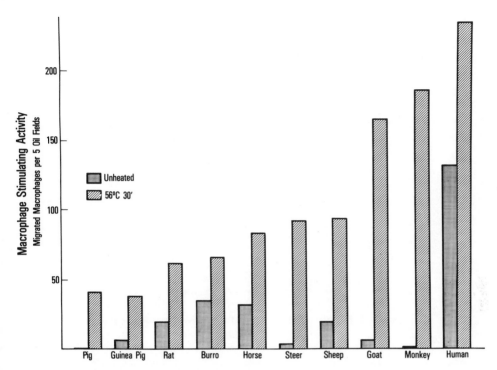

Fig. 2.   Effect of sera from different species on chemotactic
response of mouse resident peritoneal macrophages to endotoxin-
activated mouse serum.   Heated or unheated sera, in a final concentration of 12.5%, were added to the cell compartment of the
chemotaxis chamber.

dried and stained. Macrophages that had spread onto the underside
of the membrane were then counted. We found that macrophages did
not migrate toward the chemotactic factor unless serum was present
in the cell suspension (2).   The active factor in the serum was a
macromolecule and its effect was concentration dependent. When
the cells were suspended in tissue culture medium with MSP, there
was no migration. MSP sometimes caused migration of a small number of macrophages in the absence of a chemo-attractant. MSP was
found in the serum of all mammalian species tested, including mice
Comparison of a number of sera, all tested on aliquots of a single
pool of mouse macrophages, is shown in Fig. 2.   The results do not
necessarily reflect the absolute amount of MSP in the sera.   The
effects of heating, for example, suggest that the activity in
whole serum is determined in part by heat-labile inhibitors.

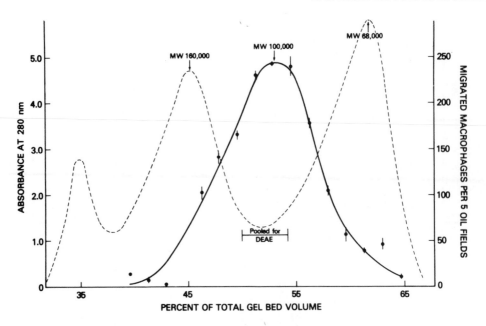

Fig. 3. Elution of human serum MSP from Sephadex G-200. Dashed line: A$_{280}$. Solid line: MSP activity.

We chose human serum as starting material for the isolation of MSP because of availability and high activity. The purification schema for MSP has been published (3). Sephadex G-200 gel filtration was the first step since the peak MSP activity is precisely where the protein concentration of the eluted fractions is at a minimum (Fig. 3). This corresponds to a MW of 100,000. Modification of our published procedure for large scale preparation involves lyophilization of serum or plasma, reconstitution to 1/3 the original volume, precipitation of unwanted protein by 8% sodium sulfate, crystallization and removal of part of the sodium sulfate at 0 C and gel filtration of the concentrated protein supernatant. The MSP fractions from 10 Sephadex G-200 runs were pooled for further purification. As shown in Fig. 3, the 2 major contaminants are 160,000 MW IgG and 68,000 MW serum albumin. Albumin was readily removed by addition of the G-200 pooled fractions of DEAE-cellulose. MSP was completely separated from albumin by stepwise elution (Fig. 4). A large amount of protein was then removed by isoelectric focusing; note the precipitous drop in A$_{280}$ values as the region of MSP activity is approached (Fig. 5). The pI of MSP is 7.0, an unusually high value for non-IgG serum proteins. Since the concentration of IgG in serum is about 1 x 10^7 times that of MSP and their isoelectric points are similar, traces of IgG were present at this stage. A second gel filtration (Fig. 6) shows a

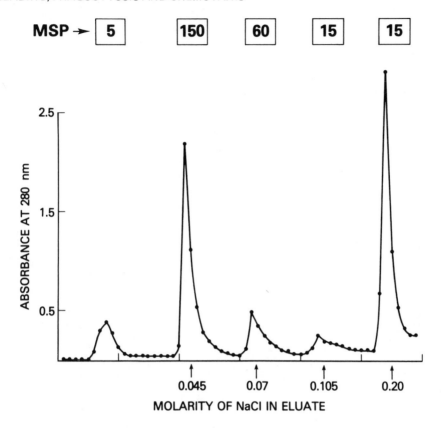

Fig. 4. Elution of G-200 pool from DEAE-cellulose. Solid line: A_{280} of eluted fractions. Albumin is the last peak. Boxes: MSP activity of pooled fractions.

symmetrical protein peak with a maximum corresponding to IgG and an MSP activity peak beyond. The amount of MSP is so small that it does not cause detectable asymmetry on the protein concentration curve. Residual IgG was removed by absorption with protein-A present on the surface of Cowan strain Staphylococcus aureus. Formalin-treated S. aureus is a convenient solid phase absorbent for trace amounts of IgG. A final step for preparation of MSP antigen was polyacrylamide gel electrophoresis. Although this was the third method in the purification schema based on protein charge, a rapidly migrating protein that stained strongly in the gel was separated from the MSP. The region of the polyacrylamide gel with MSP activity was cut out and emulsified with complete Freund's adjuvant to induce antibody production in rabbits. The starting material for MSP antigen production was about 2500 ml of human plasma, in which we estimate the MSP concentration to be less than 100 ng/ml. The final product, distributed in 10 gels for

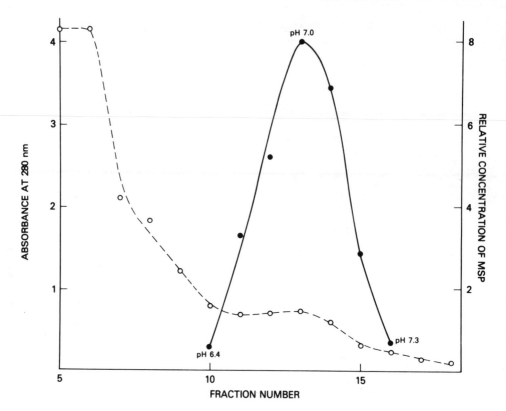

Fig. 5.   Isoelectric focusing of DEAE-cellulose MSP pool.   Dashed
line: A_{280}.   Solid line: relative concentration of MSP, calculated
from bioassay dose-response curves.

immunization and boosting, was purified about 3000x.   However, MSP
is still not purified to homogeneity.   In the MSP region of the
stained gell, 4-5 separate thin bands could be distinguished.

The effects of MSP on the morphology of mouse macrophages are
shown in Fig. 7.   Mouse peritoneal cells in Dulbecco's modified
Eagle medium without fetal calf serum were added to polystyrene
tissue culture wells, with or without MSP.   Within 1-2 hr, the
cells in MSP formed long cytoplasmic processes.   This did not occur in the controls during the same time period.   The percentage
of macrophages with extended cell processes depends on the concentration of the MSP fraction (Fig. 7, upper curve).   An anti-MSP
column, with antibody to PAGE-purified MSP, absorbed out the activity (Fig. 7, lower curve).

We also studied the effect of the MSP fraction on phagocytosis
of erythrocytes coated with the IgG fraction of antibody directed

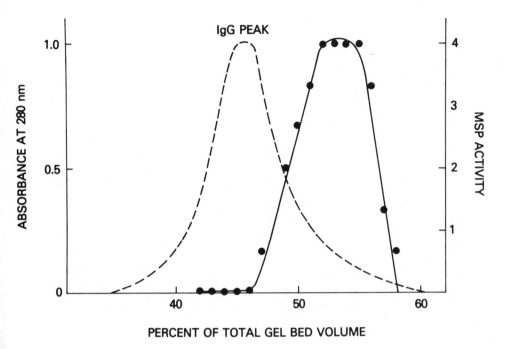

Fig. 6. Elution of isoelectric focusing pool from Sephadex G-200.
Dashed line: A_{280}. Solid line: MSP activity.

against erythrocyte Forssman antigen. The phagocytosis schema is
shown in Fig. 8. Mouse peritoneal cells were added to polystyrene tissue culture wells, allowed to adhere and then washed. MSP
or other reagents were added. At various times thereafter, ^{51}-Cr-
labeled antibody-coated erythrocytes were added. One hr later
erythrocytes bound to macrophage surfaces were lysed with a buffer
that left the macrophage intact. Thus, after washing only the
erythrocytes ingested by macrophages remained in the monolayer.
The cells were then solubilized with SDS and the ^{51}Cr was counted.
Fig. 8 shows the MSP increased phagocytosis of ^{51}CrEA. As in the
experiments on cell process formation, MSP eluted from an anti-MSP
column had no effect, whereas MSP eluted from a control column had
a progressively increasing effect on phagocytosis over the concentration range shown.

    Since MSP caused macrophages to put out long cell processes,
the amount of cell surface available for erythrocyte binding might
be increased. We found that MSP increased the number of ^{51}CrEA
bound to macrophage monolayers. It also increased ingestion of EA,
which was shown by delaying addition of MSP until after EA were
bound. The results are shown in Fig. 9. In the first part of the

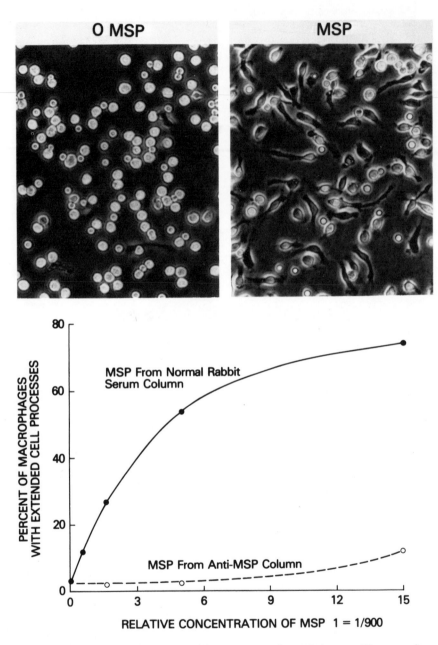

Fig. 7. Effect of MSP on cell process formation. Phase microscopy photographs were taken after 2 hr in culture with or without MSP.

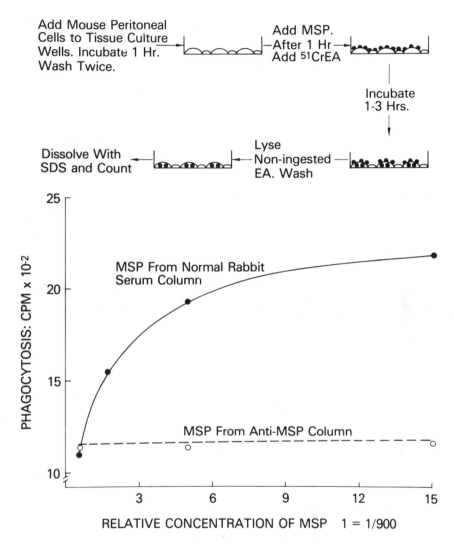

Fig. 8.   Effect of MSP on phagocytosis of [51]CrEA.

experiment, [51]CrEA were added with or without MSP. After an interval of 30 min, unbound erythrocytes were washed away, then the
adherent erythrocytes were lysed and the ^{51}Cr in the lysis fluid.
was counted. The data show that MSP increased the number of bound
EA. In the second part of the experiment, EA were added before
MSP and after an interval of 30 min unbound EA were removed by
washing. MSP was then added to the experimental wells and after
1 hr ingested EA were determined in the usual way. The results
show that MSP also increased ingestion of bound EA.

A. MSP INCREASED THE NUMBER OF EA BOUND TO MACROPHAGES.

MONOLAYER → ^{51}CrEA with → Wash out → Lyse
                or without   non-adherent   non-ingested
                MSP, 30 min   EA   EA and
                                                          Count ^{51}Cr.

                                 0 MSP: 1540 ± 110

                                 MSP: 2380 ± 70

**B. ADDITION OF MSP TO EA-MACROPHAGES, AFTER UNBOUND EA
WERE WASHED AWAY, INCREASED PHAGOCYTOSIS OF BOUND EA.**

MONOLAYER → ^{51}CrEA → Wash out → Incubate → → Count
                without   non-adherent   with or   ingested
                MSP, 30 min   EA   without ^{51}Cr
                                               MSP

                               0 MSP: 220 ± 10

                                 MSP: 430 ± 10

**MSP STIMULATION OF PHAGOCYTOSIS IS DUE BOTH TO INCREASED
BINDING OF EA AND TO INCREASED INGESTION OF BOUND EA.**

Fig. 9. Effect of MSP on ^{51}CrEA binding and phagocytosis.

The experiment outlined in Fig. 10 shows that a 20 min exposure of macrophage monolayers to MSP (third row) caused less stimulation of phagocytosis than a 60 min exposure (second row). Thus it appears that MSP must be in contact with the cells for a period of time for its maximum effect to be manifest.

To summarize our conclusions from this series of experiments, the MSP fraction enhances 3 aspects of macrophage function: chemotaxis, cell process formation and phagocytosis. It is likely that all these effects are mediated by the same protein, since antibody produced in response to the polyacrylamide gel purified fraction abolished all 3 activities. Despite the differences in these 3 macrophage functions, motility or contractile activity are common to all 3. For example, formation of a phagosome and the extension of a cell process both involve translational movement of a portion of the cell. The increasing effect on phagocytosis with time of exposure to MSP suggests that MSP stimulates formation of an intermediate, the concentration of which regulates these motility functions.

Additional insight into the nature of the MSP stimulation pathway may be gained by the use of drugs or inhibitors. As an example, Fig. 11 shows the effect of dithiothreitol (DTT), a potent agent in reducing disulfide bonds. Although DTT had some effect on phagocytosis in the absence of MSP, its more striking

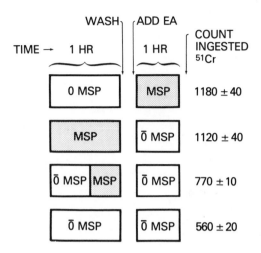

Fig. 10. Time course of MSP action. Four experimental conditions are represented by the 4 rows.

action was elimination of the stimulating effect of MSP on phagocytosis. It also decreased MSP-induced cell process formation. These results suggest that there is a DTT-sensitive step (probably involving a compound with a disulfide bridge) in the MSP stimulation pathway.

All the above experiments were on resident peritoneal macrophages. When we studied the effect of MSP on activated peritoneal macrophages, we obtained the remarkable results shown in Fig. 12. Macrophages were collected by peritoneal lavage of mice previously infected by intraperitoneal inoculation of living BCG. Under these conditions, the non-cytotoxic, peroxidase-negative resident peritoneal macrophage was almost completely replaced by a population of peroxidase-positive macrophages that are cytotoxic to tumor cells. This figure shows that when these macrophages were suspended in tissue culture medium without serum they did not migrate toward chemotactic factor. The addition of purified MSP had no effect. Thus the response to MSP is another aspect of the difference between resident and activated macrophages. Like the resident macrophage, the activated macrophage required a factor or factors from serum to support chemotactic responses and that factor is different from MSP. Fig. 13 shows that whereas human serum is an excellent source of MSP, it is a poor source, compared to FCS, of the stimulus required by BCG-activated macrophages.

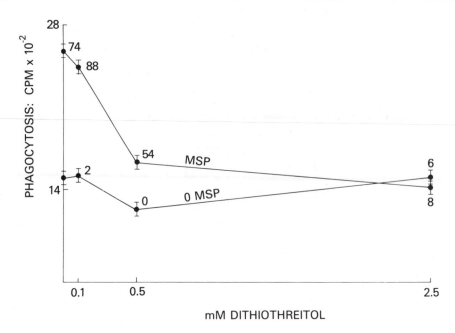

Fig. 11. Effect of dithiothreitol on phagocytosis and cell process formation. Dithiothreitol was added to the cell monolayers and then washed out before addition of MSP and ^{51}CrEA. Numerals at each point on the graph are percentages of macrophages with extended cell processes after 2 hr with or without MSP.

Our increasing knowledge of the complexity of regulation of macrophage function brings to mind 2 extensively studied serum protein systems, complement and blood clotting. Both are designed to respond to critical events in the life of the organism. The need for controls is no more evident than with the blood clotting system, balanced between the dangers of intravascular coagulation and hemorrhage. At the cellular level, the mononuclear phagocyte system is to some extent analogous: at the right time and place a large number of macrophages must appear, capable of a rapid shift to intense metabolic and destructive activity. Inappropriate activation would result in needless production of macrophage-induced damage at the site of cell accumulation.

Since the molecular weight of MSP is 100,000 the steady state concentration in the tissues is probably low. At sites of inflammation with increased capillary permeability, its concentration would rise and approach that of the serum; it could thus affect resident tissue macrophage activity. It should be noted, however, that the role of the resident macrophage in inflammation is unknown. The cells recovered by lavage of the peritoneal cavity of the mouse 18 hr after injection of a stimulus as mild as phosphate-

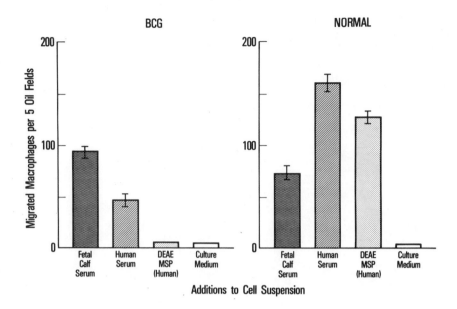

Fig. 12.   Effects of MSP or 12% serum on chemotactic responses of BCG-activated and normal resident peritoneal macrophages.

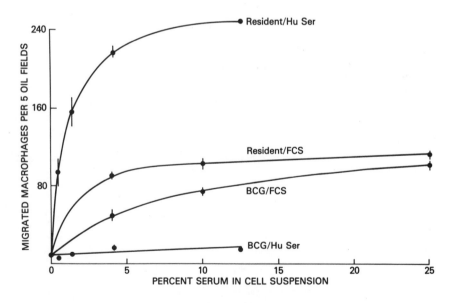

Fig. 13.   Comparison of chemotaxis promoting effects of heat-inactivated human and fetal calf serum on resident and BCG-activated macrophages.

buffered saline are newly arrived peroxidase–positive cells. Have
the residents fled the site, or are they spread out and attached
to peritoneal surfaces, like the MSP–stimulated cells on the polystyrene surface shown in Fig. 7? The controls that determine the
development and function of the activated macrophage appear to be
even more complex. They involve not only the serum factors to
which we have already alluded, but a multi–step activation pathway.

REFERENCES

1. Leonard, E. J., Ruco, L. P. and Meltzer, M. S. Cellular
    Immunol. (1978) In press.
2. Leonard, E. J. and Skeel, A. H. Exp. Cell Res. 102 (1976) 434.
3. Leonard, E. J. and Skeel, A. H. Exp. Cell Res. 114 (1978) 117.
4. Ruco, L. P. and Meltzer, M. S. J. Immunol. 119 (1977) 889.
5. Ruco, L. P. and Meltzer, M. S. J. Immunol. (1978) In press.
6. van Furth, R. (Ed) In: Mononuclear phagocytes in immunity,
    infection and pathology. Blackwell (1975) 1.

BCG-ACTIVATED MACROPHAGES: COMPARISON AS EFFECTORS IN DIRECT
TUMOR-CELL CYTOTOXICITY AND ANTIBODY DEPENDENT CELL-MEDIATED
CYTOTOXICITY

D. O. ADAMS and H. S. KOREN

Department of Pathology and Division of Immunology
Duke University, Durham, North Carolina (USA)

Multiple cellular and humoral elements of the host's immune
system act independently and in concert to destroy tumors (2).
Macrophages, now recognized as an important element in these defenses, destroy foreign cells in at least two circumstances (3).
Macrophages alone directly and selectively lyse neoplastic but
not normal cells if the macrophages are activated (3). We refer
to this as direct tumor-cell cytolysis (DTC). Second, macrophages
lyse a variety of cells when the targets are coated with antibody
(6,7) (antibody dependent cell-mediated cytotoxicity - ADCC). It
is now established that ADCC is mediated by a variety of mononuclear phagocytes including monocytes, resident tissue macrophages
and inflammatory macrophages (6). Immunostimulants such as BCG
can increase the total ADCC activity in tissues such as the spleen
(8,10). It is not known, however, whether activation of macrophages for DTC alters their effectiveness for ADCC. Since these
two effector mechanisms could interact in the inflammatory response
within tumors, we tested the effectiveness of BCG-activated peritoneal inflammatory macrophages in DTC and in ADCC and here report
that macrophages activated for DTC have greatly augmented capacity
for ADCC.

MATERIALS AND METHODS

Macrophages. Peritoneal exudate cells (PEC) were obtained
from C57BL6/J mice. Thioglycolate (TG) stimulated macrophages
were harvested three days after intraperitoneal injection of 1.0
cc of Brewer's thioglycolate broth (Difco Mfg. Co., Detroit, MI).
BCG-activated macrophages were harvested three days after intra-

peritoneal injection of 1×10^8 viable bacilli Calmette-Guerin
(BCG) (Phipps strain, Trudeau Institute, Saranac Lake, N. Y.) into
animals previously immunized intradermally and intraperitoneally
against BCG as described (1).

The cellular composition of the exudates and of their fractions was studied by preparation of smears on a cytocentrifuge
and subsequent staining with Wright's stain.

Separation of macrophages. Separation by adherence to plastic is described below. Separation on columns of G-10 Sephadex
was performed as previously described (5).

Assay for DTC. Direct tumor cell cytotoxicity was assayed as
described (1). Briefly, cytolytic activity was quantified by
co-cultivating purified macrophages with syngeneic fibrosarcoma
targets (MCA1) or syngeneic embryo fibroblasts (MEF) prelabelled
with 3H thymidine. To prelabelled targets in 16 mm wells (linbro Plastics, New Haven, Conn., Catalogue #FB16-24), PEB were
added and washed free of non-adherent leukocytes 4 hr later. The
cultures were incubated for 48 hr in Eagle's MEM containing 10%
heat inactivated fetal calf serum (TCM). The resultant released-
radioactivity in the supernatants (over 95% non-pelletable) and
the total radioactivity per well after digestion in 0.2% SDS
were quantified. All assays were performed in triplicate.

Net cytotoxicity =

$$\frac{\text{Supernatant CPM in wells} - \text{supernatant CPM in wells}}{\text{with macrophages} \qquad \text{with medium along}} \text{ X } 100$$
$$\text{Total radioactivity per well}$$

Assay for ADCC. ADCC was quantified as previously described
(9). In brief, PEC were added to 6 mm round-bottomed microtiter
plates (Linbro Plastics, New Haven, Conn. Catalogue #ISMRC96).
After 2 hr, the filled wells were vigorously washed three times.
To the resultant purified macrophages, 3×10^4 51Cr labelled
TNP-modified chicken erythrocytes (CRC-TNP) were added. Rabbit
anti-TNP at a dilution of 1:500 was added to appropriate wells,
and the microtiter plates incubated for 2 hr at 37 C. The plates
were then spun at 800 g for 5 min and the supernatants harvested
and counted.
Specific lysis =

$$\frac{\text{CPM experimental} - \text{CPM spontaneous release}}{\text{CPM released by hypotonic lysis} - \text{CPM spontaneous release}} \text{ X } 100$$

Spontaneous release from the CRC-TNP ranged between 0.5-5% over
the two hr assays.

RESULTS

Composition of the PEC. The thioglycolate stimulated PEC
were: 75 to 85% macrophages; 4 to 10% small mononuclear cells;
and 12 to 20% polymorphonuclear leukocytes. The BCG-activated
PEC were: 65 to 75% macrophages; 4 to 12% small mononuclear cells;
and 16 to 25% polymorphonuclear leukocytes.

DTC by stimulated and activated macrophages. We compared
macrophages stimulated by TG and activated by BCG. The effectors
were highly purified macrophages (<98%) as determined by morphology, staining for non-specific esterase and phagocytic uptake of
latex beads (1). The activated macrophages extensively lysed the
syngeneic tumor targets in a dose-dependent fashion. Lysis was
selective for the neoplastic targets as syngeneic embryo fibroblasts were not lysed. Stimulated macrophages did not significantly lyse either target (Table I).

Comparison of ADCC in microtiter and macrotiter wells. To
compare the activity of macrophages in ADCC and DTC, we needed
to exclude any possibility that differences were due to variations
in size and geometry of the assay wells. We thus performed the
ADCC assay simultaneously in the microtiter (6 mm) and macrotiter (16 mm) wells in which the ADCC and DTC assays were routinely
performed. Almost identical results were obtained under both
experimental conditions (Table II). Consequently, any difference
between the ADCC and DTC assays did not result from differences
in the assay plates.

Comparison of DTC and ADCC. We next compared the effectiveness of BCG-activated macrophages and TG-stimulated macrophages
in DTC and ADCC. The activated macrophages were consistently
potent effectors of both DTC and ADCC (Table III). The stimulated
macrophages were not effective in DTC but did express modest
activity in ADCC. However, the activated macrophages were consistently much more effective in expressing ADCC than the stimulated. In over 20 experiments, the BCG-activated macrophages
lysed 2 to 7 times (mean of 3.0 times) more targets at a given
dose of PEC than did TG-stimulated macrophages.

Nature of effectors. The above observations were obtained
with macrophages purified by adherence to plastic. To determine
if other methods of separation gave similar results, we employed
adherence to columns of G-10 Sephadex. DTC and ADCC activity of
the G-10 adherent, BCG-activated, peritoneal exudate cells were
considerably enhanced. (Table IV). Concomitantly, the effector
populations were enriched in macrophages. The non-adherent cells
had almost no ADCC activity but did express significant activity
in DTC. The TG-stimulated peritoneal cells were too low in DTC to
test. Their ADCC activity was almost exclusively in the adherent
fraction.

D. O. ADAMS AND H. S. KOREN

TABLE I

Direct Cytotoxicity of BCG-Activated and TG-Stimulated
Macrophages From C37B/6J Mice to Syngeneic Embryo Fibroblasts
and MCA Sarcoma Cells (Net CPM = SEM)

Effectors		Targets
	Released Label (Total % Cytotoxicity)	
#PEC Added X 1.0 X 10^6	Embryo Fibroblasts	MCA-I Sarcoma-Cells
1.0 X BCG-Activated	568 ± 33 (16%)	1561 ± 48 (68%)
.75 BCG-Activated	434 ± 21 (12%)	1509 ± 16 (66%)
.50 BCG-Activated	288 ± 8 (8%)	1400 ± 4 (61%)
.25 BCG-Activated	230 ± 17 (6%)	984 ± 11 (43%)
1.0 TG-Stimulated	302 ± 15 (9%)	190 ± 11 (8%)
Medium Alone	223 + 1 (6%)	50 + 6 (2%
Total CPM/well	3540 + 69	2303 + 49

TABLE II

Effect of Culture Vessel on ADCC by
TG-Stimulated and BCG-Activated Macrophages

	% Specific Lysis (CRC - TNP)							
Effectors	Microtiter[a]				Microtiter[b]			
	5:1	2.5:1	1.25:1	0.6:1	5:1	2.5:1	1.2:1	0.6:1
BCG	47.2	32.0	28.1	19.5	48.7	37.6	27.7	20.2
TG	15.2	8.7	11.3	10.3	9.2	5.0	3.1	3.1

[a]Linbro-96 round bottom wells, 3 x 20^4 targets/well (0.28 cm^2).

[b]Linbro-24 flat bottom wells, 2 x 10^5 targets/well (2.01 cm^2).

TABLE III

ADCC and Direct Tumor Killing by TG-Stimulated
and BCG-Activated Macrophages

Expt. No.	Effector Cells	% Specific Lysis					
		CRC – TNP			MCA – 1		
		10:1	5:1	2.5:1	1.5	1.0	.50[a]
1	TG	13.4	10.2	9.5	NT	6	NT
	BCG	72.6	67.9	47.3	74	73	66
2	TG	9.6	7.6	5.2	NT	1	NT
	BCG	27.9	20.9	12.2	55	55	27
3	TG	18.3	11.1	11.8	NT	2	NT
	BCG	57.1	43.3	33.3	69	69	62

[a]No. PEC 1×10^6 added before adherence

TABLE IV

Localization of Effector Cells
in Adherent and Non-adherent Fractionations of PEC

Effectors	Target	Percent Cytotoxicity	Percent Macrophages
BCG-unfractionated	MCA-I	46	67
BCG-G-10 adherent	MCA-I	81	83
BCG-Plastic adherent	MCA-I	56	98
BCG-G-10 non-adherent	MCA-I	30	10
BCG-unfractionated	CRC-TNP	38	67
BCG-G-10 adherent	CRC-TNP	48	83
BCG-Plastic adherent	CRC-TNP	42	98
BCG-G-10-non-adherent	CRC-TNP	3	10
TG-unfractionated	CRC-TNP	16	83
TG-G-10 adherent	CRC-TNP	15	93
TG-Plastic adherent	CRC-TNP	18	98
TG-G-10-non-adherent	CRC-TNP	2	12

DISCUSSION

We compared BCG-activated and TG-stimulated peritoneal exudate cells in effecting DTC and ADCC. The BCG-activated leukocytes expressed potent DTC and ADCC. Principal activity for both functions resided in the adherent, highly-purified macrophages. Since the non-adherent fraction of resident tissue leukocytes has been reported to have the major activity for ADCC of non-erythroid targets, (6,7), we are currently examining the potency of the BCG-activated macrophages in lysing antibody-coated tumor targets. Significant activity for DTC was expressed by the non-adherent fraction of the BCG-activated inflammatory cells, an intriguing observation in light of augmented natural killing by the leukocytes in such exudates (11). By contrast, TG-stimulated exudates had little lytic potential. They had no appreciable capacity for DTC and less than 1/3 the capacity of the activated macrophages for ADCC. Activity of these cells lay almost exclusively in the adherent macrophages. The development and augmentation of capacity for ADCC in relationship to the maturation and to the inflammatory stimulation and activation of mononuclear phagocytes warrants further study.

Although we observed parallel augmentation of DTC and ATC in BCG-activated macrophages, the two functions are not necessarily synonymous. They differ in mechanisms of target recognition and in persistence after prolonged culture (4). We are currently investigating whether these disparities are attributable to differences in fundamental recognition and effector mechanisms or to differences in sub-population of effector macrophages. The study of cytolytic functions of inflammatory macrophages may provide useful information as to how various inflammatory elements within tumors interact to destroy the neoplasm.

ACKNOWLEDGEMENT

Supported by U.S.P.H.S. Grants Nos. CA16784, CA14235, and CA14236.

REFERENCES

1. Adams, D. O., and Farb, R. M., (1978) submitted for publication.
2. Cerottini, J. C., and Brunner, K. T., Adv. Immunol., 18 (1974) 67.
3. Fink, M. A., Ed., The Macrophage and Neoplasia., Academic Press, New York, (1976).
4. Koren, H. S., Adams, D. O., (1978) manuscript in preparation.
5. Koren, H. S. and Hodes, R. J., Eur. J. Immunol., 7 (1977) 394.

6. Lovchik, J. C. and Hong, R., Prog. Allergy, 22 (1977) 1.
7. Perlmann, P., Clin. Immunobiol., 3 (1976) 107.
8. Pollack, S. B., Cellular Immunol., 29 (1977) 373.
9. Snyderman, R., Pike, M. C., Fischer, D. G. and Koren, H. S.,
    J. Immunol., 119 (1977) 2060.
10. Tagliabue, A., Mantovani, A., Polentarutti, Vecchi, A. and
    Spreafico, F., J. Nat. Cancer Inst., 59 (1977) 1019.
11. Tracey, D. C., Wolfe, S. A., Durdik, J. M. and Henny, C. S.,
    J. Immunol., 119 (1977) 1145.

ACTIVATION OF MACROPHAGES ASSESSED BY IN VIVO AND IN VITRO TESTS

J. M. RHODES and J. BENNEDSEN

Statens Seruminstitut

Copenhagen (DENMARK)

Activated and stimulated macrophages have certain features in common, such as increased vacuolization, spreading on glass and increase in hydrolases (4), but there are certain differences. Thus it has been shown that proteose-peptone (PP) stimulated and BCG activated peritoneal exudate (PE) macrophages from mice had an increased $1-^{14}C$ glucose oxidation in vitro (9), whereas the former cells had a higher digestive capacity than the latter (7). On the other hand, BCG activated macrophages inhibited the intracellular growth of Listeria monocytogenes, whereas PP macrophages did not. PE macrophages obtained from mice injected with a dead bacterial vaccine, TAB, yielded results intermediate between BCG and PP macrophages (1). Based on these results, we define macrophages as activated when they show an enhanced ability to kill facultative intracellular bacteria in vitro when compared with normal PE macrophages.

BCG and TAB immunized mice were found to be resistant to in vivo infection with L. monocytogenes but mice injected with PP were not (8), which is in agreement with the in vitro results that immunization with BCG and TAB activates macrophages. There have also been reports that mice undergoing a graft versus host (GVH) reaction (2) and tumor bearing mice (5) exhibit non-specific resistance towards L. monocytogenes.

A pertinent question was whether other means of immunological activation of macrophages, such as GVH reaction, skin transplantation and tumor cell implantation would yield the same type of in vitro results as those obtained after immunization with BCG and correspondingly, whether the in vitro assays could again be correlated with resistance in vivo towards a challenge with L.

monocytogenes. Since a simpler method for detecting activation of
macrophages was desirable, a staining technique for β-galactosidase was included because according to Dannenberg et al.(3) an
increase in this enzyme might be a marker for immunologically
activated macrophages.

MATERIALS AND METHODS

C3H mice were immunized with 1.5×10^7 viable units BCG intravenously (i. v.) or grafted with full-thickness skin from C3H
or C57Bl mice or injected subcutaneously with cells from primary
mammary tumors arisen spontaneously in C3H mice. F_1 hybrid mice
(C3H/C57Bl) were injected with either parental spleen cells to
induce a GVH reaction or with syngeneic spleen cells. The last
3 groups of mice were treated in 2 ways:

1. Challenge with a virulent strain of L. monocytogenes i. v.
on the following days: skin transplantation (7 and 11 days),
tumor implantation (21 and 56 days) and GVH reaction (18 days).
Resistance towards L. monocytogenes was expressed as survival
times in days after injection of a lethal dose of multiplication
of bacteria in the spleen 24 hr after challenge with a sublethal
dose.

2. PE cells were harvested from mice treated as above on the
specified days and the following in vitro tests were carried out:
(a) $1-^{14}C$ glucose oxidation in monolayers as described by Riss-
gaard et al.(9).
(b) Degradation of ^{125}I-labeled HSA/anti-HSA complexes in cell
suspensions as described by Rhodes et al.(7).
(c) Inhibition of intracellular multiplication of L. monocytogenes
in monolayers as described by Bennedsen et al.(1).
(d) Staining for β-galactosidase using 5-bromo-4-chloro-3-indolyl-
β-D-galactoside as substrate according to the method of Pearson
et al.(6). PE cells from BCG immunized mice were also tested for
the presence of this enzyme.

RESULTS

In vivo. Resistance to in vivo challenge i. v. is shown
in Fig. 1. Resistance is expressed as median survival times in
days and for bacterial multiplication in the spleen as log infection dose x 100/spleen count.

These results show that non-specific resistance towards L.
monocytogenes was induced after injection of parental cells into
F_1 hybrids (GVH) and that injection of syngeneic cells also af-
forded resistance, but this did not reach the same magnitude as

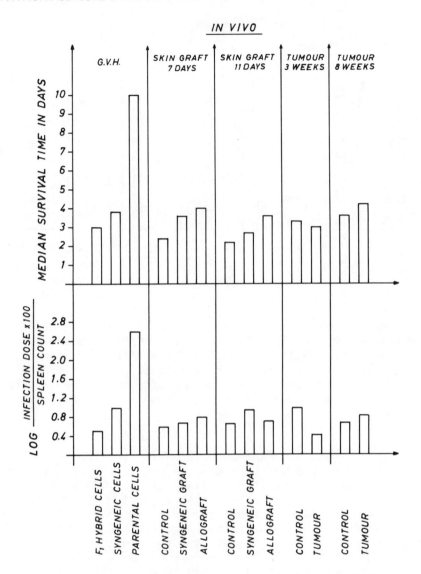

Fig. 1.   In vivo resistance of mice undergoing GVH reaction, skin grafting and tumor cell implantation towards L. monocytogenes after i. v. challenge.   Resistance is expressed as median survival times in days and log injection dose x 100/spleen count 24 hr after challenge.

that seen in the GVH reaction.   Neither skin transplantation nor the injection of tumor cells increased resistance to L. monocytogenes above that of normal values; on the contrary 21 days after injection of tumor cells there was a decrease in resistance.

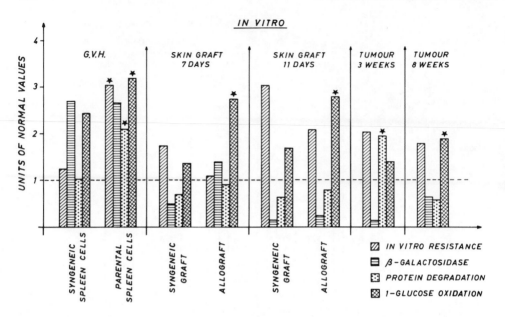

Fig. 2. Results of in vitro functional tests carried out on PE
macrophages harvested from mice undergoing GVH reaction, skin
grafting and tumor cell implantation. Asterisks: GVH denotes
where the values after parental cell injection differ from those
after syngeneic cell injection. Skin graft: where the allograft
differs from the syngeneic graft. Tumor cell implantation: where
PE cells differ from normal PE cells.

In vitro. Fig. 2 illustrates results from the in vitro
tests. All the values are expressed as units of normal values
which are indicated by the broken line. In the GVH reaction, the
asterisks denote values obtained after injection of syngeneic
spleen cells. In the skin graft the asterisk indicates where the
allograft differs from the syngeneic graft. The asterisks in the
tumor group are calculated in relation to normal values.

It is obvious that the injection of parental cells into F_1
hybrids (GVH) enhances the reaction of the PE macrophages in all
the assays. PE macrophages from these mice are thus capable of
enhanced killing of L. monocytogenes, degradation of antigen/anti-
body complexes and $1-^{14}C$ oxidation and they show increased staining for β-galactosidase. Injection of syngeneic cells caused an
increase in $1-^{14}C$ oxidation and the majority of PE macrophages
were stained for β-galactosidase but not as intensely as in the
GVH reaction (not indicated in Fig. 2). $1-^{14}C$ oxidation was also
enhanced after skin transplantation of tumor cells. There was no
evidence that PE cells from mice receiving skin graft or tumor

TABLE I

Reaction for β-galactosidase After
Intravenous Immunization with BCG

Injected With	PE Cells Harvested on Day	Intensity of Reaction	Percent Macrophages Stained
Control	–	$\pm$	26.3
BCG i. v. 1.5 x 10^7 viable units	12	$\pm$	28.2
	13	+++	54.3
	16	++++	42.1
	19	++++	46.3

$\pm$ = weakly positive; + and ++ = positive; +++ and ++++ = intense
reaction

cells could inhibit the growth of L. monocytogenes in vitro and
in only one instance were the PE cells capable of degrading
antigen/antibody complexes to a greater extent than normal cells,
i. e., 3 weeks after injection of tumor cells.

The increase in β-galactosidase after injection of parental
cells (GVH) is of the same order of magnitude as that found after
immunization of mice with BCG i. v. (Table I). Enhanced staining
for β-galactosidase was observed 13 days after the immunization
which persisted up to 19 days. This test has been carried out on
PE macrophages from many different groups of mice injected with
approximately the same dose of BCG and enhanced staining for β-
galactosidase was only seen on day 13.

DISCUSSION

These experiments have shown that, in our hands, injection
of both parental and syngeneic spleen cells into F_1 hybrids gave
rise to non-specific resistance towards L. monocytogenes injected
i. v., although resistance caused by syngeneic cells was not of
the same magnitude as that induced by parental cells.

The in vitro assays were all positive for the GVH reaction
but only 1-^{14}C glucose oxidation was increased after injection of
syngeneic cells. This indicates that PE macrophages from mice injected with syngeneic spleen cells were not activated but were
stimulated, since increase in oxidative metabolism is also a characteristic of stimulated cells. Thus, it appears that in vivo
resistance does not always correspond to the inhibition of growth
of intracellular L. monocytogenes in vitro. This difference
might be more apparent than real because it might be due to a
lack of sensitivity of the in vitro method.

The degree of staining for β-galactosidase in the PE macrophages from mice undergoing a GVH reaction is reminiscent of that
seen after immunization with BCG. PE cells harvested from mice
13 days after infection with BCG i. v. showed an intense reaction
for β-galactosidase and they also inhibited the intracellular
growth of L. monocytogenes in vitro (1). Onset of in vivo resistance towards L. monocytogenes occurs on the 12-13 day after infection and thus resistance coincides with activation of macrophages, as tested in vitro by staining for β-galactosidase.
Dannenberg et al. (3) observed that there was an increase in β-
galactosidase in local BCG lesions in rabbits, and we have now
shown that BCG exerts an effect on systemic macrophages.

If an intense reaction for β-galactosidase, and not the
percentage of cells stained, is considered as a sign of activation then only PE macrophages from mice injected with parental
cells (GVH) are positive by this criterion, whereas those obtained after injection of syngeneic cells would only be denoted
stimulated. This result would then be in agreement with the in
vivo assays and the other in vitro assays.

The results from the skin transplantation are a little difficult to interpret since there was no in vivo resistance, no
inhibition of growth of L. monocytogenes and no degradation of
antigen/antibody complexes, but there was an increase in 1-^{14}C
glucose oxidation and an intense staining for β-galactosidase
in PE macrophages from mice receiving both allograft and syngeneic grafts. It is possible that stimulation (increase in
oxidative metabolism) and increase in β-galactosidase could
occur following post-surgical operation due to the onset of inflammation and this might be an explanation for our results.

North (5) has demonstrated that there is initially decreased
resistance towards L. monocytogenes following injection of tumor
cells, but that resistance is enhanced with tumor progression.
We were able to confirm the former but not the latter result.

We conclude that the GVH reaction can give rise to activated
macrophages as assessed by in vivo and in vitro tests, that tumor

cell implantation does not activate macrophages and that skin grafting, in our hands, does not yield conclusive results. Furthermore, β-galactosidase might be a marker for activated macrophages, but the test requires more intensive investigation.

REFERENCES

1. Bennedsen, J., Riisgaard, S., Rhodes, J. M. and Olesen, L. S. Acta Pathol. Microbiol. Scand. Sect. C 85 (1977) 246.
2. Blanden, R. V. Transplantation 7 (1969) 484.
3. Dannenberg, A. M., Meyer, O. T., Esterly, J. R. and Kambara, T. J. Immunol. 100 (1969) 931.
4. David, J. R. Fed. Proc. Fed. Am. Soc. Exp. Biol. 34 (1975) 1730.
5. North, R. J., Kirstein, D. P. and Tuttle, R. L. J. Exp. Med. 143 (1976) 574.
6. Pearson, B., Wolf, P. L. and Vazques, J. Lab. Invest. 12 (1963) 1249.
7. Rhodes, J. M., Nielsen, G., Olesen Larsen, S., Bennedsen, J. and Riisgaard, S. Acta Pathol. Microbiol. Scand. Sect. C 85 (1977) 239.
8. Rhodes, J. M. and Bennedsen, J. Unpublished observations.
9. Riisgaard, S., Bennedsen, J. and Rhodes, J. M. Acta Pathol. Microbiol. Scand. Sect. C 85 (1977) 233.

A NOVEL BIOLOGICAL FUNCTION OF MACROPHAGES ASSOCIATED WITH ANTIGEN DISCRIMINATION PROPERTIES

R. M. GORCZYNSKI

Ontario Cancer Institute

Toronto, Ontario (CANADA)

There is now unequivocal evidence that the macrophage plays an essential role in the induction of both antibody and cell-mediated immune responses in culture (6, 8, 10). Moreover, there are data suggesting that the mechanism of action of this cell lies both in its ability to release immunostimulatory factors (1, 11) and probably in terms of its capacity to act as an antigen-presentation cell (7, 9). Perhaps the most convincing evidence for the latter lies in the recent work of Resenthal et al.(7) who have shown that the immunogenic determinants of the α-loop or the β-chain of insulin molecules are immunogenic to responding lymphocytes only when presented by macrophages from defined inbred strains of guinea pigs.

An understanding of the complex function of the macrophage in immunological reactions is made yet more difficult by the recent studies which have established the heterogeneity of this pool of cells (3). Thus, by analyzing either the presence/absence of cell surface determinants (Ia, Fc receptors, etc.) or the ability to reconstitute immune responses in macrophage depleted spleen cells evidence has been obtained for many different subsets of biologically active cells of this "accessory cell type". Recent findings from this laboratory have indicated that peritoneal exudate accessory cells taken directly from barrier-mixed mice can be subdivided into various pools responsible for reconstituting antibody or cell-mediated responses in lymphocyte-enriched spleen cell preparations (3). In the data presented below, one activity of these macrophage subpopulations in immune induction, namely that of antigen-presentation, has been examined by assessing the immune response generated from mixtures of antigen-pulsed macrophages and whole spleen cell preparations. In addition, this

particular antigen presentation function has been followed by a
variety of protein and saccharide antigens over a period of 14 days
in tissue culture, with the activity measured being correlated with
other known biological properties of macrophages (ADCC and phagocytosis of antibody-coated sheep erythrocytes, SRBC). The experiments described show that during this type of culture many changes
in the macrophage populations occur. These changes are most well-
defined with reference to the ability of the cells to bind to
lymphocytes and to present to them complex saccharide antigens in
immunogenic form.

MATERIALS AND METHODS

All experimental techniques have been described in detail in
previous publications (3). In essence, the protocol used has been
to obtain peritoneal exudate cells from 10 to 15 normal C3H/He
mice, to sediment these cells at 4 C for 3 hr and to collect them
with differing sedimentation rates (in the range of 4 to 14 mm/hr).
These cells were then cultured in Linbro microtiter plates for
periods of time ranging from 2 hr to 14 days. After the times
described, the medium above the cells was washed off and the cells
pulsed for 1 hr at 37 C with the appropriate antigen (TNP-carrier
conjugates) (10^{-1} µg/ml) or irradiated C3B6F$_1$ stimulator cells
(1×10^5 cells/well). The wells of the plates were washed 3 times
with a total of 300 volumes of PBS and 1.5×10^6 TNP-KLH immune
spleen cells (from mice primed 10 weeks earlier with 100 µg TNP-KLH
in bentonite) added to each well (final culture volume 0.3 ml).
After 5 days either TNP-specific PFC or CTL to 1×10^4 ^{51}Cr-labeled
EL$_4$ targets were assayed in the appropriate fashion. All data
shown subsequently represent the arithmetic mean (S. E. M. for PFC
assays: $\leq 12\%$; for ^{51}Cr assays: $\leq 6\%$) of 3 antigen-pulsed cultures.
Data to the left of each panel represent the response from pulsed
unfractionated cells (•) or unfractionated cells receiving no
antigen (Δ).

In addition, ADCC and phagocytic activities of the macrophage
populations used were studied as described in the legend to Fig. 1.

RESULTS

The data of Fig. 1 show the effect of long term culture in
fetal calf serum-containing medium on the ADCC and phagocytic activity of peritoneal exudate cells. The most striking results,
which were seen consistently, were the rapid fall of ADCC activity
(o-o) in the first 24 hr of culture and the re-emergence of such
activity at later times in fractions (especially large cells, e. g.,
12 to 14 mm/hr sedimentation velocity) that were quite inactive
initially. In contrast, phagocytic activity (o-o) though waning

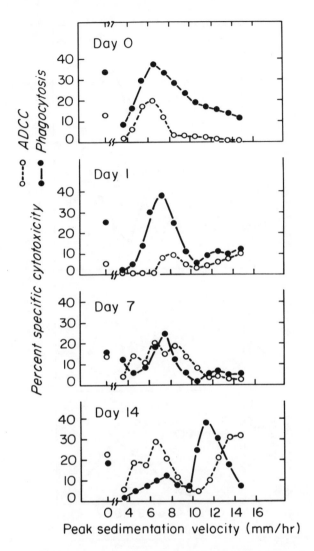

Fig. 1.   Sedimentation velocity (at day of sacrifice) of cultured
peritoneal exudate cells responsible for ADCC (o-o) or phagocytic
activity (●-●) for 1 x 10[6] antibody coated, ^{51}Cr-labeled sheep
erythrocytes.   ADCC was measured from the c. p. m. released into
the medium in 4 hr at 37 C from triplicate cultures of macrophages
and antibody-coated erythrocytes.   Phagocytosis was estimated from
the c. p. m. released by NH$_4$Cl lysis of the washed cells obtained
from the ADCC assay.   All data represent arithmetic means (S. E. M.
≤ 5.0% in all cases) of three determinations.

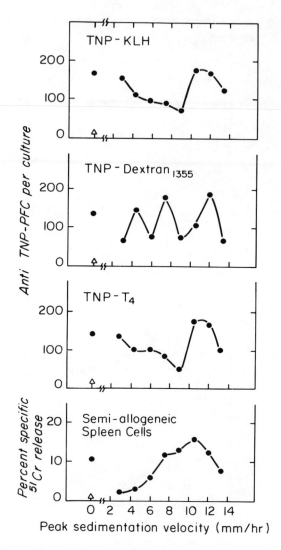

Fig. 2. Ability of freshly harvested, velocity sedimented macrophages to handle different TNP-carrier conjugates for subsequent
antibody formation by B cells or to handle C3B6F$_1$ spleen cells
for induction of cytotoxic cells.

during culture, was always present in cells derived from the 6 to
8 mm/hr peritoneal exudate pool. Again, the marked increase in
activity at 14 days of culture was predominantly due to the appearance of activity in previously inactive larger cells (in this
case 10 to 12 mm/hr cells).

When the ability of freshly harvested macrophages to present
a variety of immunogens (TNP-conjugates or irradiated semi-allogeneic spleen cells) to B/T cells to induce antibody formation or
cytotoxic T lymphocytes (CTL) was compared interesting results
were obtained (Fig. 2). Binding of TNP carbohydrate carrier for
antibody formation (TNP-Dextran$_{1355}$) or binding of a protein-
carbohydrate moiety (in the form of cell-bound MHC determinants)
for induction of CTL were not properties of the same macrophage
cell types. This may in part be explained by the fact that the
antigens concerned were subsequently presented to B or T lymphocytes in these instances. However, binding of TNP-protein conjugates, whether for presentation to T-dependent or T-independent
B lymphocytes, was clearly not a function of the same cell pool
which handled the TNP-carbohydrate antigen (i. e., compare data
for TNP-T$_4$ or TNP-KLH antigen presentation with that for TNP-
Dextran$_{1355}$). These data, which are reported in greater detail
elsewhere (5), suggested a hitherto unexpected role of the macrophage in the discrimination of different classes of carrier molecules.

In order to examine whether the antigen handling capacity of
macrophages (like their phagocytic/ADCC activities) varied upon
long-term culture, the experiments described in Fig. 2 were repeated with macrophage fractions obtained by sedimentation on the
day of sacrifice but pulsed with the different antigen at various
times after culture in fetal calf serum (FCS)-containing medium.
These data are shown as the series of figures from Figs. 3 to 6,
in each of which the ADCC (---) and phagocytic (——) activity of
the cultured cells are graphically depicted for comparison.

It seemed that a good case could be made for the notion that
antigen handling of semi-allogeneic cells for induction of CTL was
a function of cells with demonstrable phagocytic activity, a point
which was perhaps best made by comparing phagocytosis and antigen-
handling of the various fractions at day 14 of culture (lower
panel, Fig. 3). There was no such clear-cut correlation apparent
when presentation of protein antigens (T-dependent, TNP-KLH (X-X),
TNP-CGG (o-o) or T-independent, TNP-T$_4$ (●-●), for antibody formation by B lymphocytes was investigated (Fig. 4). However, one
of the most interesting features of these data, for which only
representative samples are given for the sake of clarity, was that
a given cultured macrophage subpopulation handled each of the
antigens in a similar fashion, which was in no way correlated with
the ability of those cells to handle C3B6F$_1$ spleen cells (Fig. 3).

In marked contradistinction to these latter data were those
shown in Fig. 5, in which are compared the ability of cultured
macrophage subpopulations to present TNP on two different saccharide carriers (TNP-Dextran$_{1355}$ (o-o) or TNP-Levan (●-●) to T-
independent B cells. Not only were the antigen-binding cells in

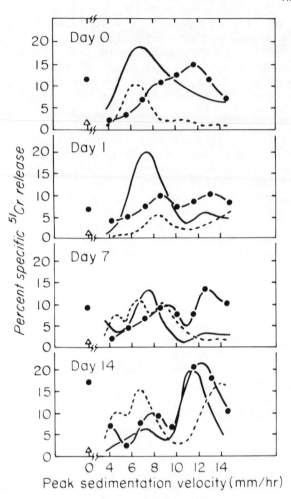

Fig. 3. Comparison of ADCC (---)/phagocytic (——) activity of cultured, velocity sedimented macrophages with their ability to present irradiated semi-allogeneic (C3B6F$_1$) spleen cells (o-o) to C3H spleen cells for a subsequent CML response.

this case quite different from those depicted in Fig. 4 (and seemingly more like those for Fig. 3) but they were also clearly not identical for the two different TNP-conjugates. Once again, as noted in Fig. 2, it seemed that different macrophage subpopulations were able to detect (recognize) subtle differences in carbohydrate structure while allowing perhaps a relatively passive binding (charge mediated) or protein antigens for antigen presentation.

The data of Fig. 6 were obtained from an experiment in which

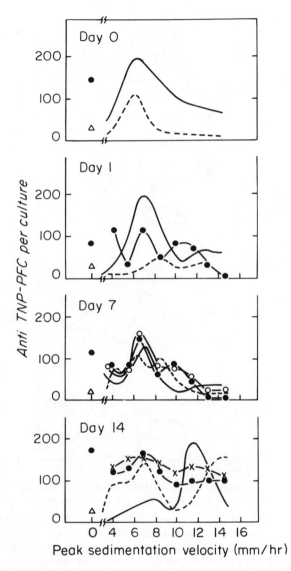

Fig. 4. Comparison of ADCC (---) and phagocytic (——) activity of cultured, veolcity sedimented macrophages with their ability to present TNP-T4 (●-●), TNP-KLH (X-X) or TNP-CGG (o-o) to TNP-KLH primed C3H spleen cells for an anti-TNP-antibody response.

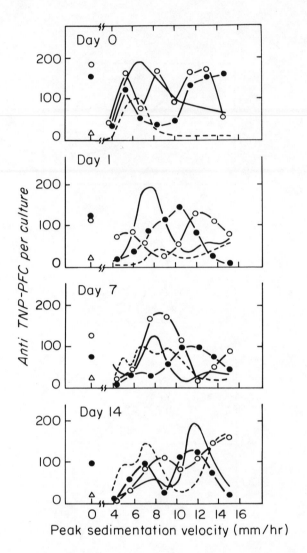

Fig. 5. Comparison of ADCC (---) and phagocytic (——) activity of
cultured velocity-sedimented peritoneal exudate cells with their
ability to present TNP-Levan (•-•) or TNP-Dextran$_{1355}$ (o-o) to TNP-
KLH immune C3H spleen cells for an antibody response to TNP.

the inferred specificity attached to the "recognition" of carbohydrate carrier moieties by the cultured macrophage populations
was investigated. In this case macrophages at various times of
culture were pulsed with 10^{-1} µg/ml TNP-Dextran$_{1355}$ or TNP-Levan
in the presence (right hand panels) or absence (left hand panel)
of an excess of unconjugated Levan (25 µg/ml). It was evident

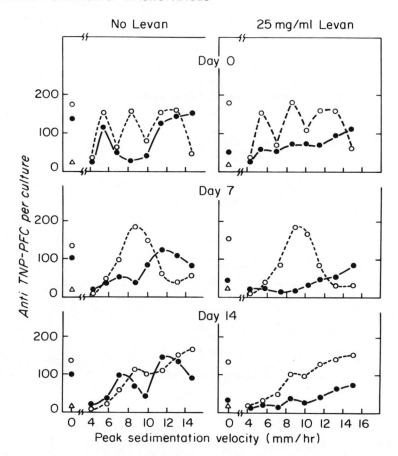

Fig. 6. Ability of unconjugated Levan (25 µg/ml added during a 1 hr antigen pulse) to inhibit the binding (for subsequent antigen presentation to B cells) of TNP-Dextran$_{1355}$ (o-o) or TNP-Levan (•-•) to cultured, velocity sedimented macrophages.

that the unconjugated carrier Levan specifically inhibited the binding of TNP-Levan to all of the relevant antigen-binding cells seen, while having no effect on the capacity of those same cells to bind TNP-Dextran$_{1355}$. In a similar experiment TNP-BSA (but not BSA or KLH) was found to be an ineffective means of inhibiting the ability of cultured cells to bind TNP-KLH in an immunogenic form. Presumably, as suggested, this was indicative of an inhibition of a predominantly charge-mediated binding for this conjugate.

The data shown in Table I indicated that similar heterogeneity in antigen-handling properties of cultures peritoneal exudate

TABLE I

Induction of Antibody or Cytotoxic Responses
in Tumor-Bearer Spleen Cells by Fresh or
Cultured Antigen-Pulsed Macrophages
Derived from Normal or Tumor-Bearer Mice

Source of Peritoneal Exudate Cells	Anti-TNP PFC in Response to:		Percent Cytotoxicity after Challenge with $C3B6F_1$ Cells
	TNP-Dextran$_{1355}$	TNP-KLH	
Normal: Fresh	106 ± 19	168 ± 17	29 ± 1.7
Cultured	129 ± 21	209 ± 25	32 ± 1.6
Tumor-Bearer: Fresh	21 ± 4	160 ± 11	$0.4 \pm .2$
Cultured	131 ± 14	186 ± 19	7.8 ± 1.2

cells could be seen when such cells were taken from tumor-bearer
versus age-matched normal animals. It was apparent from these
studies that the relative inability of freshly prepared unfractionated tumor-bearer peritoneal cells (compared to normal peritoneal cells) to present TNP-Dextran$_{1355}$, TNP-KLH or $C3B6F_1$ antigens to tumor-bearer spleen cells was changed after culture for
48 hr in fetal calf serum containing medium. At such a time the
tumor bearer-derived macrophages were now capable of promoting
immune responses in tumor bearer spleen lymphocytes to a similar
degree to that shown by cultured normal macrophages. The relevance such findings have to the host anti-tumor response remains
to be determined.

In conclusion, it has been shown that long term culture of
peritoneal exudate cells alters the readily detectable (phagocy-
tosis/ADCC) biological activities of those cells in a dramatic
and reproducible fashion. In addition, the differential ability
of subpopulations of peritoneal exudate cells to present a variety of carbohydrate antigens to murine lymphocytes, which is
already evident with freshly prepared peritoneal cells, becomes
even more pronounced with time in culture. With the auxillary
data (to be published elsewhere) (5) showing that this "recognition" capacity of macrophages for carbohydrate antigens is a

temperature dependent function, it is tempting to speculate that the techniques described detect the vestige of a primitive antigen-discrimination property of a primordial defense mechanism. However, alternative explanations in terms of a differential susceptibility of the various responses to suppressor cells (2) (induced perhaps by unique populations of TNP-specific B cells for TNP-Dextran$_{1355}$ and TNP-Levan) (4, 5) remain to be ruled out.

SUMMARY

The ability of fresh or cultured subpopulations of adherent peritoneal exudate cells to perform discrete biological functions commonly associated with macrophages, namely antibody dependent cytotoxicity (ADCC) and phagocytosis, has been compared with the ability of the same cells to present TNP coupled to carbohydrate or protein carriers for a subsequent antibody response, or semi-allogeneic cells for T cell cytotoxic responses, in tissue culture. Data are presented to show that ADCC reactivity rapidly disappears on cultures of peritoneal cells, though phagocytic activity is more persistent throughout the 14 days of culture. When ADCC activity reappeared it was no longer restricted to those fractions active initially. Antigen handling of different TNP-protein conjugates was pronounced throughout the culture period and was not easily explained in terms of the ADCC/phagocytic activity of the macrophage subpopulation concerned. In contrast, however, antigen handling of carbohydrate antigens for presentation to T or B lymphocytes by the different macrophage populations varied during the culture period in fashions which were in some degree correlated with the phagocytic activity of the various cells but were also a function of the antigen under consideration. These data are interpreted in terms of a novel role for the macrophage in discrimination of carbohydrate antigens for presentation to lymphocytes.

ACKNOWLEDGEMENTS

Supported by the Canadian Medical Research Council (Grant No. 5440) and the National Cancer Institute of Canada. The author would like to thank Ms. F. Sochasky and Ms. S. MacRae for their excellent assistance and Dr. G. Price for his many helpful suggestions.

REFERENCES

1. Beller, D. I., Farr, A. G. and Unanue, E. R. Fed. Proc. 37 (1978) 91.
2. Cantor, H. and Boyse, E. A. J. Exp. Med. 141 (1975) 1376.

3. Gorczynski, R. M.   Scand. J. Immunol. 5 (1976) 1031.
4. Gorczynski, R. M.   Immunology 32 (1977) 717.
5. Gorczynski, R. M., MacRae, S. and Jennings, J.   (1978)
    Submitted for publication.
6. Mosier, D. E.   Science 158 (1967) 1573.
7. Rosenthal, A. S., Barcinski, M. A. and Rosenwasser, J. J.
    Fed. Proc. 37 (1978) 791.
8. Shortman, K., Diener, E., Russell, R. P. and Armstrong, W. D.
    J. Exp. Med. 134 (1970) 461.
9. Unanue, E. R.   Adv. Immunol. 15 (1972) 95.
10. Wagner, H., Feldman, M., Boyle, W. and Schroeder, J. W.
    J. Exp. Med. 136 (1972) 331.
11. Waksman, B. H. and Namba, Y.   Cell. Immunol. 21 (1976) 161.

MACROPHAGE-LIKE PROPERTIES OF HUMAN HYALOCYTES

G. BOLTZ-NITULESCU, G. GRABNER and O. FÖRSTER

Institute of General and Experimental Pathology and
Second Department of Ophthalmology, University of
Vienna, Vienna (AUSTRIA)

Hyalocytes from the vitreous body of adult human eyes were
isolated after hyaluronidase treatment. They are mononuclear
cells, adhere to glass and plastic surfaces and stain intensely
for α-naphthylacetate-esterase. They differ from blood monocytes
by lack of inhibition of non-specific esterase staining by NaF.
After incubation with latex particles 50-80% of the cells showed
phagocytosis. The hyalocytes express on their surface receptors
for rabbit IgG and mouse complement. Our results strongly suggest that hyalocytes are mature macrophages.

Hyalocytes are a population of polymorphic cells with vacuoles
and basophilic, PAS-positive granules in vitreous body of the eyes
of mammals and birds (2, 8). They were first described by Hannover
in 1840 (9) and subject of many studies during the last century
(14). Recent publications consider them to be macrophage-like
cells (7). It is unclear, however, if all hyalocytes have common
precursors. There are indications that they are able to proliferate locally (5, 7) but under certain conditions an immigration
of cells or precursors seems to occur (6). These immigrating cells
could be blood monocytes (7) or glial cells (10, 16).

The fact that hyalocytes are mononuclear phagocytes has never
been convincingly demonstrated. We have, therefore, performed
studies to test cells obtained from human autopsy eyes for some
properties commonly ascribed to mononuclear phagocytes: adherence
to glass or plastic surfaces, phagocytosis, presence of surface
receptors for latex-beads, for immunoglobulin G (rabbit IgG) and
for complement (mouse-complement, probably C3) and content of nonspecific esterase in their cytoplasm.

223

MATERIALS AND METHODS

Cell preparations. For this study we used isolated cells
from the vitreous body of adult human eyes. More than 60 autopsy
eyes without pathological changes other than senile cataract were
used. To obtain a sufficient quantity of cells the vitreous body
of up to 6 eyes were pooled. Four to twelve hr post mortem the
eyes were enucleated under sterile conditions, washed with Hanks-
Balanced Salt Solution containing 100 µg/ml gentamicin (Flow
Laboratories, Irvine, Scotland). The bulbs were opened by a
corneal trepanation (66 mm diameter), the ciliary body separated
from the scleral spur with a blunt instrument and the sclera cut
four to six times in meridional direction up to the optic nerve.
In all cases choroid and retina except for the part adhering to
the vitreous base could be easily removed from the cortical gel.
The remaining part and the lens were completely cut away. The
vitreous gel was then incubated in Hepes buffered RPMI 1640 medium
(Flow Laboratories) containing testicular hyaluronidase (Boehring-
er Mannheim, West Germany) 300 µg/ml + gentamicin (100 µg/ml) at
37 C for 15 min. After filtration through a stainless steel sieve,
centrifugation and washing, the cells were resuspended in tissue
culture-medium RPMI 1640 supplemented with 1% L-glutamine (200 mM
Flow Laboratories) and 10% fetal calf serum (FCS) (Flow Laboratories) and gentamicin (100 µg/ml). The cells were cultivated one to
two hr in cell culture plastic Petri dishes (Nunclon, A/S Nucn,
Roskilde, Denmark) in an atmosphere of 95% air and 5% CO_2. After
this time non—adherent cells, dead cells, and other particles
were removed by vigorous shaking and rinsing. The adherent cells
were recovered from the surface of the Petri dishes with a rubber
policeman. In some experiments, cover slips (20 x 20 mm) were
placed into plastic Petri dishes. After cultivation, they were
removed and stained with Giemsa or Diff Quik (differential Wright-
Giemsa staining, Harleco, Merz and Dade, Bern, Switzerland). They
were used for studying or morphological characteristics and phagocytosis properties in light microscopy. The viability of cells
was tested with trypan blue before and after cultivation.

Phagocytosis procedure. The cells were incubated with latex
particles (1.1 µm diameter; Dow Diagnostics, Indianapolis, Indiana)
30-60 min under tissue culture conditions (15). Afterwards the
phagocytosis rate was determined either by phase contrast microscopy on the inverted microscope or after staining by light microscopy.

Non-specific esterase staining. For this histochemical
method we used ∝-napthylacetate (British Drug Houses Ltd.) as a
substrate (13). In addition, experiments with sodium flouride
(1.5 mg/ml) were performed and compared with human blood monocyte
preparations.

Rabbit anti-Forssman antibodies. These were prepared in the
following manner: rabbits were immunized i. v. three times a week
for several weeks with boiled sheep red blood cells (SRBC)-stro-
mata (11). Animals were bled 10 days after the last injection by
cardiac puncture. The antisera were heat-inactivated (56 C/30
min) and stored frozen until use. From these antisera IgG- and
IgM-fractions were separated by ion exchange chromatography on
QAE-Sephadex (Pharmacia, Uppsala, Sweden) equilibrated with 50 mM
ethylenediamineacetate buffer, pH 7.2. Antiserum dialyzed against
this buffer was applied and the protein containing fractions
eluting with starting buffer were collected, concentrated and
dialyzed against phosphate buffered saline, pH 7.2 (PBS). This
preparation contained pure IgG. The IgM was obtained together
with other proteins by further elution using 340 mM Na-acetate,
pH 4.0. The protein containing fractions were pooled, adjusted to
pH 7.2, concentrated and the macroglobulin obtained by gel-
filtration on porous glass beads (4) followed by absorption of
remaining IgG on Protein A-Sepharose (Pharmacia). The IgG and IgM
containing fractions were tested in immunelectrophoresis, SRBC-
agglutination, antiglobulin reaction and mixed agglutination with
IgG-sensitized chicken red blood cells. There was no cross-con-
tamination of the preparations by these criteria. They were not
tested, however, for presence of other immunoglobulin classes.

Demonstration of Fc-receptors. One volume of 2% SRBC was
sensitized with one volume of a non-agglutinating amount of pure
IgG (1:400 dilution of IgG in PBS). The mixture was washed 3
times and resuspended in PBS. One part of 1% IgG-sensitized SRBC
(EA) was added to one part of hyalocytes (2 x 10^6/ml). The mixture was centrifuged in Kahn tubes (3 min, 150xg, room temperature)
and stored at 4 C. On the next day cells were resuspended by
rotating for one min at low speed (22xg), one drop of the cell
suspension was stained with one drop toluidine blue, mounted on a
siliconized glass slide with cover slips and sealed with paraffin
wax. The slides were kept in humidified atmosphere on ice until
counting. For each experiment at least 500 hyalocytes were counted
in a light microscope and the percentage of rosette forming cells
(RFC) was determined. Cells binding 3 or more erythrocytes were
considered as rosettes. Control samples with unsensitized SRBC
were processed in the same manner.

Demonstration of complement receptors. A 2% SRBC suspension
was incubated 30 min at room temperature with an equal volume of
a non-agglutinating dilution of rabbit IgM. Afterwards, the
erythrocytes (EA-IgM) were centrifuged, washed and finally resuspended in PBS. As complement source we used mouse serum diluted 1:5 in complement fixation buffer (Flow Laboratories).
Equal volumes of 1% EA-IgM and of mouse complement were incubated
10 min at 37 C. After washing 0.2 ml of 1% erythrocytes (EAC) was
added to 0.2 ml of hyalocytes (2 x 10^6/ml). The mixture was

centrifuged 3 min, 90xg at 4 C, and kept overnight on ice. RFC
were counted in the same manner as for Fc-receptors. As controls
we used IgM-sensitized erythrocytes without complement for incubation with hyalocytes.

RESULTS

Using the above described methods we were able to isolate a
sufficient quantity of hyalocytes from the vitreous body of human
eyes for our in vitro investigations. However, the number of cells
isolated from one vitreous body of an adult human eye was very low.
In our experiments it was dependent on the time interval between
death and enucleation, and the degree of bacterial contamination
which was frequently observed despite sterile conditions and addition of gentamicin to the medium. After hyaluronidase treatment,
we obtained under optimal conditions between 2-5 x 10^6 cells per
eye. Less cells were isolated in some initial experiments using
hyaluronidase and collagenase or collagenase alone. The cell
viability was different from experiment to experiment with a range
between 30-85%. The cells isolated from the vitreous body adhered
to glass and plastic surfaces. This property was used to purify
them from other cell types, dead cells and cell debris. The adherence was better after treatment with a low dose of hyaluronidase
(300 µg/ml) than after treatment with higher doses (500-1000 µg/ml)
or a combination of hyaluronidase and collagenase. However, a
really good spreading was scarcely observed. For morphological
characterization the native cells were examined by phase contrast
microscopy. On the cover slips adherent hyalocytes were inspected
in light microscopy after Giemsa or Diff Quik staining. More than
90% of cells showed the morphological characteristics of hyalocytes
as described by Balazs et al.(2) and Hamburg (8).

Phagocytosis. Fifty to eighty percent of hyalocytes showed
phagocytosis after incubation with polystyrene-latex beads. The
number of ingested particles exhibited quantitative differences.
Some cells contained just a few, in others the cytoplasm was
stuffed with latex beads. Phagocytosis of bacteria, which occasionally contaminated our preparation, was also observed.

Non-specific esterase staining. Hyalocytes incubated with
α-naphthylacetate showed strong black or dark brown staining
throughout the cytoplasm, which is typical for mononuclear phagocytes. To differentiate hyalocytes from blood monocytes sodium
fluoride was used as inhibitor. An inhibition of staining was
observed for blood monocyte preparations but not for hyalocytes.

Fc-receptors. With the rosette technique we could demonstrate the presence of a receptor for IgG. Between 60-70% of

hyalocytes formed EA-rosettes. In the control samples no binding
of unsensitized erythrocytes (E-rosettes) was observed.

Complement-receptor. About 30% of hyalocytes incubated with
IgM-sensitized SRBC and complement formed EAC-rosettes. No
rosetting was found in control samples using IgM-sensitized erythrocytes (EA-IgM rosettes).

DISCUSSION

Cells in the cortical layer of the vitreous body of mammalian
and avian eyes, termed hyalocytes by Balazs (1), have been frequently thought to be mononuclear phagocytes. Some authors described them as macrophages (2, 7), others as blood monocytes (6)
or microglial cells (10, 16), which have immigrated into the
vitreous. Certainly one has to distinguish between resting or
resident hyalocytes, present in the normal eye, which have the
property of proliferation to mild stimuli (5), and reactive cells
in the vitreous with the appearance and properties of hyalocytes,
which are recently immigrated cells in response to more severe
injuries (6).

The subject of our studies was the population of resting
hyalocytes isolated from normal human autopsy eyes. These cells
had many of the properties of mononuclear phagocytes. They adhered
to plastic surfaces, phagocytized latex-spheres of 1.1 μm diameter
and formed rosettes with IgG (EA)- and with IgM +complement (EAC)-
sensitized sheep erythrocytes.

Previous studies with india ink (8) or saccharated iron oxide
(2) have not beyond any doubt established the phagocytic properties
of these cells. The size of the ingested particles was not reported in these publications and the possibility of having observed
macropinocytosis still exists. The ingestion of 1.1 μm-sized particles, as seen in our experiments definitely identifies this
process as true phagocytosis. The presence of Fc (IgG)-receptors
and complement-receptors on hyalocytes is shown here for the first
time.

ACKNOWLEDGEMENTS

We wish to thank Drs. Erich Neumann and Helmut Rumpold for
their invaluable help in esterase staining and Miss Irene Kothbauer
for her excellent technical assistance.

REFERENCES

1. Balazs, E. A. Acta XVIII Concilium Ophthal. II (1959) 1296.
2. Balazs, E. A., Toth, L. Z. J., Eckl, A. E. and Mitchell, A. P. Exp. Eye Res. 3 (1964) 57.
3. Blakemore, W. F. Acta Neuropath. (Berlin) Suppl. VI (1975) 273.
4. Frisch-Niggemeyer, W., Heinz, F. and Stemberger, H. Immunitat Infektion 2 (1974) 231.
5. Gloor, B. P. Invest. Ophthal. 8 (1969) 633.
6. Gloor, D. P. Mod. Probl. Ophthal. 10 (1972) 41.
7. Gloor, B. P. Graefes Arch. Klin. Exp. Ophthal. 187 (1973) 21.
8. Hamburg, A. Ophthalmologica 138 (1959) 81.
9. Hannover, A. Muller's Arch. (1840) 1.
10. Kolmer, W. von Mollerdorff's Hb. Mikr. Anat. Menschen vol. III/2 (1936) 372.
11. Mayer, M. M. In: Experimental immunochemistry, 2nd edition. (Eds. E. A. Kabat and M. M. Mayer) C. C. Thomas Publishing, Springfield, Ill. (1961) 150.
12. Oehmichen, M. In: Mononuclear phagocytes in immunity, infection and pathology. (Ed. R. van Furth) Blackwell Scientific Publications, Oxford (1975) 223.
13. Schmalzl, F. and Braunsteiner, H. Klin. Wochenschr. 46 (1968) 642.
14. Szirmai, J. A. and Balazs, E. A. A. M. A. Arch. Ophthal. 59 (1958) 34.
15. Winchester, R. J. and Ross, G. In: Manual of clinical immunology (Eds. N. R. Rose and H. Friedman) American Society for Microbiology, Washington (1976) 64.
16. Wolter, J. R. Amer. J. Ophthal. 49 (1960) 1185.

CORRELATION OF B CELL ACQUISITION OF DIFFERENTIATION ANTIGENS

WITH CAPACITY TO INTERACT WITH ALLOGENEIC EFFECT FACTOR (AEF)

J. R. BATTISTO, J. H. FINKE AND B. YEN

Department of Immunology, Research Division, Cleveland
Clinic Foundation
Cleveland, Ohio (USA)

Differentiation and maturation of lymphoid precursor cells to
the stage at which they are competent to synthesize antibody is an
area of active interest. When bone marrow cells, used to reconstitute x-irradiated animals, fully develop this humoral immunological
capacity has been of primary concern (1, 7, 19, 26, 32). Furthermore, descriptions of various membrane markers on mature B cells
have added new dimensions to differentiation studies by providing
pivotal points to correlate with the appearance of functional
competency. Detection of cell surface immunoglobulins (6, 21, 32),
Fc receptors (3, 10, 22, 23), complement receptors (4, 12, 23), Ia
(9, 13), Lyb-3 (5, 15) and Ly-4 (30) antigens are foremost examples
in this regard.

Recently, two differentiation antigens on adult B cells of
CAB/J mice have been delineated as being responsible for stimulating blastogenesis in isogeneic lymphocyte culture (ILC) (14,
24). During differentiation antigen 1 (MDA-1) provokes replication of neonatal thymic cells while MDA-2 triggers blastogenesis
of adult lymph node T cells as well as neonatal thymic cells.
Maturation of these antigens on B cells, obtained from bone marrow (BM) reconstituted, x-irradiated mice, has revealed that MDA-
1 makes its appearance at approximately 12 weeks and MDA-2 at
about 5 weeks (11, 24).

In the present study, we have sought to determine when
splenic B cells of x-irradiated, BM reconstituted mice become
capable of interacting with allogeneic effect factor (AEF) so as
to produce IgM and IgG antibodies. Furthermore, we have sought to
correlate the acquisition of these synthesizing capabilities with
the times of appearance of MDAs on the B cell surface.

METHODS

Animals. Mice used in these experiments were of the CBA/J strain (purchased from Jackson Laboratories, Bar Harbor, Maine) and of the CBA/H strain obtained from Dr. B. Helyer (Case Western Reserve University, Cleveland, Ohio). Neonates from the two strains were derived from matings in our quarters.

Preparation of cell suspensions. Splenic, BM, and neonatal thymic cells were teased in supplemented RPMI-1640 medium (Grand Island Biological Co., Grand Island, N. Y.) and single cell suspensions were obtained following removal of sedimented clumps. Viable cell counts were performed using the trypan blue dye (0.5% solution) exclusion method.

Reconstitution of X-irradiated mice. Syngeneic bone marrow cells (2×10^7) were injected intravenously into mice that had 8 to 24 hr previously been x-irradiated with 950R. At various times after reconstitution, spleens from these mice were used as a source of stimulator cells in both types of ILC and as a source of B cells for in vitro immunizations.

Isogeneic lymphocyte cultures (ILC). ILC were set up using both neonatal thymocytes (Type 1 ILC) and adult lymph node cells (Type 2 ILC) as responders while adult spleen cells served as stimulators. Spleen cells were treated with 25 μg/2×10^6 cells of mitomycin-C (Nutritional Biochemical Co., Cleveland, Ohio) prior to culturing to prevent their replication. Triplicate cultures with an equal number of responder and stimulator cells were placed in microtiter plates at a final concentration of 2.5×10^5 cells/ 0.2 cc and incubated for 96 hr in a humidified 5% CO_2 incubator at 37 C. The medium was RPMI-1640 supplemented with 5% fetal calf serum and 100 units of penicillin plus 100 mcg of streptomycin per cc of medium. Controls consisted of responder or stimulator cells which were cultured alone at twice the number used in mixed cultures. Cultures were pulsed with tritiated thymidine (^{3}HT, Schwarz-Mann Co., Orangeburg, N. Y.) 8 hr before harvesting on a multiple automated sample harvester (MASH II, Microbiological Associates, Walkersville, Maryland). Cells were then placed in a scintillation cocktail (14 grams omnifluor per liter toluene) and the amount of incorporated ^{3}HT was determined on a Mark I counter (Nuclear-Chicago Corp., Des Plaines, Ill.) All results are expressed in counts per min (CPM) and by a stimulation index (S. I.) that is calculated by the following formula:

$$\text{S. I.} = \frac{\text{CPM of experimental cultures}}{\frac{1}{2} \text{ CPM of responder cells alone} + \frac{1}{2} \text{ CPM of stimulator cells alone}}$$

Separation of splenic cells. B cells were separated from spleen cells of mice that had earlier been x-irradiated and reconstituted with BM cells. Crude purification of B cells was accomplished by fractionation on nylon wool columns according to the method of Julius, et al.(17). Thereafter, adherent fractions were treated with anti-Thy 1.2 serum and complement (C) to eliminate the remaining T cells. The anti-Thy 1.2 serum was prepared according to the method of Reif and Allen (25). When used at a dilution of 1:30, 0.4 ml incubated with 2×10^7 thymus cells and 1:12 C (agarose absorbed guinea pig serum) was effective in killing 95% of the cells.

For treatment of nylon wool adherent cells the following conditions were used: 5×10^7 cells in 0.4 ml medium, 0.4 ml antiserum and 0.3 ml C. Killing was assessed by the trypan blue exclusion method. Furthermore, the effectiveness of serological treatment on the adherent cells was assessed by culturing the cells with and without various mitogens. Typically 2.5×10^5 cells with or without mitogen were cultured in triplicate for 72 hr and pulsed with tritiated thymidine (^{3}HT) 8 hr prior to harvesting on a MASH II. Thereafter, incorporated ^{3}HT was read on a Mark I counter. The CPM that resulted when purified B cells were cultured in medium alone were 1415; in Concanavalin A (Miles Laboratories, Kankakee, Ill.) 1936; and in lipopolysaccharide (LPS from E. coli 055:B5, Difco Laboratories, Detroit, Michigan) 6651. These data attest to the fact that the purification of B cells had been effective.

In vitro immunizations. Splenic B cell populations in supplemented minimal essential medium as described by Mishell and Dutton (20) were immunized in Marbrook vessels (Bellco Glass, New Jersey) for 5 days. These cells (2×10^7/ml) were combined with 40 µl of a 1% suspension of washed SRBC at time 0. Allogeneic effect factor (AEF), prepared as described by Hunter and Kettman (16) was added to the dialysis bag (50% of the total volume) at 48 hr, the optimal time for a primary immunization (28).

PFC assay. SRBC-specific PFC of the IgM and IgG classes were detected on day 5 by the method of Cunningham and Szenberg (8). IgM and IgG PFC were determined according to the method of Silver and Winn (29). For further details see Yen and Battisto (34).

RESULTS

Thus far, two types of ILC have been described (14, 24). The first type (Type 1) is that in which neonatal thymocytes respond blastogenically when co-cultured with Mitomycin-C treated adult splenic cells. The second (Type 2, ILC) is that in which lymph node B cells of adult mice replicate in response to adult splenic

TABLE I

Typical Results of Two Types of
Isogeneic Lymphocyte Cultures (ILC)

Responder Cells From:	Stimulator Cells From:[a]	CPM at 72 hr			Assigned Type of ILC
		Exptl.	Backgrnd.[b]	S.I.	
Neonatal thymus	Adult spleen[c]	13,425	424	29.2	1
Neonatal thymus	Adult lymph nodes	3,445	421	8.1	1
Adult lymph nodes	Adult spleen	1,021	306	3.3	2
Adult lymph nodes	Adult lymph nodes	423	350	1.2	-

[a]Treated with mitomycin-C
[b]Sum of responder and stimulator cells grown alone
[c]At least 10 weeks of age

B cells. Typical data generated by the two types of ILC are shown in Table I. When neonatal T cells were stimulated by splenic cells, the stimulation index was 29.2 whereas when they were triggered by lymph nodal cells, the index was 8.1. Adult lymph node cells that were co-cultured with adult spleen cells yielded a stimulation index of 3.3, while adult lymph node cells were unable to cause replication of other lymph node cells.

Since BM cells have been described as being unable to cause replication in either type of ILC (11), a study was initiated to determine when BM cells, used to repopulate x-irradiate mice, would develop the requisite stimulating markers (11). Mice that had been lethally x-irradiated and given 2×10^7 BM cells were sacrificed at intervals so that their splenic cells could be used as a source of stimulator cells for adult lymph node cells and neonatal thymic cells. Spleen cells from normal mice were used as controls. Shown in Table II are the times at which the differentiation antigens that trigger the two types of ILC are acquired by the BM cells. The data given are the percents of the original stimulation indices seen in each of the ILC types. As can be seen, the marker that causes Type 2 ILC (i.e., MDA-2) is only fully detected on BM cells after 5 weeks in an x-rayed splenic environment. That antigen

TABLE II

Acquisition of Murine Differentiation Antigens
(MDA) by BM Cells in Spleens of X-rayed Mice

Weeks Following BM Reconstitution	% of Original Stimulation Index Triggered by MDA's in ILC of:		Type 2
	Type 1		
	MDA 1	MDA 2	MDA 2
0	3.2	22.8	5.7
1	2.4	17.1	14.3
5	11.2	80.0	137.0
9	9.2	65.7	N. D.
12	215.0	N. D.	N. D.

which triggers Type 1 ILC (i.e., MDA-1) is only fully detected on
B cells 12 weeks following BM reconstitution. Furthermore, we
observed that MDA-2 also caused replication of neonatal T cells
in Type 1 ILC.

Next we decided to determine whether B cell function could in
any way be correlated with appearance of MDAs on B cell surfaces.
Accordingly, spleen cells were obtained from mice that had been
x-rayed and reconstituted with BM cells for varying time periods.
The spleen cells were passed through nylon wool columns to re-
cover adherent cells, which were then treated with anti-Thy 1.2
plus complement to eliminate all remaining T cells; the resulting
B cells were put into Marbrook vessels for in vitro immunization
to SRBC. To half of such cultures allogeneic effect factor was
added. As control, splenic B cells from adult, normal animals
were purified and immunized in parallel. The averaged results of
two such experiments are shown in Table III. In keeping with the
observation that SRBC is a T cell dependent antigen our common
experience has been that splenic B cells respond to SRBC with IgM
PFC and few if any IgG PFC. With the addition of AEF at 48 hr
after antigen we routinely have noted a doubling in the IgM PFC
and the appearance of one to three hundred IgG PFC (Table III).
By comparison with the control splenic B cells, those B cells derived from mice reconstituted with BM cells for 3 to 4 weeks showed
a minimal number of IgM PFC (a non-significant number of IgG PFC)

TABLE III

Correlation of B Cell Acquisition of
Differentiation Antigens with Capacity
to Interact with Allogeneic Effect Factor (AEF)

Splenic B Cells[a] from BM Reconstituted, X-rayed Recipients Sacrificed at Week:	AEF Added at 43 hr	SRBC-specific PFC/10^6		
		M	G	Total
Control adult splenic B cells	0	623	0	623
	+	1309	189	1498
3-4	0	87	42	130
	+	98	0	98
6	0	396	0	396
	+	378	7	385
12	0	1099	91	1190
	+	1607	336	1943

[a]Splenic B cells were purified by nylon wool adherence followed by
treatment with anti-Thy 1.2 plus complement, then washed and put
into Marbrook cultures

with or without added AEF. At 6 weeks, however, the number of IgM
PFC had increased by 3 to 4-fold over that value seen at 3 to 4
weeks. Still, no increase in IgM PFC and no appearance of IgG
PFC developed as a consequence of adding AEF. Thus, acquisition
of MDA-2 is not correlated with interaction of B cells with AEF.
Yet at 12 weeks after reconstitution, the B cells showed capacity
to respond to antigen and to AEF with an increase in IgM PFC and
IgG PFC attesting to the fact that they were fully competent.
These data suggest that appearance of MDA-1 on B cells is correlated with the capacity to interact with AEF so as to cause an
increase in IgM PFC as well as IgG PFC.

DISCUSSION

In this study we have shown that as BM cells mature in an x-
irradiated splenic environment and acquire differentiation antigens
1 and 2 they also become capable of interacting with AEF to produce
the maximal number of cells synthesizing antibodies of IgM and IgG

classes. Both of these events occurred at 12 weeks following
reconstitution of the x-irradiated mice with BM cells. By contrast, at 5 to 6 weeks following reconstitution, when such cells
first displayed MDA-2, the cells remained incapable of receipt of
the AEF signal to cause increased numbers of IgM PFC or the appearance of IgG PFC. The increase in the number of IgM-type
plaques seen at 6 weeks after reconstitution over the number observed at 3 to 4 weeks (Table III) could be ascribed simply to
time-dependent clonal expansion.

The fact that acquisition of MDA-1 is so closely correlated
in time with the capacity for cells to be triggered by AEF suggests that MDA-1 may be a receptor for AEF. Still, the fact that
MDA-2 is acquired prior to MDA-1 may also allow it to have some
function in this regard that is not now apparent.

We have already reported that MDA-1 can be made to appear on
BM cells sooner than 12 weeks (i.e., by 4 to 5 weeks). This is
accomplished simply by incorporating splenic T cells along with
BM cells (11). We have not yet completed tests with splenic B
cells that have matured more speedily in the presence of splenic
T cells for their capacity to interact with AEF, but these are
currently in progress.

Others have suggested that the B cell marker designated as
Lyb-3 may serve as a receptor for a T cell signal (5, 15). In
those studies, the antiserum to the Lyb-3 antigen served to enhance the number of IgM and IgG SRBC-specific PFC, and thus
mimicked the T cell signal. Thus, no functional test of whether
Lyb-3 antigen actually interacts with T cell replacing factor or
AEF was performed. Whether Lyb-3 antigen bears any relationship
with MDA-1 remains to be determined.

Another surface moiety that has been described as interdigitating with a T cell signal, T cell replacing factor (TRF),
may be the Fc receptor of B cells (28). Free Fc portions of immunoglobulin molecules have been shown to inhibit the TRF-dependent
anti-SRBC response in nu/nu spleen cell cultures.

We have reported that MDAs are either Ia antigens or they are
closely associated with Ia antigens on B cell membranes based on
studies in which Type 1 ILC was completely inhibited by anti-Ia
serum (11). Recently two types of helper T cells, Ia(-) and Ia(+),
have been described as being involved in the cooperative aspect of
antibody responses (31). Furthermore, AEF has been reported to
possess Ia determinants (2) but indications are that TRF does not
(28), despite the fact that synthesis of TRF, just as AEF, can be
triggered by mixtures of allogeneic cells. Thus, while some aspects
of helper factors remain in a state of flux, speculation about
which factor in our preparation termed AEF interacts with MDA would
be premature.

Many investigators have studied the maturation of BM cells in x-irradiated environments (1, 7, 19, 26, 32). Some have looked at the maturation of antibody synthesizing capacity and have reported that full capability is not acquired by BM in the absence of thymic influences for as long as 60 to 100 days in an x-rayed environment (5). Our observations confirm these results while pointing to a rational explanation for the prolonged delay. What appears to be contradictory to these observations is the finding that mouse BM small lymphocytes contain competent precursors for a primary PFC response to heterologous RBC and trinitrophenyl-coupled RBC (27). The response of such cells in vitro was found dependent on T cooperative factors evoked from irradiated spleen cells and Con A. Many aspects of this study differ from our own and from those of others, thus close comparisons of the data are not possible.

Whether the appearnace of MDAs can in any way be correlated with appearance of precursor cells that eventually synthesize IgM, IgG and IgA is at this point conjectural.

SUMMARY

We have sought to determine whether the acquisition of certain differentiation antigens by B cell precursors in BM could be correlated with capacity of such cells to interact with allogeneic effect factor during primary immunization. The murine differentiation antigens (MDA) are those that are detectable on B cells by two types of isogeneic lymphocyte culture (ILC). MDA-1 is responsible for causing replication of neonatal thymic cells (Type 1 ILC) whereas MDA-2 triggers blastogenesis of adult lymph node T cells (Type 2 ILC) and of neonatal T cells.

Bone marrow cells known to lack both MDAs were used to reconstitute x-irradiated CBA/J mice and splenic cells were removed from these mice at intervals to determine when they became capable of stimulating replication of neonatal T cells in Type 1 ILC and adult lymph node cells in Type 2 ILC. Other portions of such purified splenic B cells were exposed in Marbrook cultures to sheep erythrocytes and allogeneic effect factor.

We found that splenic B cells of mice that had been reconstituted with BM cells for 12 weeks acquired MDA-1 and at the same time became capable of interacting with AEF to product the maximum number of cells synthesizing SRBC-specific IgM and IgG. BM cells that acquired MDA-2 at 5 to 6 weeks following reconstitution were still unable to interact with AEF in this manner. Whether MDA-1 may be a receptor on B cells for AEF and whether MDA-2 may have a contributory function in this regard have been discussed.

REFERENCES

1. Aisenberg, A. C. and Davis, C. J. Exptl. Med. 128 (1968) 1327.
2. Amerding, D., Sachs, D. H. and Katz, D. H. J. Exptl. Med. 140 (1974) 1717.
3. Basten, A., Miller, J. F. A. P., Sprent, J. and Pye, J. J. Exptl. Med. 135 (1972) 610.
4. Bianco, C., Patrick, R. and Nussenzweig, V. J. Exptl. Med. 132 (1970) 702.
5. Cone, R. E., Huber, B., Cantor, H. and Gershon, R. K. J. Immunol. 120 (1978) 1733.
6. Cooper, M. D., Lawton, A. R. and Kincade, P. W. Clin. Exp. Immunol. 11 (1972) 143.
7. Cross, A. M., Leuchars, E. and Miller, J. F. A. P. J. Exptl. Med. 119 (1964) 837.
8. Cunningham, A. J. and Szenberg, A. Immunology 14 (1968) 599.
9. Dickler, H. B., Kubicek, M. T., Arbeit, R. D. and Sharrow, S. O. J. Immunol. 119 (1977) 348.
10. Dickler, H. B. and Kunkel, H. G. J. Exptl. Med. 136 (1972) 191.
11. Finke, J. H. and Battisto, J. R. In: Immuno-aspects of the spleen. (Eds. J. R. Battisto and J. W. Streilein) Elsevier/ North Holland Biomedical Press, Amsterdam, The Netherlands, p. 89 (1976).
12. Gelgand, M. C., Elfenbein, G. J., Frank, M. M. and Paul, W. E. J. Exptl. Med. 139 (1974) 1125.
13. Hammerling, U., Chin, A. F., Abbott, J. and Scheid, M. P. J. Immunol. 115 (1975) 1425.
14. Howe, M. L., Goldstein, A. L. and Battisto, J. R. Proc. Nat. Acad. Sci. 67 (1970) 613.
15. Huber, B., Gershon, R. K. and Cantor, H. J. Exptl. Med. 145 (1977) 10.
16. Hunter, P. and Kettman, J. R. Proc. Natl. Acad. Sci. (USA) 71 (1974) 512.
17. Julius, M., Simpson, E. and Herzenberg, L. A. Eur. J. Immunol. 3 (1973) 645.
18. Lamon, E. W., Andersson, B., Whitten, H. D., Hurst, M. M. and Ghanta, V. J. Immunol. 116 (1976) 1199.
19. Melchers, F. and Andersson, J. In: Cellular selection and regulation of immune response. (Ed. G. M. Edelman) Raven Press, New York, p. 217 (1974).
20. Mishell, R. I. and Dutton, R. W. J. Exptl. Med. 126 (1967) 423.
21. Owen, J. J. T. In: Ontogenesis of lymphocytes in B and T cell in immune recognition. (Eds. F. Loors and G. E. Roelants) John Wiley and Sons, New York, p. 21 (1977).
22. Parakevas, F., Lee, S. T., Orr, K. B. and Israels, L. G. J. Immunol. 108 (1972) 1319.
23. Parish, C. R. Transpl. Rev. 25 (1975) 98.
24. Ponzio, N. M., Finke, J. H. and Battisto, J. R. J. Immunol.

114 (1975) 971.

25. Reif, A. E. and Allen, J. M.   Cancer Res. 26 (1966) 123.
26. Rozing, J., Brons, H. C. and Benner, R.   Cellular Immunol. 29 (1977) 37.
27. Ryser, J. E. and Dutton, R. W.   Immunology 32 (1977) 811.
28. Schimpl, A., Wecker, E., Hubner, L., Hunig, T. H. and Muller, G.   In: Progress in immunology. III.   p. 397 (1977).
29. Silver, D. and Winn, H. J.   J. Immunol. 111 (1973) 1281.
30. Snell, G. G., Cherry, M., McKenzie, I. F. C. and Bailey, D. W. Proc. Natl. Acad. Sci. 70 (1973) 1108.
31. Tada, T., Takemori, K., Okumura, M., Nonokaand, T. and Tokuhisa, T.   J. Exptl. Med. 147 (1978) 446.
32. van Musiwinkel, W. B., van Beek, J. J. and van Soest, P. L. Immunology 29 (1975) 327.
33. Vitetta, E. S., Cambier, V. C., Kettman, J. R., Strober, S., Yuan, D., Zan-bar, I. and Uhr, J. W.   Aust. Acad. Sci. (1977) 65.
34. Yen, B. and Battisto, J. R.   J. Immunol. 119 (1977) 1655.

PARTIAL IMMUNOCHEMICAL CHARACTERIZATION OF HUMAN B-LYMPHOCYTE

DIFFERENTIATION ANTIGEN (BDA-1)

E. W. ADES, P. A. DOUGHERTY, and C. M. BALCH

Cellular Immunobiology Unit, University of Alabama
Birmingham, Alabama (USA)

Antisera prepared for identifying cell surface antigens on human B cells are useful for comparing phenotypic expression of subsets of normal and neoplastic lymphocytes. This type of analysis can be done with greatest precision, however, if the number and nature of the reacting antigens can be identified immunochemically, since it is known that even specific antisera can contain a multiplicity of antibodies (1,3).

We have prepared xenogeneic antisera from monkey spleen B lymphocytes that cross-react with one or more human B-cell differentiation antigens (BDA) using direct immunofluorescence and cytotoxicity assays (4,5). The antigen(s) reacting with anti-BDA was distinct from other known cell surface constituents on human B cells, including surface immunoglobulin (sIg), Fc receptors, complement receptors, and DR (Ia-like) antigens (5). Anti-BDA sera did not react with T lymphocytes or monocytes. In this study, we used immunochemical techniques to further define the number and nature of surface membrane antigens reacting with this specific antiserum.

MATERIALS AND METHODS

Cell sources and preparation. Human B lymphocytes were isolated from peripheral blood of healthy donors by incubation in plastic petri dishes (for removal of adherent monocytes) and E-rosette depletion as previously described (8). Both E-rosette positive and E-rosette negative lymphocyte populations were then washed twice with RPMI 1640 and resuspended at a concentration of 1.5×10^7 cells in 130 µl of phosphate buffered saline pH 7.2

(PBS) and 100 µl of 10^{-5}M potassium-iodide (KI) for iodination.

B lymphoblastoid cell lines (RAJI, SB) and a T lymphoblastoid cell line (MOLT-3) were maintained as suspension cultures in RPMI 1640 supplemented with 10% heat inactivated fetal calf serum (FCS), 0.05 mg/ml gentamicin (Schering Corp., Kenilworth, N. J.) and 0.3 mg/ml glutamine. Viable lymphoblastoid cells were separated over a Ficoll-Hypaque gradient, washed twice RPMI 1640, and resuspended at a concentration of 1.5 x 10^7 cells in 130 µl of PBS and 100 µl of KI. Viability of all cell preparations was greater than 98%.

Anti-B-cell antiserum (anti-BDA). Spleen cells from Rhesus monkeys were teased gently from their stroma and washed twice in Hanks balanced salt solution (HBSS). Erythrocytes were removed either by passage over a Ficoll-Hypaque gradient or by hypotonic lysis. Adherent cells were removed by incubating the cell suspension on a plastic surface for 1 hr at 37 C. Nonadherent cells were diluted to a concentration of 1 x 10^7/ml in HBSS with 10% fetal calf serum (FCS) and incubated with sheep erythrocytes (E) by a standard procedure (2). Nonrosetting cells were separated from rosetting cells by passage over a Ficoll-Hypaque gradient at 400 x G for 40 min at room temperature. B cells (greater than 90% sIg positive) remaining at the interface were collected by aspiration, washed twice with HBSS and injected intravenously (2-4 x 10^7) into three rabbits on days 0 and 14. The immune serum, designated anti-BDA, was collected on day 21, heat inactivated at 56 C for 30 min and stored at -20 C. All data described in these experiments were obtained with immune sera from one rabbit (#574).

Anti-BDA was adsorbed once with human erythrocytes and twice with each of the following: human thymocytes, a cultured T lymphoblastoid cell line (MOLT-4), fetal liver cells, and insolubilized human IgG and IgM. All adsorptions were carried out as previously described (3,4). Preimmunization serum from the same rabbit (#574) was used as a normal rabbit serum (NRS) control. The specificity of this antiserum (anti-BDA) is as described in Table I.

Radioiodination of cell surface proteins. External surface proteins were iodinated with carrier free ^{125}I)-iodide (200 mCi/ml; New England and Nuclear, Boston, MA.) by the lactoperoxidase method (11). To 1.5 x 10^7 cells were added 4 mCi of ^{125}I, 50 µl of lactoperioxidase (2.0 mg/ml) and 20 µl of 0.03% H_2O_2. The cells were vigorously mixed and incubated at 30 C for 5 min; 50 µl of lactoperioxidase and 20 µl of 0.03% H_2O_2 were added again, mixed and incubated. Iodination was performed in 50 ml conical polystyrene centrifuge tubes and the reaction was stopped by the addition of 10 ml of chilled PBS. The cells were centrifuged at 1200 rev/min for 15 min at 4 C and washed twice more with PBS.

TABLE I

Characteristics of Anti-BDA Xenogeneic Antisera on Human Cells

1. FITC-conjugated anti-BDA double-labeled virtually all lymphocytes reactive with RITC-conjugated anti-Ig.
2. No reactivity with T-cells labeled with RITC-conjugated anti-t cell serum.
3. No inhibition of spontaneous E-rossette formation.
4. Unreactive with cultured human fibroblasts, T lymphoblastoid cell lines (MOLT-3, HSB-2), melanoma cell lines and a macrophage cell line (U9340).
5. No immunoprecipitation with human Ig.
6. No blocking of FITC-conjugated anti-BDA reactivity on B lymphocytes by prelabeling cells with unconjugated anti-Ig, anti-DR (Ia-like), or anti-T-cell antisera or with aggregated Ig.
7. Independent surface modulation of BDA and sIg, HLA, B_2-microglobulin or DR antigens by immunofluorescence or lysostrip assays.
8. No reactivity with purified human DR (Ia-like) antigen by a radiolabeled immunoprecipitation technique.
9. No reactivity with acute or chronic myelogenous leukemia cells.
10. Reacts with acute and chronic lymphocytic leukemia cells from a majority of patients, including those with a "pre-B" cell phenotype.

Solubilization of labeled cell-surface proteins. Radioiodinated cells were disrupted in 0.5 ml of 0.5% sodium deoxycholate (DOC), 10 mM Tris-HCl pH 8.2 with 100 µl of 0.1 M phenylmethyl-sulphanylfluoride (PMSF) for 30 min on ice with vigorous agitation. After incubation the lysate was centrifuged at 15,000 rev/min at 4 C for 15 min and the supernatant retained.

Immunoprecipitation of B-cell antigens with specific antiserum. Radioiodinated cell-surface protein was isolated by co-precipitation with anti-BDA and formalin-fixed Staphylococcus aureus Cowan strain I (SOA) (9). Controls included co-precipitation of a radioiodinated human T lymphoblastoid cell line (MOLT-3) and E-rosette positive T-cells using either anti-BDA serum or NRS. Also, a B cell line was examined with NRS.

Conditions for co-precipitation were optimized with anti-BDA and SPA such that more than 90% of the anti-BDA was precipitated. Generally, 100 µl of radioactive cell-surface protein was mixed with 15 µl of anti-BDA for 30 min at 4 C with constant shaking in a 30 ml round-bottom tube. 0.8 ml of a 10% (v/v) solution of SPA was then added for an additional 30 min at 4 C. The co-precipitation mixture was then centrifuged at 4,000 rev/min for 15 min at 4 C. The precipitate was washed with solubilizing media twice more.

Antigen separation by slab electrophoresis in polyacrylamide gels. Specific co-precipitates of radioiodinated cell-surface proteins were resolved on 5-10% gradient sodium dodecyl sulfate-polyacrylamide slab gel electrophoresis (SDS-PAGE) in a discontinuous buffer system by the method of Laemmli (10). Samples were prepared for electrophoresis by dissolving precipitates in 100 µl of sample dilution buffer containing 10% (v/v) glycerol-2% (v/v) mercaptoethanol-3% (w/v) SDS in 0.125 M-Tris-Hcl, pH 6.8. The samples were heated for 3 min in a boiling water bath or at 56 C for 10 min. Samples to be subjected to electrophoresis without reduction were dissolved in a similar buffer minus the mercapto-ethanol. The gels were sliced into 85-95 fractions and counted for radioactivity in plastic tubes with the Beckman Biogamma counter. Molecular weight (M.W.) markers were run internally with each gel. Mobilities (F_f) are expressed as distance migrated relative to that of a Bromophenol Blue dye marker.

RESULTS

Radiolabeled membrane proteins were immunoprecipitated from DOC solubilized cell extracts of paired cultured B and T lympho-blastoid cell lines using rabbit anti-BDA serum. SDS-PAGE of the precipitates from the B cell line (SB) gave three peaks of radio-activity with molecular weights of 65,000, 17,000 and 12,000 daltons (Fig. 1). The 17,000 dalton peak was present on the paired T cell line (HSB-2) while both the 17,000 and 12,000 dalton peaks were present on another T cell line (MOLT-3). The 65,000 dalton peak was obtained with or without reduction using 2-mercapto-ethanol or by heating the samples to 100 C.

PAGE profile analysis of precipitates from enriched preparations of normal blood B and T lymphocytes gave similar results. Labeled proteins precipitated by anti-BDA serum from enriched B cells (E^-, sIg^+) had three peaks (p65, p17, p12) corresponding with those identified on B-lymphoblastoid cell line (SB), while precipitates from enriched T cells (E^+, sIg^-) did not possess the p65 antigenic peak (Fig. 2). The pre-immune normal rabbit serum also precipitated two lower molecular weight peaks (p17, p12) corresponding to those identified with anti-BDA serum.

Immunodepletion experiments were then performed to determine if the p17 and p12 peaks reacting with NRS and anti-BDA serum

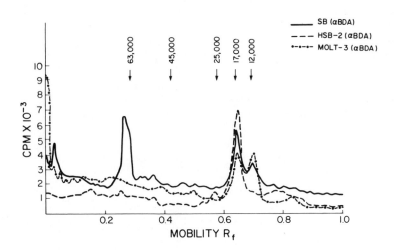

Fig. 1.   SDS-PAGE gel profiles of cultured lymphoblastoid cell lines demonstrating a 65,000 dalton peak on SB cells.

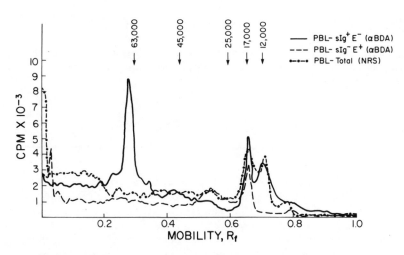

Fig. 2.   SDS-PAGE gel profiles of blood lymphocyte subpopulations.   A 65,000 dalton peak was identified on enriched B cells.

were similar. Solubilized SB cell membranes were first precipitated with NRS and SPA. After the precipitated antigens had been cleared from the solution by centrifugation (4000 rev/min for 15 min), the remaining soluble proteins were precipitated with anti-BDA and SPA. Only the p65 peak was present when this second precipitate was analyzed on PAGE gels (Fig. 3). Anti-B_2-microglobulin (obtained from Dr. Ralph Reisfeld, Scripps Clinic and Research Foundation, La Jolla, CA) also failed to precipitate any cell membrane constituents corresponding to the 65,000 dalton peak precipitated by anti-BDA (data not shown).

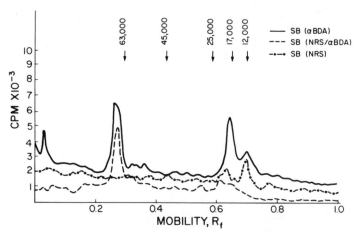

Fig. 3. Immunodepletion experiments demonstrating that NRS removes the lower molecular weight peaks without altering the 65,000 dalton peak.

DISCUSSION

A B cell differentiation antigen with a molecular weight of 65,000 daltons was identified using anti-BDA xenogeneic antiserum. We have designated this antigen as BDA-1. The two lower molecular weight peaks (17,000 and 12,000 daltons) are probably nonspecific antigens since they were recognized by anti-BDA on both T and B cell sources and because the preimmunization normal rabbit serum reacted with the same two peaks. BDA-1 does not appear to be associated with B_2-microglobulin and does not appear to be comprised of subunits held together by disulfide bonds since its migration profile on SDS-PAGE gels was not appreciably altered by 2-mercaptoethanol.

Other investigators have identified antigen peaks with molecular weights in the range of 55,000 to 70,000 daltons from papain or detergent solubilized lymphocyte membranes (7,12-14). It has been postulated that this protein represents a dimer of DR antigen that dissociates into a bimolecular complex when heated to 100 C (13,14) or is solubilized in deoxycholate (7,12). In contrast to these findings with putative DR antigens, the BDA-1 antigen identified in this study was not dissociated either by heating to 100 C or by detergent solubilization. Furthermore, preliminary immunodepletion experiments using anti-DR antisera (obtained from Ferrone, Scripps Clinic and Research Foundation, La Jolla, CA) has indicated that BDA-1 is antigenically distinct from the bimolecular complex (p28,35) characteristic of DR antigen (unpublished observation).

These immunochemical observations corroborate previous studies (5) comparing BDA and DR antigens using immunofluorescence and cytotoxicity assays (Table I). Anti-BDA failed to react with human DR antigens as detected by either alloantisera or xenoantisera in blocking or in lysostrip experiments. In the latter assay, removal of BDA surface antigens by modulation techniques (6) did not alter susceptibility of target cells to complement-mediated lysis by subsequent treatment with anti-DR antiserum and vice versa. By immunofluorescence assays, BDA expression was restricted to normal B lymphocytes and some lymphocytic leukemia cells, whereas DR antigen has a broader representation, being found on normal monocytes and on some myelogenous leukemia cells as well. Finally, anti-BDA did not precipitate immunochemically purified DR antigen in a radioimmunoprecipitation assay (Dr. Peter Cresswell, Duke Medical Center, Durham, N. C., personal communication).

BDA-1 antigen thus appears to be a unique differentiation antigen expressed on human B lymphocytes that is distinct from DR antigen and other known B cell membrane surface constituents.

ACKNOWLEDGEMENTS

This work was supported by grants from the Medical Research Service of the Veteran's Administration and from the National Institute of Health (CA 13148, CA 16673). Dr. Ades is recipient of a Special Fellowship from the Leukemia Society of America and Dr. Balch is recipient of a Faculty Fellowship in Oncology from the American Cancer Society. We wish to thank Barbara Yarber, ART, for her skillful typing.

REFERENCES

1. Ades, E. W., Bukacek, A., Zwerner, R., Dougherty, P. A. and Balch, C. M., J. Immunol. (1978) in press.
2. Ades, E. W., Dougherty, P. A., Shore, S. L., and Balch, C. M., (1978) submitted for publication.
3. Balch, C. M., Dougherty, P. A., Dagg, M. K., Diethelm, A. G. and Lawton, A. R., Clin. Immunol. and Immunopath. 8 (1977) 448.
4. Balch, C. M., Dougherty, P. A., and Vogler, L. B., J. Surg. Res. 22 (1977) 636.
5. Balch, C. M., Dougherty, P. A., Vogler, L. B., Ades, E. W. and Ferrone, S., (1978) submitted for publication.
6. Bernoco, D., Cullen, S., Scudeller, G., Trinchieri, G. and Ceppelleni, R., In: Histocompatibility Testing. (Eds. J. Dausset and J. Colambani), Munksgaard, Copenhagen, (1973) 527.
7. Billing, R. J., Safani, M. and Patterson, P., J. Immunol. 117 (1976) 1589.
8. Dougherty, P. A., Ades, E. W., and Balch, C. M., (1978) submitted for publication.
9. Kessler, S. W., J. Immunol. 117 (1976) 1482.
10. Laemmli, V. K., Nature (London) 227 (1970) 680.
11. Marchalonis, J. J., Cone, J. J., and Santer, V., Biochem. J. 124 (1971) 1589.
12. Snary, D., Barnstable, C. J., Bodmer, W. F., Goodfellow, P. N., and Crumpton, M. J., Scand. J. Immunol. 6 (1977) 439.
13. Springer, T. A., Kaufman, J. F., Terhost, C., and Strominger, J. L., Nature, 268 (1977) 213.
14. Winchester, R. J., Rosa, G. D., Jarowski, C. I., Wang, C. Y., Halper, J., and Broxmeyer, H. E., Proc. Natl. Acad. Sci. 74 (1977) 4012.

THE EFFECT OF XENOANTISERA ON T-LYMPHOCYTE FUNCTIONS IN THE

ABSENCE OF COMPLEMENT

R. RABINOWITZ, R. LASKOV and M. SCHLESINGER

Department of Experimental Medicine and Cancer Research
The Hebrew University-Hadassah Medical School
Jerusalem, (Israel)

Alloantigenic markers have been useful for the delineation of subpopulations of murine T lymphocytes (26,27). The Ly-1, Ly-2, Ly-3 and Ly-5 antigens were shown to be present on thymus cells as well as on peripheral T lymphocytes, while the Ly-6 alloantigen system seems to be expressed exclusively on peripheral T cells (16). The differential expression of the Ly-1, Ly-2, and Ly-3 antigens on subsets of T lymphocytes has led to the identification of three subpopulations of T cells (4,26,27). Cytotoxic T cells and suppressor T cells possess the Ly-2, 3 antigens, while T cells containing the Ly-1 antigen, function as helper cells. Cells possessing the Ly-1, Ly-2 and Ly-3 antigens seem to be precursors of Ly-1 and Ly-2,3 cells and act as helper-amplifiers and as suppressor-amplifiers. Subsets of T cells could also be identified by quantitative differences in the expression of Thy-1 antigenicity (21,24.28).

Relatively little is known on the relationship between cell surface alloantigens and functional receptors. Antisera to H-2 antigens have been shown to inhibit antigen binding ty T cells (10). Anti-Ia sera seem to bind to Fc receptors on T cells (29) and to block MLR-stimulating antigens (17). However, alloantibodies specific for T cell surface alloantigens, such as Thy-1 and Ly alloantibodies, were not found to exert any consistent effect on T cell functions in the absence of complement (25).

In view of the limited information available on the interaction of alloantisera with functional T cell receptors, attention has been given to the use of xenoantisera against T cell surface constituents (20,30). Xenoantisera against mouse immunoglobulins

have been reported to partially inhibit antigen binding by T cells
(10,11,22), but failed to exert any effect on MLR (1) and on the
cytotoxic activity of effector T cells (8,31). Kimura provided
evidence that xenoantisera prepared against effector T-lymphocytes
may block their cytotoxic activity (12).

In previous studies we characterized the specificity of xenoantisera raised by immunization of rabbits with various murine
lymphoid cells (13,20). The aim of the present study was to determine whether any of the xenoantisera tested contain antibodies
specific for T cell receptors. Accordingly, mouse lymphoid cells
were exposed to various xenoantisera in the absence of C' and
tested for their capacity to carry out various T cell functions.

MATERIALS AND METHODS

Mice and tumors. Mice aged 8-12 weeks of the inbred strains
AKR/J and BALB/c were used as donors of lymphoid cells. A cloned
cell line of the MPC-11 myeloma producing IgG$_2$b (14) was kept by
s.c. transfers in BALB/c mice. The lymphosarcoma 6C3HED (6) and
a C3H-B cell lymphoma (38C-13) (2) kindly provided by Dr. J.
Haimovich and Dr. N. Haran Ghera were maintained by s.c. transfer
in C3H mice. The EL-4 leukemia (9) was carried as ascites tumors
in C57BL/6 mice.

Antisera. Xenoantisera were elicited as described previously
(13,20) by immunizing rabbits at weekly intervals. Rabbits were
immunized by injections of either BALB/c thymus cell suspensions
to elicit rabbit anti-thymus serum (RAT), or boiled thymus homogenates to elicit the production of rabbit anti-boiled thymus
serum (RABT). Rabbit antibrain serum (RABR) was raised by injections of BALB/c brain homogenate, while rabbit anti-bone-marrow
serum (RAB) was elicited by injections of BALB/c bone-marrow cell
suspensions in PBS.

The immunized rabbits were bled from the ear-vein after the
last challenge. All rabbit sera were heat inactivated for 30 min
at 56 C and kept at -20 C until use.

Absorptions. Unless otherwise indicated, normal and immune
rabbit sera were absorbed with washed, packed BALB/c liver and
kidney homogenates at 1:1 volume ratio of serum to absorbent
tissue. In some experiments, following absorption with liver and
kidney, rabbit antithymus serum and rabbit anti-boiled thymus serum
were absorbed with various tissues at a 1:1 V/V ratio. The absorbent tissues were washed with cold RPMI-1640 medium (GIBCO, Grand
Island, N. Y.) at 15 x g until clear supernates were obtained.
Rabbit sera were added to the washed, packed tissue homogenates.
The absorption mixtures were kept for 1 hr at 4 C, mixed occasion-

ally, centrifuged at 1500 x g for 10 min, and the sera in the
supernates were collected.

Mixed lymphocyte reactions (MLF) and lectin stimulation.
Mixed lymphocyte cultures and lectin stimulation experiments were
performed with suspensions of peripheral and mesenteric lymph-
node cells, as described previously (21).

Lymphocyte-mediated cytotoxicity (CML). The CML assay was
performed with minor modifications according to the method of Berke
et al. (3). The peritoneal exudates were harvested from BALB/c
mice 14 days after the i.p. injection of 20 x 10^6 EL-4 tumor cells.
Purified peritoneal exudate lymphocytes (PEL) were obtained by
incubating the cells for 30 min on plastic petri dishes and passage
of the non-adherent cells through a nylon wool column. Mixtures
of PEL and ^{51}Cr labeled EL-4 target cells were incubated with
rocking in 35 mm plastic petri dishes at 37 C in a humidified
atmosphere containing 5% CO_2. Each mixture contained 1 x 10^6 PEL
and 5 x 10^4 ^{51}Cr labeled EL-4 cells in 1 ml RPMI-1640 supplemented
with 10% heat-inactivated FCS. Control cultures contained labeled
tumor cells in the absence of PEL. At the end of 2 hr incubation
1 ml of cold PBS was added to each mixture and the mixtures were
transferred to plastic tubes (Packard). The tubes were centrifuged
at 2,500 x g for 5 min, and 1.0 ml aliquots of the supernates were
collected. The supernates as well as the target cell suspensions
remaining in the original tubes were counted in a gamma spectrometer
(Packard).

Exposure of cells to antisera. In order to assay the effect
of heat-inactivated xenoantisera on the MLR and the response of
lymph-node cells to lectins, 12 x 10^6 lymphocytes in a final volume
of 1.0 ml were exposed to 0.25 ml of various dilutions of either
xenoantisera or normal rabbit serum (NRS) for 60 min at 37 C. In
most experiments at the end of the incubation period the antiserum
was not removed but fresh medium was added so as to adjust the
suspensions to the appropriate cell concentration.

The effect of antisera on CML was assayed by incubating
either PEL (2.5 x 10^6) cells/ml per test tube) or labeled tumor
cells (7.5 x 10^6) cells/ml per test tube) with 0.2 ml of various
dilutions of antisera for 60 min at 37 C. Antiserum-treated cells
were washed once and resuspended again to the appropriate concentration. The inhibitory effect of the antisera was calculated by
comparing the activity of antiserum-treated cells with that of
cells exposed to NRS serum, following deduction of background
values as described previously (21,24).

RESULTS

The effect of xenoantisera on mixed lymphocyte reactions.
Rabbit anti-brain serum (RABR). Prolonged exposure of lymph-node
cells to heat-inactivated RABR markedly increased the background
proliferation as compared with that of cells exposed to NRS (Fig.
1). RABR treatment also increased the thymidine incorporation of
cells involved in MLR as compared with NRS-treated cells, although
the augmentation of the MLR was less pronounced than that of background proliferation (Fig. 1).

Rabbit anti-boiled thymus serum (RABT). RABT, which like
RABR contains a high concentration of heterologous Thy-1 antibodies,
had the opposite effect of RABR. It caused a marked decrease of
the background proliferation and inhibited the MLR to an even
greater extent (Fig. 2). Absorption of RABT with spleen, thymus,
or bone marrow cells completely eliminated the inhibitory effect
of the serum on MLR, while absorption with brain only partially
reduced the inhibitory activity (not shown).

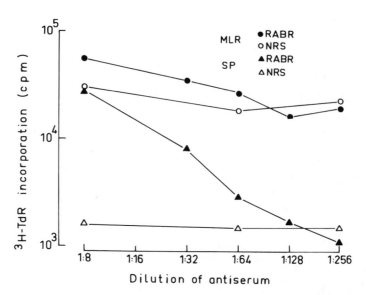

Fig. 1. The effect of rabbit anti-brain serum on the proliferation of BALB/c lymph-node cells. The incorporation of ^{3}H-thymidine
was determined in BALB/c lymph-node cells cultured either in the
presence of mitomycin-C treated AKR/J lymph-node cells (▲) or in
the absence of allogeneic stimuli (Δ). Responder cells treated
with rabbit anti-brain serum (●). Responder cells treated with
normal rabbit serum (o).

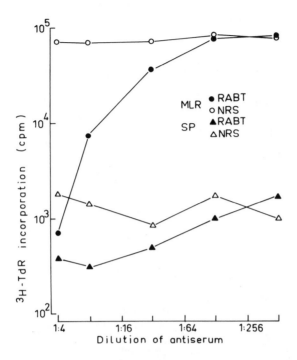

Fig. 2.   The effect of rabbit anti-boiled thymus serum on the proliferation of BALB/c lymph-node cells.   BALB/c lymph-node cells
cultured either in the presence of mitomycin-C treated AKR/J
lymph-node cells (▲) or in the absence of allogeneic stimuli (Δ).
Responder cells exposed to antiserum (●).   Responder cells exposed
to normal rabbit serum (o).

    Rabbit anti-thymus serum (RAT).   The addition of RAT strik-
ingly increased the background proliferation of lymph-node cells.
In the absence of allogeneic stimuli the thymidine incorporation
into lymph-node cells exposed to high concentrations of RAT was
higher than that into NRS-treated cells (Fig. 3).   High concentrations of RAT regularly inhibited the MLR (Fig. 3).   The stimulatory effect of RAT on background proliferation could be eliminated
by absorption with brain.   High concentrations of RAT absorbed
with brain inhibited the MLR much more effectively than unabsorbed
sera (Fig. 4).

    In order to characterize the antigen responsible for the in-
hibitory effect of RAT on MLR the serum was absorbed with a
variety of tissues and the residual inhibitory activity on MLR

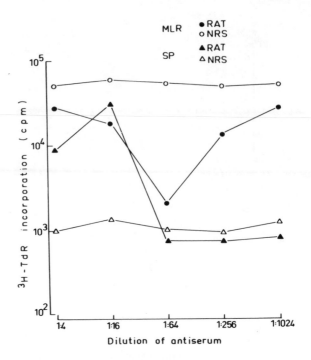

Fig. 3.   The effect of rabbit anti-thymus serum on the proliferation of BALB/c lymph-node cells.   (Symbols as in Fig. 2).

was determined.   The inhibitory activity of RAT, elicited by
immunization with BALB/c thymus cells, could be readily eliminated
by absorption with thymus cells from either BALB/c or AKR/J mice.
Absorption with either spleen cells or bone marrow cells caused a
partial reduction of the inhibitory activity of RAT (Table I).   A
number of tumors were tested for their absorptive capacity.   The
C3H B-lymphoma tested showed clear absorptive capacity.   EL-4 and
6C3HED showed a weak absorptive capacity, while MPC-11 myeloma
cells showed no absorptive capacity whatsoever.

Rabbit anti-bone marrow serum (RAB).   Exposure of lymphocytes
to RAB absorbed with brain inhibited the MLR (Fig. 5).   Following
absorption with liver and kidney RAB failed to exert any inhibitory
effect on the MLR (Fig. 5).   The effect of RAB following various
absorptions on the background proliferation paralleled its effect
on MLR.

The effect of xenoantisera on the response to lectins.   Exposure to BALB/c lymph-node cells to either RAT or RABT almost

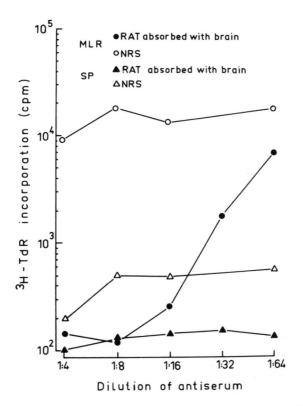

Fig. 4. The effect of rabbit anti-thymus serum absorbed with brain on the proliferation of BALB/c lymph-node cells (Symbols as in Fig. 2).

completely inhibited their mitotic response to either phytohemag-glutinin (PHA) or concanavalin A (Con A), while RABR had no such effect (Table II). Absorption experiments indicate that neither brain nor bone marrow cells removed the inhibitory effect of RAT (Table III). Absorption with two T-lymphomas, EL-4 and 6C3HED, completely removed the inhibitory effect of the serum while ab-sorption with myeloma (MPC-11) was without effect.

The effect of xenoantisera on cell mediated lympholysis. Ex-posure of sensitized peritoneal lymphocytes to either RAT or RABT completely prevented their cytotoxic activity on EL-4 target cells. RABR and RAB had no such inhibitory effect (Table II).

TABLE I

The Effect of Various Absorptions on the Inhibition of
Mixed Lymphocyte Reactions by Rabbit Anti-Thymus Serum

Tissue Used for Absorption	Inhibition by Various Dilutions of Antiserum (%)		
	1:8	1:16	1:32
Unabsorbed[a]	98[b]	92	84
BALB/c thymus	23	−23	
BALB/c spleen	49	44	
BALB/c bone marrow	64	48	39
BALB/c brain	99	86	61
BALB/c liver & kidney[c]	96	96	75
AKR/J thymus	−89	−25	−54
AKR/J bone marrow	53	37	−5
EL-4	86	44	33
6C3HED	92	30	
MPC-11	99	94	76
C3H B-lymphoma	46	−18	

Rabbit anti-thymus serum was treated for its inhibitory activity
on the reaction of BALB/c lymph-node cells against AKR/J mitomycin-C treated cells. The serum was either absorbed with liver
and kidney only, or additionally with various other tissues.

[a]RAT absorbed with liver and kidney only.

[b]Mean of three absorption experiments.

[c]RAT absorbed twice with liver and kidney.

        The inhibitory activity of RAT was entirely attributable to
its reaction with effector cells. Exposure of target cells to the
serum for 60 min did not prevent their lysis by sensitized PEL.
Absorption of RAT with thymus, spleen, or bone marrow cells removed the inhibitory effect of RAT on cytotoxic effector cells.
EL-4, 6C3HED and C3H B-lymphoma absorbed the inhibitory activity
of RAT on CML while MPC-11 myeloma cells failed to do so (Table IV).
A mixture of RAT absorbed with bone marrow and RAT absorbed with
EL-4 failed to inhibit CML, thus indicating that each of the absorption procedures remove the same antibody.

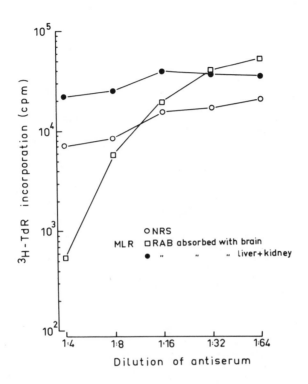

Fig. 5. The effect of rabbit anti-bone marrow serum on the proliferation of BALB/c lymph-node cells. Responder cells were exposed to normal rabbit serum (o), rabbit anti-bone marrow serum
absorbed with brain (□) or rabbit anti-bone marrow serum absorbed
with liver and kidney (●).

DISCUSSION

     In the present study various rabbit antisera were tested
for their effect on the activity of T lymphocytes in mice. The
attachment of antibodies to the cell surface of lymphocytes, in
the absence of C', may have different effects. Antibodies may
inhibit the activity of lymphocytes either by blocking specific
functional receptors or by interfering with the activity of the
cells in a nonspecific way. Alternatively, the attachment of
antibodies to the cell membrane may have the opposite effect and
lead to mitotic triggering of the cells (18). The findings in
the present study indicated that, indeed, the various xenoantisera
tested differed markedly in their effect on thymidine incorporation.

TABLE II

The Effect of Various Antisera on the Response of Lymph-Node Cells
to Lectins and on Cell-Mediated Lysis by Peritoneal Exudate Cells

Serum [a]	PHA Response [b]		Con A Response [b]		CML	
	c.p.m.	Inhibition (%)	c.p.m.	Inhibition (%)	^{51}Cr Release (%)	Inhibition (%)
NRS	49,916		69,790		71	
RAT	285	100	356	100	24	87
RABT	4,237	90	8,630	88	25	85
RABR	72,735	-41	76,925	-7	74	-6

[a] All the sera were absorbed with kidney and liver only and used
at a 1:8 dilution.

[b] The concentration of PHA used was 2 μl/ml while that of Con A
was 2 μg/ml.

TABLE III

The Effect of Various Absorptions on the Inhibitory Activity of
RAT on the Mitotic Response of BALB/c Lymph-Node Cells to Lectins

Serum	Tissue Used for Absorption	Mitotic Response			
		PHA		Con A	
		c.p.m.	Inhibition (%)	c.p.m.	Inhibition (%)
NRS	Unabsorbed [a]	59,768		155,255	
RAT	"	523	99	777	100
RAT	EL-4 [b]	58,588	2	127,588	18
RAT	6C3HED [b]	67,984	-14	144,097	7
RAT	MPC-11 [b]	516	100	881	100
NRS	Unabsorbed [a]	125,255		227,351	
RAT	"	638	100	443	100
RAT	Brain [b]	9,647	93	7,085	97
RAT	Bone marrow [b]	16,618	87	19,018	92

[a] Serum absorbed with liver and kidney only.
[b] The serum was first absorbed with liver and kidney and then
with the other tissues indicated.

TABLE IV

The Effect of Various Absorptions on the Inhibition of
Lymphocyte Reactivity by Rabbit Anti-Thymus Serum

Tissue Used for Absorption	Absorptive Capacity for:			
	CML	MLR	Con A	PHA
Thymus	+++ (a)	+++	+++	+++
Spleen	+++	++		
Bone marrow	+++	+	−	−
Brain	+	−	−	−
6C3HED	+++	+	+++	+++
EL-4	+++	+	+++	+++
MPC-11	−	−	−	−
C3H B lymphoma	+++	++		

(a)Arbitrary values for relative absorptive capacity:
+++ complete or almost complete absorption,
++ and + partial absorption, - no absorptive capacity.

RABR and high concentrations of RAT had a marked stimulatory effect,
whereas RABT and low concentrations of RAT inhibited the background
proliferation of lymph-node cells. The effect of the xenoantisera
on the response to mitogenic stimuli (MLR, PHA and Con A) tended
to parallel their effect on "spontaneous proliferation". RABR
augmented the proliferation, while RABT and RAT had an inhibitory
effect.

RAT and RABT were shown to contain antibodies specific for
T lymphocytes of all strains of mice tested (13,20). In addition,
RAT absorbed with liver and kidney contained antibodies reactive
with B lymphocytes (13). In spite of the complexity of the sera
it became obvious that RAT affected the MLR both through inhibition
of the activity of responder T cells and by coating of antigenic
determinants on stimulator cells. The decreased activity of RAT
absorbed with either bone marrow or B-lymphoma cells may reflect
the removal of antibodies which could coat stimulator cells. Absorption with EL-4 and 6C3HED probably removed antibodies reactive with responder cells. The fact that RAT inhibited, in the
absence of complement, the response of lymph-node cells to lectins,
clearly demonstrated the presence of antibodies to receptors on
responder T cells. These antibodies could be removed by absorp-

tion with EL-4 and 6C3HED lymphoma cells but not with brain, bone
marrow or myeloma cells. It seems, therefore, that the inhibitory effect of RAT on the response of lymph-node cells to various
mitogenic stimuli resulted from interaction of the antiserum with
a T lymphocyte specific antigen. A completely different antigen
was involved in the inhibitory effect of RAT on the CML, since
here either bone marrow or C3H B-lymphoma cells eliminated the
activity. The finding that absorption with EL-4, 6C3HED, thymus
or spleen cells removed the inhibitory activity of the serum indicates that the CML is inhibited by antibodies directed against
antigenic determinants shared by T and B lymphocytes. It is unlikely that this antigen is H-2 since H-2 antibodies probably
were eliminated by absorption with liver and kidney. There is a
possibility that the activity of RAT was directed against Ia determinants expressed on activated T lymphocytes (19). This seems
unlikely, however, since allogeneic Ia antibodies have not been
shown to inhibit effector cells in the CML (15), and since EL-4
cells, which removed the activity of RAT, lack any known cell surface Ia determinants (5). Activated T lymphocytes may express
antigenic determinants which are absent from non-activated T cells
and which are shared with B cells (7,23). It seems, therefore,
that the antigenic determinants on cytotoxic T cells, with which
RAT reacts, belong to the same category of antigens which become
expressed on T cells after activation. Preliminary data (unpublished) showed that the Fab fragment of RAT inhibited CML, thus
indicating that this cell surface constituent on killer T cells
may be directly involved in their cytotoxic activity.

SUMMARY

     An attempt was made to determine whether xenoantisera can
detect functional receptors on mouse T lymphocytes. Antisera
were raised by immunizing rabbits with BALB/c thymus cells, boiled
thymus homogenate, brain homogenate or bone marrow cells. Following heat inactivation these antisera were absorbed with mouse
kidney and liver homogenates, and studied for their effect, in the
absence of C', on the activity of murine T lymphocytes. Rabbit
anti-bone marrow serum (RAB) had no effect on the mixed lymphocyte reaction (MLR) nor on cell-mediated lysis (CML). In contrast,
rabbit anti-thymus serum (RAT) and anti-boiled thymus serum (RABT)
inhibited strikingly, the MLR, CML, and the response to concanavalin A and phytohemagglutinin. Rabbit anti-brain serum (RABR)
caused a marked increase of the proliferation of lymphocytes both
in the presence or absence of various stimuli and had no effect
on the CML. Absorption experiments indicated that a number of
antigens are involved in the inhibitory activity of RAT. Antibodies to a T cell specific antigen interfere with the response
of T lymphocytes to mitogenic stimuli, while the activity of cy-
toxic T cells is inhibited by antibodies to a determinant shared
by B and T lymphocytes.

ACKNOWLEDGEMENTS

This study was supported by grants from the US-Israel
Binational Science Foundation (No. 714) and from the DKFZ.

REFERENCES

1. Abbasi, K., Festenstein, H., Verbi, W. and Roitt, I. M.,
   Nature (Lond.) 251 (1974) 227.
2. Bergman, Y. and Haimovich, J., Eur. J. Immunol. 7 (1977) 413.
3. Berke, G., Sullivan, K. A. and Amos, D. B., J. Exp. Med. 135
   (1972) 1334.
4. Cantor, H. and Boyse, E. A., Cold Spring Harbor Symp. quant.
   Biol. 41 (1977) 23.
5. David, C. S., Transpl. Rev. 30 (1976) 299.
6. Dunham, L. C. and Stewart, H. L., J. Nat. Cancer Inst. 13
   (1953) 1299.
7. Feeney, A. J. and Hämmerling, U., J. Immunol. 118 (1977) 1488.
8. Feldman, M., Cohen, I. R. and Wekerle, H., Transpl. Rev. 12
   (1972) 57.
9. Gore, P. A. and Amos, D. B., Cancer Res. 16 (1956) 338.
10. Hämmerling, G. J. and McDevitt, H. O., Isr. J. Med. Sci. 11
    (1975) 1331.
11. Hogg, M. N. and Greaves, M. F., Immunology 22 (1972) 967.
12. Kimura, A. K., J. Exp. Med. 139 (1974) 88.
13. Laskov, R., Rabinowitz, R., Haimovitz, A. and Schlesinger,
    M., Isr. J. Med. Sci. 13 (1977) 767.
14. Laskov, R. and Scharff, M. D., J. Exp. Med. 131 (1970) 515.
15. Lonai, P. In: Immune Recognition (Ed. A. S. Rosenthal),
    Academic Press, New York, (1975) 683.
16. McKenzie, I. F. C., Cherry, M. and Snell, G. D. Immunogene-
    tics 5 (1977) 25.
17. Meo, T., David, C. S., Rijnbeek, A. M., Nabholz, M., Miggiano,
    V. C. and Shreffler, D. C., Transpl. Proc. 7 (1975) 127.
18. Ochiai, T., Ahmed, A., Grebe, S. C. and Sell, K. W., Transpl.
    Proc. 9 (1977) 1049.
19. Plate, J. M. D., Eur. J. Immunol. 6 (1976) 180.
20. Rabinowitz, R., Cohen, A., Laskov, R. and Schlesinger, M.,
    J. Immunol. 112 (1974) 683.
21. Rabinowitz, R., Laskov, R. and Schlesinger, M., Immunology
    34 (1978) 959.
22. Roelants, G. E., Ryden, A., Hagg, L. B. and Loor, F., Nature
    (Lond.) 247 (1974) 106.
23. Schirrmacher, V. and Festenstein, H., J. Immunogen. 2 (1975)
    337.
24. Schlesinger, M., Israel, E. and Gery, I., Immunology 30
    (1976) 865.
25. Shiku, H., Kisielow, P., Bean, M. A., Takahashi, T., Boyse, E.
    A., Oettgen, H. F. and Old, L. J., J. Exp. Med. 141 (1975)
    227.

26. Simpson, E. and Beverley, P. C. L., Progress in Immunology
    3 (1978) 206.
27. Snell, G. D., Immunol. Rev. 38 (1978) 4.
28. Stobo, J. D. and Paul, W. E., J. Immunol. 110 (1973) 362.
29. Stout, R. D., Murphy, D. B., McDevitt, H. O. and Herzenberg,
    L. A., J. Exp. Med. 145 (1977) 187.
30. Waksman, B. H., Transpl. Rev. 6 (1971) 30.
31. Wigzell, H. and Häyry, P., Curr. Topics Microbiol. Immunol.
    67 (1974) 1.

EFFECT OF IMMUNE SERA UPON ENHANCED IN VITRO ANTIBODY RESPONSES

S. J. FRANK, S. SPECTER, A. NOWOTNY and H. FRIEDMAN
Albert Einstein Medical Center, Temple University School
of Medicine and University of Pennsylvania School of
Dental Medicine, Philadelphia, Pennsylvania and University of South Florida, Tampa, Florida (USA)

Both the intact Serratia marcescens lipopolysaccharide (LPS)
and a small molecular weight non-mitogenic polysaccharide (PS)-
rich derivative stimulate specific and nonspecific antibody plaque
forming cell (PFC) responses of mouse spleen cells cultures to
sheep erythrocytes in vitro (2, 3). These stimulatory effects
appear due to the adjuvanticity of the material, which can be
demonstrated both in vivo and in vitro. In order to determine
whether there is a relationship between immunostimulatory activity
of the intact LPS and the PS derivative, antisera were prepared in
rabbits to the LPS and examined in the present study for their
ability to affect the immunomodulating activities of LPS and/or PS.
The effects of the antisera were found to be markedly different
depending upon the method of immunizing the rabbits to obtain the
sera and the endotoxin type used for immunomodulation.

MATERIALS AND METHODS

The S. marcescens LPS was prepared by the trichloroacetic acid
extraction method from overnight cultures of the organisms and
purified as described previously (4). The S. marcescens PS was
prepared from the endotoxic LPS by hydrolyzation in 1N HCl at 100 C
for 30 min by the methods of Chang et al. (1).

For obtaining antisera, New Zealand white rabbits were injected
with varying concentrations of either heat-killed Serratia or intact LPS in either saline or Freund's incomplete adjuvant following
an immunization schedule with the preparations injected subcutaneously on day 0, intravenously on day 4, and intramuscularly on day 8.

261

The development of antibody to the LPS and PS was determined
by counterimmunoelectrophoresis whereby the rabbit antisera were
placed in one well and LPS or bacterial suspensions in the other
well. Agglutinin tests were performed by determining the ability
of the antisera to agglutinate heat-killed Serratia.

The effects of the antisera on in vitro immunostimulation by
LPS and PS were determined using the hemolytic plaque assay described previously (3). For this purpose, 5 x 10^6 mouse spleen
cells were cultured in vitro in Linbro plates together with 2 x 10^6
SRBC. The PFC number developing in each well was determined 5 days
later using the microplaque assay.

Addition of 25 or 10 µg LPS or PS, respectively, to the cultures at the time of initiation induced a marked increase in the
PFC response. In order to determine the effects of the antisera
on the response, the sera were first mixed with either LPS or PS
in vitro for 30 min at 37 C. The mixture was then added directly
to the cultures. The PFC response was then determined for cultures
containing untreated SRBC immunized spleen cells, or spleen cells
treated with LPS or PS, with or without prior antiserum treatment.

RESULTS

Production and counterimmunoelectrophoresis of antisera to
LPS. Rabbits were immunized with either LPS, LPS in mineral oil,
S. marcescens heat-killed bacteria, or S. marcescens heat-killed
bacteria in mineral oil. Their sera were electrophoresed with
either the LPS or bacteria as Ag, and patterns were obtained. In
almost all cases, pattern lines of Ab-Ag reaction were obtained
with the bacteria used as Ag (Table I). Heaviest banding was
obtained when bacteria in oil were used as the immunizing agents,
although higher bacterial agglutination titers were also obtained
when bacteria alone were used as the immunizing agents. In several cases, the sera obtained were not monospecific, as two bands
appeared in the patterns. Only immunization of rabbits with bacteria in oil resulted in antisera reactive against the LPS preparation. Again, in one case the electrophoresis patterns resulted
in two bands, suggesting some antigenic heterogeneity. In one
case each, using LPS in oil or bacteria as immunizing agents, the
animals failed to respond, as measured by serum electrophoresis
patterns, although the former did exhibit a small Ab agglutination.

Effect of anti-LPS antiserum of LPS-stimulated specific PFC
response to SRBC in vitro. The anti-LPS antiserum raised by immunization of rabbits with S. marcescens bacteria in oil further
enhanced the PFC directed against SRBC that were stimulated by LPS
(Table II). This stimulation was greatest at 1:10 dilution of antiserum, where a 410% stimulation was obtained, versus a 177% stimu-

TABLE I

Counterimmunoelectrophoresis with Antisera from
Rabbits Immunized with Heat-killed Serratia or LPS

Immunogen Name[a]	Rabbit Number	Precipitin Bands[b]		Agglutinin Titer
		Bacteria	LPS	
Bacteria				
(saline)	1	2	0	1:256
	2	$\underline{+}$	0	1:8
	3	2	0	1:256
(oil)	4	2	2	1:256
	5	1	1	1:256
	6	1	1	1:256
LPS				
(saline)	7	1	0	<1:8
	8	1	0	1:128
	9	1	0	1:64
(oil)	10	0	0	1:32
	11	1	0	1:32
None	12	0	0	<1:2

[a]Rabbits infected with either LPS or heat-killed Serratia in
saline or mineral oil
[b]Number of precipitin bands using antisera and either suspension
of bacteria or LPS

lation resulting from LPS treatment alone. The anti–LPS antiserum
alone as control never resulted in more than a marginal 129% enhancement of PFC number. Also, normal rabbit serum as a control
did not stimulate PFC more than 15% above LPS alone. Greater
dilutions of antiserum over a 10-fold range still yielded enhancement, but less than 30% lower than the 1:10 dilution. Thus the
anti–LPS serum and LPS, when added to culture together, exhibited
a synergistic enhancement of PFC.

Effect of anti–LPS antiserum on PS-stimulated specific PFC
response to SRBC in vitro. The anti–LPS antiserum raised by immunization of rabbits with S. marcescens heat-killed in oil did not
further enhance the PFC directed against SRBC that were stimulated

TABLE II

Effect of Anti-LPS Antiserum on S. marcescens
LPS Stimulated Hemolytic PFC Response In vitro by
Normal Balb/c Spleen Cell Cultures Immunized with SRBC

Endotoxin Preparation[a]	Anti-LPS Antiserum[b]	Normal Serum[c]	PFC Response Per 10^6 Spleen Cells[d]	Percent of Control
None			734 ± 69	—
		1:50	760 ± 82	104
	1:10		950 ± 102	129
	1:50		836 ± 71	114
	1:100		810 ± 84	110
S. marcescens LPS			1297 ± 117	177
		1:50	1412 ± 141	192
	1:10		3013 ± 172	410
	1:50		3028 ± 148	413
	1:100		2280 ± 192	382

[a] 5×10^6 viable spleen cells from normal mice cultured in vitro for 5 days at 37 C in 10% CO_2 and immunized with 2×10^6 SRBC; 25 µg S. marcescens LPS added to cultures

[b] Anti-LPS serum from rabbits immunized with LPS

[c] Normal serum from unimmunized rabbits added to cultures

[d] Average PFC response (± S. E.) for 6-9 cultures per group

TABLE III

Effect of Anti-LPS Antiserum on S. marcescens
PS Stimulated Hemolytic PFC Response In vitro by
Normal Balb/c Spleen Cell Cultures Immunized with SRBC

Endotoxin Preparation[a]	Anti-LPS Antiserum[b]	Normal Serum[c]	Antibody PFC Response Per 10^6 Spleen Cells[d]	Percent of Control
None			734 ± 69	104
		1:50	760 ± 82	129
	1: 10		950 ± 102	114
	1: 50		836 ± 71	110
	1:100		810 ± 84	
S. marcescens PS			1075 ± 101	146
		1:50	1136 ± 88	155
	1: 10		1070 ± 93	146
	1: 50		1096 ± 74	149
	1:100		1072 ± 89	146

[a] 5×10^6 viable spleen cells from normal mice cultured in vitro for 5 days at 37 C in 10% CO_2 and immunized with 2×10^6 SRBC; 10 μg S. marcescens PS added to cultures

[b] Anti LPS serum from rabbits immunized with LPS in oil

[c] Normal serum from unimmunized rabbits added to cultures

[d] Average PFC response ($\pm$ S. E.) for 6-9 cultures per group

by PS (Table III), as compared to the increased stimulation obtained beyond that resulting with LPS (Table II). Normal rabbit
serum controls did not stimulate PFCs more than 9% above PS alone,
while anti-LPS never resulted in more than 3% additional enhancement of PFC number for any of the three dilutions studied when
used in conjunction with the immunostimulatory PS.

DISCUSSION AND CONCLUSION

In the present study, the effect of antisera prepared in
rabbits against Serratia marcescens on the immunostimulatory
properties of the Serratia LPS or PS on the in vitro immune
response to SRBC was examined. Rabbits immunized with heat-
killed Serratia or LPS in saline or mineral oil developed agglutinating antibody to the intact bacteria (Table I). However,
only immunization with heat killed Serratia in mineral oil resulted in antisera capable of reacting to LPS, as shown by
countercurrentimmunoelectrophoresis. This antisera had marked
effects on the immunomodulating activity of the intact Serratia
LPS added to cultures of normal spleen cells immunized in vitro
with SRBC (Table II). Such cultures generally showed a marked
increase in antibody responsiveness in the presence of LPS with
or without SRBC as the immunogen. When the LPS was first treated
with graded amounts of the anti-Serratia serum there was an increasing stimulatory effect on the antibody response rather than
the expected decrease. Thus, instead of "neutralizing" the LPS
stimulatory activity, the anti-Serratia serum appeared to augment
the effect. This could be due to development of antigen-antibody
complexes with the relatively large molecular weight LPS and the
specific anti-Serratia antibody. Normal sera did not have such an
effect. However, such complexes, even if formed in vitro, did not
appear to affect the background antibody response in cultures without SRBC (not reported here). Such cultures showed an increased
background response to SRBC in the presence of LPS and there was
no significant alteration of this response when the anti-Serratia
serum was used to neutralize the stimulatory activity of the LPS.

It is noteworthy that similar effects did not occur when PS
was used as the immunostimulator in vitro. Earlier studies in
this laboratory had shown that PS, a relatively much smaller
molecular weight material derived from Serratia LPS without a
detectable lipid moiety, was equivalent to the LPS in stimulating
PFC responses in vitro (2, 3). Those studies indicated that the
lipid moiety was not a necessary component for the immunoadjuvant
activity of the LPS extracts. Furthermore, since PS was non-
mitogenic, those studies indicated that mitogenicity was not a
necessary prerequisite for immunostimulatory activity. Very little
difference, however, could be observed during the cytokinetics of
the enhanced immune response of normal spleen cell cultures incu-

bated with PS <u>versus</u> LPS (3). In the present study, however, it
was evident that addition of the anti-Serratia sera prepared in
rabbits immunized with Serratia bacteria did not affect the immunostimulatory activity of this small molecular weight derivative,
either in a positive or negative manner. Thus it seems likely
that PS, as compared to LPS, may not form an immune complex with
the antisera or that the antisera <u>per</u> <u>se</u>, although induced in
rabbits with intact Serratia did not contain sufficient amounts of
antibody to recognize the immunologic or serologic determinants of
the PS. Regardless of the mechanism involved, it appears that the
antisera used in this study, although capable of enhancing the
immunostimulatory activities of LPS, did not do so with PS, both
in regard to antigen specific and nonspecific responses. These
results, therefore, point to a possible difference between PS and
LPS in terms of immunoadjuvant activities <u>in</u> <u>vitro</u>.

SUMMARY

Immunization of rabbits with <u>S. marcescens</u> bacteria in Freund's
incomplete adjuvant resulted in development of anti-Serratia sera
with bacterial agglutinating properties as well as LPS modulating
properties. The antisera reacted with the LPS in counterimmuno-
electrophoretic assays. Such antisera also stimulated the LPS
induced enhancement of specific anti-SRBC responses from normal
spleen cell cultures but did not further enhance the stimulated
responses of similar cultures incubated with the smaller molecular
weight PS-rich derivative. The antisera had no effect on LPS or
PS enhanced nonspecific background anti-SRBC response as compared
to normal rabbit serum-treated controls. These results point to
a possible role for immune complexes as an enhancer of the immuno-
stimulating activities of LPS antibody-treated cultures and also
indicate a difference between LPS and PS as immunomodulators.

REFERENCES

1. Chang, H., Thompson, J. J., Nowotny, A. Immunol. Commun. 3
    (1974) 401.
2. Frank, S. J., Specter, S., Nowotny, A. and Friedman, H. J.
    Immunol. 119 (1977) 855.
3. Frank, S. J., Specter, S., Nowotny, A. and Friedman, H. Abstr.
    Ann. Meet. ASM E119 (1976).
4. Nowotny, A., Cundy, K. R., Neale, N. L., Nowotny, A. M.,
    Radvany, P., Thomas, S. P. and Tripodi, D. J. Ann. N. Y. Acad.
    Sci. 133 (1968) 586.

GROWTH OF HUMAN T-CELLS FOLLOWING IN VITRO ALLOGRAFT SENSITIZATION

J. L. STRAUSSER and A. ROSENBERG

Surgery Branch, National Cancer Institute, National
Institutes of Health, Bethesda, Maryland (USA)

Sensitization of human lymphocytes to alloantigens and tumor
in vitro permits close examination of the mechanisms of immune reactivity. Use of such sensitized cells for in vivo experiments
or therapy, however, has been limited to date, by the small numbers
of cells generated with mixed lymphocyte culture and the finite
survival of these cytotoxic lymphocytes. Gallo, et al. (5) recently
demonstrated maintenance of non-cytotoxic human thymus derived
lymphocytes in long-term culture by growth on a lymphocyte conditioned medium. Gillis and Smith (1) subsequently used a modified
form of this medium to continuously culture cytotoxic murine lymphoid cell lines. The continuous proliferation of allosensitized
human cytotoxic T cells provides a potential source of material
for passive adoptive immunotherapy. We herein describe conditions
under which fresh or cryopreserved human lymphocytes sensitized
in vitro to alloantigens can be continuously cultured in exponential proliferation while maintaining specific cytotoxicity.

Lymphocytes from leukophoresis of normal human volunteers were
prepared by Ficol-Hypaque gradients. Cells which were not used
immediately in culture were cryopreserved by the method of Sears
(8). The secondary mixed lymphocyte culture (2° MLC) technique of
Bach (10) was used to sensitize lymphocytes to alloantigen. For
the primary sensitization procedure 4×10^{6} lymphocytes were co-
cultured with 6×10^{6} allogeneic lymphocytes which had previously
received 2,000 rads. Cells collected from the primary cultures at
day 10, after the peak of their cytotoxic activity, then underwent
secondary sensitization by co-culture of 4×10^{6} of these cells
with 1×10^{6} irradiated cells from the same allogeneic source.
Cells from the secondary sensitization were harvested on day 2, at
the peak of their cytotoxic activity, and cryopreserved. Cells

from secondary MLC were used for growth on human conditioned medium (HCM) rather than those from primary MLC as we have found that higher levels of cytotoxicity and specificity generally can be obtained with these cells.

HCM was prepared by culture of pooled human 0 positive peripheral mononuclear cells in RPMI 1629 with 0.1% PHA-P and 1% autologous plasma at 10^6 cells/cc. Cells were prepared by one to two hr incubation with plasma-gel followed by harvest of the leukocyte rich supernatant and passage through nylon-wool columns. After 72 hr of culture of 37 C, the cells were centrifuged and the supernatants were harvested and frozen. Conditioned media was concentrated five-fold by filtration (Amicon Corporation, Lexington, Massachusetts) prior to usage.

Lymphocytes were grown on HCM in 15 cc round bottom tube cultures with 1.5×10^5 cells/cc seeded into a total volume of 2 cc consisting of 20% HCM plus 10% fetal calf serum in RPMI 1640 and antibiotics. Cultures were incubated at 37 C, 5% CO_2 and high humidity and were routinely split and re-seeded at 1×10^5 cells/cc when cell numbers had increased to approximately 1×10^6 cells/cc. All cell counts were done by the trypan blue exclusion technique in triplicate. Data shown represent the mean of the viability counts.

Fig. 1 describes the growth of allosensitized human lymphocytes on HCM. Characteristically, there is a five to seven day cycle during which the cells expand approximately 5 to 10-fold in number with a 54 hr doubling time. Viability remains 95-100% during this period. Control cultures containing medium alone or medium supplemented with PHA-P do not proliferate greater than five-fold nor can they be maintained for longer than 12 days under similar culture conditions. If cell cultures on HCM are re-seeded on fresh medium when cell numbers have increased to approximately 1×10^6 cells per cc, the sensitized cell lines can be maintained and expanded indefinitely, (longer than four months to date). Allowing cell numbers to increase to greater than 10^6 cells/cc in tube cultures results in decreased proliferation and decreased viability as does transfer of the cells to medium not supplemented with HCM. Seeding at concentrations of as low as 5×10^4 cells/cc will allow similar growth rates.

To test whether the specific cytotoxicity of the allosensitized cells grown on HCM is maintained, cells grown as described above were tested for their lytic capacity in four hour ^{51}Cr-release assays (6). The cytotoxicity against specific, nonspecific and control targets was assessed and compared with that of: a) autologous cells sensitized against alloantigens, but not grown on HCM; b) autologous cells not sensitized, but grown on HCM; and c) autologous cells not sensitized, and not grown on HCM[*]. The results

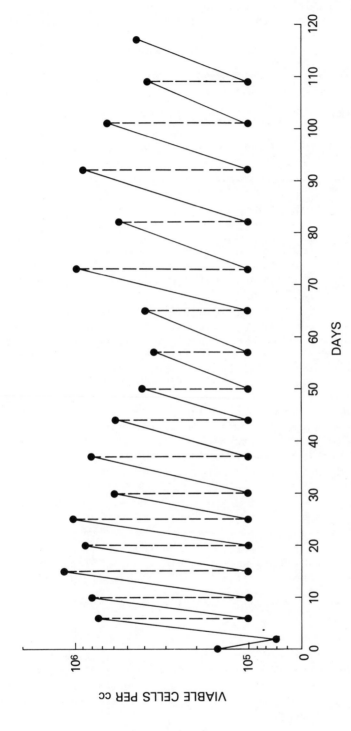

Fig. 1. Kinetics of growth of peripheral blood mononuclear leukocytes sensitized by 2° MLC in vitro and seeded on HCM. Solid line represents culture growth in the presence of HCM; vertical broken line indicates split of the culture to a lower cell density on fresh medium supplemented with 20% HCM. All points represent the means of triplicate determinations from separate cultures. Standard deviation about the points is less than 5%.

of a typical experiment are presented in Table I. While the capacity to lyse specific targets is maintained after proliferation of
the allosensitized cells on HCM, nonspecific or control lysis remains less than 10% at the effector to target ratios tested. The

TABLE I

Cytotoxicity of Allosensitized Cells Grown on HCM

Effectors	Days Grown on HCM	Percent Lysis of Targets ± SD[a]		
		α[b]	β	λ
α(non-sensitized)	0	-5.7±2.2	0.8±0.7	-0.1±2.0
	37	0.6±0.5	6.5±0.9	1.3±1.9
	92	-0.7±1.0	7.2±2.3	-0.7±0.6
α sensitized to β[c]	0	-4.1±0.5	51.7±3.9	8.6±2.3
	37	1.6±0.5	14.2±2.5	0.2±0.2
	92	5.4±1.0	26.3±2.2	2.4±1.4

[a]Freshly defrosted effector lymphocytes were added to ^{51}Cr-labelled
target lymphocytes in Linbro round bottom microtiter plates and
incubated for four hr at 37 C and 5% CO_2 at 10:1 effector : target
ratios. Supernatants from these cultures were harvested with the
Skatron-Titertek system and counted for gamma particle emission.
Maximal isotope release was produced by incubation of targets with
0.1 N HCl. Percent lysis was calculated by:

$$100 \text{ X} \quad (\frac{\text{Experimental CPM} - \text{Spontaneous CMP}}{\text{Maximal CPM} - \text{Spontaneous CPM}})$$

[b]HLA Types of Cells: $\alpha = A_2B_7B_{51}BW_4BW_6C_2$; $\beta = A_2A_3BW_{22}CW_1CW_3$;
$\lambda = A_1A_2B_7B_8$.

[c]Cells were sensitized as described in the text. All cultures
were maintained on RPMI 1640 with antibiotics and 5% plasma from
the responder cell donor. Cultures were incubated at 37 C, 5%
CO_2 and high humidity.

*Specific cytotoxicity refers to lysis of target lymphocytes to
which the effectors have been sensitized. Nonspecific cytotoxicity is directed against lymphocytes to which the effectors have
not been sensitized. Control targets are non-sensitized cells
isogenic with the effectors.

fact that virtually no lytic activity can be demonstrated against self by cells grown on the HCM is a most important control, as potential use of in vitro sensitized cytotoxic lymphocytes for adoptive immunotherapy would necessarily be hampered should the cytotoxic cells nonspecifically lyse normal donor as well as target cells.

To date we have tested the cytotoxicity of sensitized cells through greater than 10^{10}-fold proliferation on HCM. We have noted that while some cell lines retain cytotoxic specificity throughout the proliferation, others demonstrate gradual loss of cytotoxic potential with increasing expansion. All cell lines to date have maintained cytotoxic specificity through at least 10^4-fold proliferation on HCM.

Efforts are now underway to extend the observations of others (2,3,4,9) on the ability to sensitize human lymphocytes in vitro to 'tumor antigens. Hopefully, such human T cells sensitized in vitro to tumor specific transplantation antigens will provide stem cells for proliferation on HCM and thus provide a source of material for tumor immunotherapy.

In summary, it is possible to grow human cytotoxic lymphocytes in continuous culture on HCM maintaining specific cytotoxicity over the course of the culture. Cytotoxic cell lines have been expanded to over 10^{10} times their initial numbers to date in culture.

REFERENCES

1. Gillis, S. and Smith, K. A., Nature 268 (1977) 154.
2. Golub, S. H., Cellular Immun. 28 (1977) 371.
3. Golub, S. H. and Morton, D. L., Nature 251 (1974) 161.
4. Martin-Chandon, M. R., Vanky, F., Carnaud, C. and Klein, E., Int. J. of Cancer 15 (1975) 342.
5. Morgan, D. A., Ruscetti, F. W. and Gallo, R., Science 193 (1976) 1007.
6. Rosenberg, S. A. and Schwartz, S., J. Natl. Cancer Inst. 52 (1974) 1151.
7. Ruscetti, F. W., Morgan, D. A. and Gallo, R. C., J. of Immun. 119 (1977) 131.
8. Sears, H. F. and Rosenberg, S. A., J. Natl. Cancer Inst. 58 (1977) 1.
9. Sharma, B. and Terasaki, P. I., Cancer Res. 34 (1974) 115.
10. Zier, K. S. and Bach, F. H., Scand. J. of Imm. 4 (1977) 607.

Part III
Immunopathology of the Reticuloendothelial System

Recent investigations in many laboratories have indicated that immunopathologic reactions involving antibody and lymphocytes may not be due merely to "forbidden responses" but also due to loss of immunoregulatory functions. T lymphocytes have been the focus of much attention in terms of suppressor or helper activity. However, it is quite apparent that macrophages and other monocytes are directly involved in autoimmune reactivity and allergies. Altered immune responsiveness, either in a positive or negative manner, may influence a wide variety of disease states as well as the "normal" phenomenon of aging. Stimulation of the RE System may be an important factor in the so-called autoimmunity. This section deals with a wide variety of topics concerning the complex interactions of RE cells and such autoimmune phenomena as well as other immunopathologic reactions.

IMMUNOSUPPRESSION AS A HOMEOSTATIC MECHANISM IN DISEASE AND AGING

H. R. STRAUSSER and M. M. ROSENSTEIN

Department of Zoology and Physiology
Rutgers University
Newark, New Jersey (USA)

Prostaglandins (Pg) have been found to be increased in a large
variety of animal and human tumors by many investigators. For
example, Levine et al.(13) found large amounts of Pg in 5 clonal
strains of a mouse $HSDM_1$ tumor line as compared with normal cell
lines and Jaffe et al.(10) found elevated PgE levels in the plasma
of humans and rats with a veriety of tumors. In these and other
reported instances the high Pg content was considerably lowered
by treatment with indomethacin.

In our own laboratory, Humes and Strausser (9) established
that Pg of the E series were increased as much as 53 fold in a
virus-induced murine sarcoma (MSV) in BALB/c mice. Further studies
indicated that the activity of the Pg was mediated by cyclic AMP
and that indomethacin in vivo and in vitro caused a decrease in
the Pg level as well as in the cyclic AMP (7). Osteoclast activity in bones close to the tumor site was attributed to Pg accumulated in the local area (21). The administration of indomethacin
in vivo delayed and in some instances inhibited the size of the
tumor, but it should be noted that MSV tumors in the young mouse
are self-regressing. Thus, a long-term tumor-inhibitory effect
could not truly be demonstrated.

That the effect of Pg on tumors has been a contradictory and
intricate study is illustrated by experiments by Santoro et al.
(19,20). The results of these investigators, who used a B-16
melanoma in mice indicated that Pg addition to culture inhibited
tumor cell proliferation. Also, the in vivo administration of 16,
16-dimethyl PgE_2 methyl ester intratumorally on day 8 depressed

the growth of tumor on a dose-dependent basis during the 22 day
observation period.

Pelus and Strausser (15) were able to demonstrate that spleen
cells of mice with many different types of spontaneous transplanted
tumors as well as methylcholanthrene-induced tumors had depressed
spleen cell immune responses to T and B cell mitogens. Earlier,
Plescia et al. (16) were able to show plaque-forming cell activity
depression in C_{57}Bl/6 mice bearing MC-16 tumors. Further, Grinwich
and Plescia (5) indicated that following in vitro cultures of normal syngeneic spleen cells with MC-16 tumor cells, the antibody or
plaque forming cell response of the spleen cells to sheep red blood
cells was inhibited. Strausser and Pelus cooperated with Plescia
and Grinwich (unpublished) to demonstrate that Pg of the E series
were increased in these cultures. Indomethacin restored the Pg
level to almost normal values and also restored the plaque forming
response of the spleen cells.

Research in this area was further advanced by the work of
Pelus and Strausser (14) and Rosenstein et al. (18) who sought to
characterize the cell type elaborating the Pg in the spleens of
the tumor-bearing mice. Using the MC-16 tumor, they allowed dis-
persed spleen cells to adhere to plastic petri dishes. The Pg
levels of the E series were then measured by radioimmunoassay
They found an increase in the Pg levels of the adherent population,
but not in the cells of the non-adherent populations when the two
were separated. Indomethancin reduced the Pg level of the adherent
cells but had no effect on the non-adherent ones. When the two
populations were reconstituted the Pg levels again increased.
Additionally, the immune response of the non-adherent cells to
mitogens was considerably depressed in the presence of the adherent population, unless indomethancin was present. Thus, it
can be concluded from the above studies that a population of spleen
cells from tumorous mice produced large quantities of Pg which
directly or indirectly suppressed the responsiveness of T and B
cells to mitogens. Similar defects in immune responsiveness have
been observed in cancer patients and experimental or spontaneous
tumors of animals (22). Restoration of the immune responsiveness
of T and B cells can be partially accomplished in the experimental
animal, but the literature to date indicates that this procedure
only induces temporary inhibition of tumor growth.

Recently Humes et al. (6) and Bonney et al. (1) have shown that
inflammatory stimuli and immune complexes induce the production
and release of Pg from macrophages. Extrapolating from this, one
might hypothesize that Pg-induced immunosuppression in tumors may
function as a homeostatic mechanism to prevent excess T and B cell
production. The prevention of excess T and B cell production
would thereby inhibit the formation of immune complexes with con-
consequent preclusion of such diseases as glomerulonephritis (23,24)

atherosclerosis in stressed exbreeder rats (12) and enhancement of atherogenesis in rabbits induced with heterologous serum protein and an atherogenic diet (11). Other diseases in which immune complexes have been implicated as causative agents include hepatitis and poly-artheritis nodosa (17), rheumatoid arthritis (26) and adult coeliac disease, Crohn's disease and ulcerative colitis (4). Since indome-thacin only partially restored immune responsiveness in the tumor-bearing animal and had no effect in the atherosclerotic animal, it is obvious that immune suppressors other than and in addition to Pg may be involved in the suppression of immune complex disease. Glucocor-ticoids, which may inhibit T suppressor cells, also have been shown to inhibit production and release of Pg from macrophages (8) and may eventually exacerbate these immune complex diseases. On the same basis, we may suppose that stress of the type which releases adrenal steroids may be an initiator or enhancing agent in these disease states.

Another possible example of this type of homeostatic mechanism which acts to suppress the response of T and B cells is illustrated in the results of Warchalowski and Strausser (25) using EMC-M virus infected DBA/2J mice. Fifty percent of the mice infected with this virus develop hyperglycemia, glycosuria and other symptoms of diabetes. These symptoms and the pathology of the disease has been fully characterized by Craighead (3). The spleen cells of these mice exhibit considerable immunodepression prior to and following ex-posure to T and B cell mitogens as compared with non-infected con-trol mice of the same age and strain. The administration of Leva-misole in vivo caused considerable elevation of the response to Con-A but at the same time the diabetic symptoms, e.g. glycosuria, were markedly heightened. Rat anti-mouse lymphocyte serum although depressing the response to the mitogens, was effective in amelio-rating the diabetic condition. Prostaglandins appeared to be of minor importance here, since indomethacin in vitro only partially restored the suppressed response of B cells to the mitogen PWM. The fact that depressed immune responsiveness also involves T cells was shown by Buschard et al. (2) who could not produce diabetes with the EMC-M virus in thymectomized mice. The depressed response of the B cell, mentioned above, may in fact be due to lack of T hel-per cells, as well as the presence of suppressor substances, such as Pg.

In the aged BALB/c mouse (18 mo old) spleen cells there is as much as a 5-fold increase in the Pg of the E series as compared to the amount present in the spleen cells of the 2 month old mouse. The aged mouse also demonstrates depressed T and B immune respon-siveness to mitogens and to antigens, e.g. sheep red blood cells. The in vivo and in vitro administration of indomethacin partially restored the depressed immune responses of the spleen cells from the aged mice as in the tumor-bearing mouse, but had no signifi-cant effect on those from the 2 month old mice. Investigation of the particular spleen cell population in aged mice responsible for the depressed immune response, again revealed them to be adherent cells, which when removed or treated with indomethacin were prevented from producing Pg with consequent immune response depression.

In the instance of the aged mouse, it is presumed that previous exposure to viruses or other agent inducing inflammatory responses may cause increase in the amount of Pg produced as noted above. It is also postulated that this rise in Pg in the aged animals may actually be due to an accumulation of immune complexes produced by many antigenic exposures. These immune complexes might act on macrophages to increase Pg production, and this in turn results in Pg-induced immune suppression. Pg and other suppressor substances may in the aged animal act as a homeostatic mechanism which exists to suppress immune responses and thereby prevent the development of immune complex disease. We, therefore, speculate that the information derived from the investigations described in this report may be illustrative of a common immuno-suppressive factor. This factor may prove to be operative in many debilitating diseases of man.

REFERENCES

1. Bonney, R. J., Wightman, P. D., Narun, P., Richardson, T. G., Davis, P., Galavage, M. and Humes, J. L., Fed. Proc., 37 (1970) 1353.
2. Buschard, K., Rygaard, J. and Lund, E., Acta Patha Microbiol. Scanda., 84 (1976) 299.
3. Craighead, J. E., Science 162 (1968) 913.
4. Doe, W. F., Booth, C. C., Brown, D. L., Lancet 1 (1973) 402.
5. Grinwich, K. D. and Plescia, O. J., Prostaglandins 14 (1977) 1175.
6. Humes, J. L., Bonney, R. J., Pelus, L., Dahlgren, M. E., Sadowski, S. J., Kuehl, F. A., Jr. and Davies, P., Nature, 269 (1977) 149.
7. Humes, J. L., Cupo, J. J., Jr., and Strausser, H. R., Prostaglandins, 6 (1974) 463.
8. Humes, J. L., Kehl, F. A., Jr., Davies, P. and Bonney, R. J., Fed. Proc., 37 (1978) 1318.
9. Humes, J. L. and Strausser, H. R., Prostaglandins, 5 (1974) 183.
10. Jaffe, B. M., Behrman, H. R. and Parker, C. W., J. Clin. Invest., 52 (1973) 398.
11. Lamberson, H. V., Jr. and Fritz, K. E., Arch. Path., 98 (1974) 9.
12. Lattime, E. and Strausser, H. R., Science, 198 (1977) 302.
13. Levine, L., Hinkle, P. M., Voelkel, E. F. and Tashjian, A. H., Biochem. Biophys. Res. Comm., 47 (1972) 888.

14. Pelus, L. M., Rosenstein, M. M. and Strausser, H. R., (1978) in preparation.
15. Pelus, L. M. and Strausser, H. R., Int. J. Cancer, 18 (1976) 653.
16. Plescia, O. J., Smith, A. H. and Grinwich, K. K., Proc. Nat. Acad. Sci. (USA), 72 (1975) 1848.
17. Prince, A. M. and Trepo, C., Lancet I (1971) 1309.
18. Rosenstein, M. M., Pelus, L. M. and Strausser, H. R., Fed. Proc., 37 (1978) 1451.
19. Santoro, M. G., Philpott, G. W. and Jaffe, B. M., Nature, 263 (1976) 777.
20. Santoro, M. G., Philpott, G. W. and Jaffe, B. M., Prostaglandins, 14 (1977) 645.
21. Strausser, H. R. and Humes, J. L., Int. J. Cancer, 15 (1975) 724.
22. Stuttman, O., Adv. Cancer Res., 22 (1975) 261.
23. Teague, P. O., Yunis, E. J., Rodney, G., Fish, A. J., Stuttman, O. and Good, R. A., Laboratory Invest., 22 (1970) 121.
24. Unanue, E. R., Dixon, F. J. and Feldman, J. D., Experimental Immunologic Diseases of the Kidney (Ed. P. A. Meischer and H. J. Muller-Eberhard), Grune and Stratton, New York, (1976) 231.
25. Warchalowski, G. A. and Strausser, H. R., (1978) submitted for publication.
26. Winchester, R. J., Kunkel, H. G. and Agnello, V., J. Exp. Med., 134 (1971) 286s.

SUPPRESSOR MONOCYTES IN HUMAN DISEASE: A REVIEW

G. P. SCHECHTER[1], L. M. WAHL[2] and J. J. OPPENHEIM[2]

Hematology Section, Veterans Administration Hospital
and George Washington University[1], Washington, D. C. (USA)
National Institute of Dental Research, National Institute
of Health[2], Bethesda, Maryland (USA)

Recent results in experimental animals have suggested that macrophages may act as suppressors of the immune response in a wide variety of situations (12,13,18,25). Suppression of mitogen and antigen-induced lymphoproliferation by macrophages has been observed in lymphocyte cultures from animals bearing large tumor burdens, infected with bacteria and viruses, or undergoing graft vs host reactions (18). There is a growing literature describing similar suppression by monocytes and macrophages in human diseases due to an equally wide variety of causes (2,3,8,11,15,16,22,23,27, 28,30). Table I lists some of the reports which implicate suppressor macrophages in human disease. Included are the tumors of lympho-reticular origin such as Hodgkin's disease (18,23) and multiple myeloma (3), solid tumors such as lung cancer (2,30) and chronic infections and granulomatous diseases such as tuberculosis (22), disseminated fungal diseases (27) and sarcoidosis (11), and autoimmune diseases such as lupus erythematosus (16). It has also been suggested that suppressor monocytes are present in the blood of healthy individuals at lower concentrations and may increase with aging (15). Deficiences in cell mediated immunity and lymphopenia are often found, in these conditities associated with suppressor macrophages, and therefore, the cause and effect relationship of suppressive macrophages to defective cell mediated immunity will be discussed.

METHODS FOR DETECTION OF SUPPRESSOR MONOCYTES

Suppressor monocytes have been detected predominantly with assays of T cell function such as mitogen-induced blastogenesis or the mixed leukocyte reaction (Table I). An exception is

TABLE I

Suppressor Monocytes Associated with Human Diseases

Authors	Assay	Diseases
1. Twomey, 1975 Laughter, 1977	↓MLR stimulation	Hodgkin's disease (16/30) [a]
2. Schechter, 1976, 1978	Antigen-, mitogen-induced proliferation; LAF production	Hodgkin's disease (5/12) Tuberculosis (3/5)
3. Goodwin, 1977	Indomethacin sensitive inhibition of PHA-induced proliferation	Hodgkin's disease (6)
4. Broder, 1975	PWM-induced antibody synthesis	Multiple myeloma (3/6)
5. Berlinger, 1976	↓MLR stimulation	Non-lymphoid malignancy (11)
6. Zembala, 1977	Con A and PHA-induced protein synthesis of cocultures with normal cells	Non-lymphoid malignancy (15/27)
7. Stobo, 1977	Monokine inhibition of mitogen- and antigen-induced proliferation	Disseminated fungal infection (5)
8. Katz, 1978	PWM-induced antibody synthesis	Sarcoidosis (10/12)
9. Markenson, 1978	Mitogen-induced proliferation	Lupus erythematosus (14/32)

[a] Number of patients showing evidence of inhibition/number tested.

the observation by Broder et al. (3) of the in vitro suppression of pokeweed mitogen (PWM)-induced polyclonal immunoglobulin synthesis by peripheral blood monocytes of patients with myeloma. Depletion of monocytes from the peripheral blood mononuclear cells by carbonyl iron ingestion restored polyclonal immunoglobulin synthesis. Recently, Katz and Fauci (27) also reported monocyte inhibition of polyclonal antibody synthesis in sarcoidosis. Since both of these assays of B cell function are T cell dependent, it is not clear whether both T and B cells are sensitive directly to suppression by monocytes or whether the effect on B cells is an indirect result of inhibition of T helper cell function.

In many of the reports cited above suppressor monocytes have been detected by demonstrating that the mitogen-induced responses of unfractionated mononuclear cell populations are enhanced by the removal of glass-adherent or phagocytic cells (2,3,11,16,22,23,30). An example of this kind of experiment using the mononuclear cells of 2 patients with advanced active Hodgkin's disease is shown in Table II. Prior to monocyte depletion the reactivity of phytohemagglutinin (PHA)-stimulated cultures equalled that of cultures incubated without mitogen. After monocyte depletion by carbonyl iron ingestion striking enhancement of PHA-induced ^{3}H-thymidine uptake occurred in the mononuclear cell cultures from patient 1. This finding indicated that the patient's T lymphocytes were capable of responding in the normal range. Monocyte depletion resulted in a more modest increase in the PHA response of the cells from the second patient. The suppressive effect of macrophages tended to disappear when the patients were treated sucessfully with chemotherapy (Table II).

Morphological studies of the suppressed cultures correlated well with the thymidine incorporation data. Only a few lymphoblasts were found in the unfractionated mononuclear cell (monocyte-rich) cultures whereas large numbers of lymphoblasts were seen in the monocyte-depleted cultures in these patients. Therefore, it is unlikely that the decrease in thymidine uptake in the monocyte-rich cultures was due merely to excess cold thymidine in the medium, a mechanism previously suggested for macrophage suppression of lymphocyte proliferation (19).

The monocyte-depletion experiments described above offer circumstantial evidence that the suppression noted is monocyte-mediated. Further support for this hypothesis comes from the findings that the suppressing cells have been resistant to radiation (2,3,11,15,22,23,28) and corticosteroids (11). Direct evidence that the macrophage is the suppressor cell is provided by experiments in which lymphoproliferation has been inhibited by the addition of purified populations of macrophages (23,30). The suppressive effect of irradiated mononuclear leukocytes or of purified adherent cells (>99% macrophages) from 2 patients with

TABLE II

Effect of Monocyte Depletion on PHA induced
Blastogenesis of Peripheral Blood Mononuclear
Cells (MNL) in Advanced Hodgkin's Disease

Subjects	Clinical Status	^{3}H-thymidine Incorporation[a] (DPS)	
		Unfractionated MNL	Monocyte-depleted MNL
B.S.	(a) IVA, relapse	150	3450
	(b) partial response	2050	2030
C.D.	(a) IVB, untreated	230	770
	(b) partial response	2700	1220
Normal Control	– –	3110	3950

[a]Mononuclear cells containing 2×10^5 lymphocytes were cultured in 0.2 ml, with 1 μgm/ml PHA. 1 μCi ^{3}H-thymidine was added for 4 hr on the 3rd day of culture. Mean disintegrations per second of ^{3}H-thymidine uptake by triplicate cultures are shown. S.E.M. are <20% of the mean. ^{3}H-thymidine incorporation without PHA was <60 DPS (23).

Hodgkin's disease on the PHA responses of moncyte-depleted peripheral blood mononuclear cells is shown in Fig. 1.

A number of investigators (2,3,28,30) have successfully demonstrated suppressor cells in patients' mononuclear cells by their ability to inhibit the responses of normal cells (Table I). However, as illustrated in Fig. 1, we have not been able to inhibit the response of normal lymphocytes using mononuclear cells or macrophages from patients with demonstrated inhibition of autologous lymphocyte proliferation. Katz and Fauci (11), were also unable to demonstrate suppression of PWM induced antibody synthesis of allogeneic cells by mononuclear cells from patients with sarcoidosis. These contradictory findings may stem from technical differences such as differing cell concentrations or ratios. Alternatively macrophage suppression may be mediated by a number of differing mechanisms which are singled out by a particular assay. An important possibility is that impaired lymphocytes or different subpopulations may be more readily suppressed by macrophages.

CHARACTERIZATION OF SUPPRESSOR MONOCYTES

The distinctions between monocytes which suppress and those which potentiate lymphocyte responses are only beginning to be elucidated. However, it is not clear whether monocyte populations consist of a mixture of heterogeneous cells with differing functions or whether the heterogeneity of function represents differing states of activation or concentrations of a homogeneous population. Both quantitative and qualitative differences between suppressor monocytes and normal monocytes have been demonstrated. Suppressive mononuclear cell populations often contain increased concentrations of monocytes (16,23) and the suppressor activity per monocyte may be increased in comparison with equal mumbers of normal monocytes (23). Normal monocytes have also been shown to be capable of suppressing lymphocyte responses in the mixed leukocyte reaction but only when added in high concentrations (15). This finding favors the view that monocyte suppression is a quantitative phenomenon, i.e. that monocytes in excess will result in suppression. Alternatively, suppressive monocytes may be members of a very small subpopulation of monocytes in normal individuals which is stimulated to increase by certain diseases.

A number of investigators (9,16,23) have detected increased mumbers of monocytes in the leukocyte cultures from their patients with low blastogenic responses. This finding is not unexpected since many of the diseases associated with monocyte suppressive activity demonstrate a high incidence of peripheral blood lymphopenia and relative monocytosis. In our series of patients with advanced Hodgkin's disease (23) those individuals with monocyte

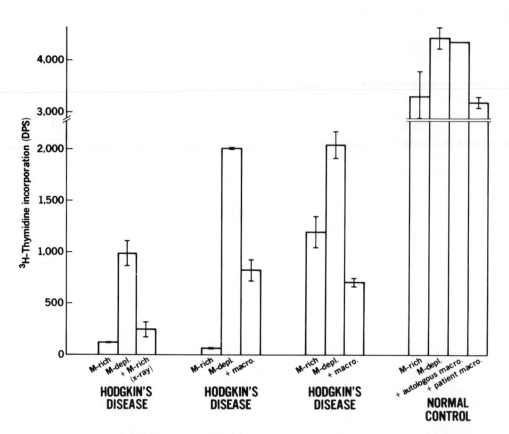

Fig. 1. PHA-induced blastogenesis of mononuclear cells before and after monocyte depletion from two patients with Hodgkin's disease and a normal control. "M-rich" refers to unfractionated mononuclear cells; "M-depl" are mononuclear cells partially depleted of monocytes by carbonyl iron treatment. The effect of the addition of autologous irradiated (3000R) to monocyte-depleted cells("+M-rich x-ray") is shown in panel 1. The effect of the addition of 3 x 10^4 autologous adherent cells (>99% macrophages) to monocyte-depleted cells is shown in panels 2 through 4 ("+Macro"). The last column in panel 4 shows the result of the addition of macrophages from the patient in panel 3 to normal monocyte-depleted cells. ^{3}H-thymidine incorporation of cells without PHA in all cases including the allogeneic mixture of normal lymphocytes and patient macrophages was less than 20 DPS. Mean DPS ± 1 SD of duplicate or triplicate cultures are shown (See Table I for method).

suppressor activity had significantly higher percentage of monocytes in their mononuclear cell preparations (38.5% vs 12.6% for
the normal subjects p<.001) (23). This monocytosis was the result of a profoundly depressed peripheral blood lymphocyte/
monocyte ratio due to marked lymphopenia. In the patients with
monocyte inhibitory activity the peripheral blood lymphocyte/
monocyte ratio was 0.6 as compared to 1.9 for patients whose cells
did not show suppressor activity (p<.01) and 4.4 for normal subjects (p<,001). Thus our findings suggest that lymphopenia may
be a contributory factor to macrophage inhibitory activity and
that the consequent increase in the ratios of macrophages to
lymphocytes may facilitate its expression.

Although a relative increase in monocytes is often found in
suppressive mononuclear cells, this is not invariable, suggesting
that suppression results from quantitative as well as quantitative differences between normal and suppressive monocytes. Several investigators have noted no differences in the percentage
of monocytes in the mononuclear cell populations of patients
with macrophage suppressor activity as compared to normal subjects (8,11,27). Furthermore, where quantitative differences
exist, qualitative differences in macrophages often can also be
demonstrated. Table III illustrates an experiment involving a
patient with tuberculosis who manifested monocyte suppressor
activity which was initially thought to be related to the high
numbers of monocytes in the cultures. However, fractionation
experiments indicated a qualitative difference as well. Whereas
the addition of 15,000 irradiated macrophages inhibited the PPD
response of the patient's monocyte depleted cells, the same number of normal macrophages potentiated the lymphoproliferative
response of cells from a PPD-skin test-positive healthy subject.
Significant suppression by normal macrophages of autologous lymphocytes was not seen until 6×10^4 normal macrophages were
added to the cultures. Fig. 1 shows similar results in two patients with Hodgkin's disease indicating qualitative differences
between suppressor and normal macrophages.

RELATIONSHIP OF LAF PRODUCTION TO MONOCYTE SUPPRESSION

In an attempt to define further the lymphocyte-macrophage
interactions in patients with monocytes which exhibit suppressor
activity we have examined the ability of their monocytes to stimulate lymphoproliferation through the production of lymphocyte
activating factor (LAF). This factor is a protein of 12,000 to
20,000 molecular weight which is found in the supernatants of
mononuclear cell cultures and is mitogenic for thymocytes (6,7).
Its production is potentiated by agents which stimulate macrophages (such as lymphokines, lipopolysaccharide, or lymphocytes
activated by PHA) suggesting that it has a potentially important

TABLE III

Addition of Irradiated Macrophages to PPD-Stimulated Lymphocyte Cultures

Cells	No. Autologous[b] Irradiated Macrophages	^{3}H-Thymidine Incorporation (DPS)	
		TB Patient	Normal Control
Unfractionated MNL[a]	–	270	1690
Monocyte-depleted MNL[a]	–	9100	580
" " "	15,000	6980	1870
" " "	30,000	1910	1530
" " "	60,000	1170	470

[a]The unfractionated MNL from the patient and control contained 35% or 210,000 and 14% or 65,000 monocytes, respectively. The monocyte-depleted fraction contained 2% or 8200 monocytes. Each culture contained 400,000 lymphocytes in 0.2 ml with 1 μgm PPD/ml, and was incubated for 4 days and ^{3}H-thymidine uptake of triplicate cultures was assayed. SEM was less than 10% of the mean.

[b]Leukocytes were irradiated with 3000R and cultured for 7 days, yielding a preparation of >99% macrophages (21).

role in the bidirectional amplification of T cell-macrophage interaction (6,7). We have found that LAF activity is severely depressed
in the mononuclear cell cultures of certain patients with monocyte
suppressor activity (24). Five of 12 patients with Hodgkin's
disease and 1 of 4 patients with tuberculosis had significantly depressed PHA-induced LAF production, and 3 of these 6 produced less
LAF in response to LPS as well. Monocytes from five of these
patients had previously been shown to suppress blastogenesis. Only
1 patient whose mononuclear cells produced normal LAF levels had
monocyte suppressor activity.

The decrease in LAF activity in the monocyte-rich cell cultures may be due a) suppression of T cell function which is required to potentiate LAF production b) primarily impaired macrophage function or c) excessive production of a soluble inhibitor.
Since PHA-induced LAF production is a T cell-dependent function,
the decrease noted in our patients may reflect the impaired T cell
function in these patients. However, LPS-induced LAF activity which
is T cell independent, was at times severely depressed, suggesting
a defect at the monocyte level as well. The profound deficiency of
LAF activity in the cultures of one such patient with Hodgkin's
disease and a second patient with tuberculosis, both of whose cultures also exhibited suppressor monocyte activity is shown in
Table IV.

Efforts to detect a soluble inhibitor of LAF have not been
successful. However, LAF production could be increased significantly in these patients' cell cultures by two maneuvers, a) decreasing the cell density and b) monocyte depletion. In contrast
when these two maneuvers were applied to normal cells there was
little change or a fall in LAF activity (Fig. 2). Monocyte-
depletion in case of the patient with Hodgkin's disease also resulted in a striking rise in LAF production by unstimulated cultures (Fig. 2) which suggests that the remaining monocytes were
in an activated state. In experimental animals such as nude mice
increased levels of spontaneously produced LAF have been noted to
be associated with certain states of activation (2). The suppression of LAF production at high monocyte density suggests that cell
contact was an important factor in this inhibition. Another possibility is that intact T cell function may be more important than
previously realized in spontaneous and LPS-induced LAF generation
in these patients' cultures. Removal of suppressor monocytes could
have allowed T cell dependent LAF production by the residual monocytes to proceed. A third consideration is the inhibitory effect
of excess prostaglandin production by the unfractionated mononuclear cell cultures of patients with suppressor monocytes.

TABLE IV

LAF Activity in Supernatants of Mononuclear Cells
From Two Patients with Macrophage Suppression[a]

Stimu-lants	Dose (ug/ml)	Mean CPM of ^{3}H-Thymidine Incorporation of Mouse Thymocytes Incubated with 1:8 Dilution of MNL Supernatants		
		Normal Control	Hodgkin's Patient	Tuberculosis Patient
None	–	2130	140	100
LPS	50	13,080	110	150
PPD	100	2350	150	110
"	10	8700	140	160
"	1	7370	–	100
PHA	2	28,470	170	410

[a]Human unfractionated mononuclear cells were cultured for 24 hr in 95% RPMI 1640/5% fetal calf serum mixture with or without a stimulant. A 1:8 dilution of the supernatant medium of the MNL cultures was then cultured with thymocytes from C_3H-H_eJ mice for 72 hr. ^{3}H-thymidine incorporation of triplicate cultures was assayed. SEM were less than 20% of the mean.

TABLE V

PGE Production By Mononuclear Cells (MNL)[a]

	Cells x 10^6	Monocytes x 10^6	PGE (pg/ml) in Supernatant Medium	
			No stimulants	LPS
Hodgkin's				
P.S.	1.5	.31	12,580	20,800
B.S.	1.5	.90	1344	20,910
Normal	1.5	.30	280	1680
Control	4.5	.90	1680	1690

[a]Unfractionated MNL were cultured for 24 hr in RPMI 1640. Supernatant medium was assayed for PGE by a radioimmunoassay sensitive to PGE_1 and PGE_2 (29).

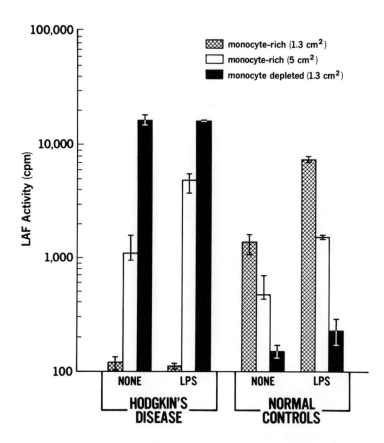

Fig. 2.   Effect of cell density and monocyte depletion of LAF
activity of mononuclear cells from a Hodgkin's disease patient
and a normal control.   "Monocyte-rich" cells are unfractionated
mononuclear cells (MNL); MNL were partially depleted on monocytes
by carbonyl iron treatment.   MNL were cultured over a 1.3 cm^2 or
5 cm^2 area.   (See Table IV for method).

ROLE OF PROSTAGLANDINS IN SUPPRESSION BY MONOCYTES

In 1977 Goodwin et al (8) demonstrated that addition of
prostaglandin synthesis inhibitors such as indomethacin to the
suppressed mononuclear cell cultures from Hodgkin's disease
patients resulted in enhancement of PHA-induced blastogenesis to
the level of normal control cultures.   They also noted elevated
levels of prostaglandin E were present in the supernatants of these
patient's cultures.   Removal of glass adherent cells blocked the

enhancement of blastogenesis by indomethacin. This finding is consistent with the data that macrophages are the main source of the secreted prostaglandins (10,14). Thus prostaglandin E secreted by macrophages became an excellent candidate for the soluble suppressive material which exerts its inhibiting influence across allogeneic lines.

Using a radioimmunoassay, we have also detected significantly elevated levels of prostaglandins of the E series in the LPS- and PHA-stimulated culture supernatants of our patients with advanced Hodgkin's disease (24). The PGE levels are greater than can simply be accounted for by the numbers of monocytes in the cultures (Table V). The relationship between the supernatant PGE levels and inhibition of blastogenesis and LAF production was reinforced by the observations that the experimental conditions that corrected the suppression were associated with decreases in PGE levels. Furthermore, the direct addition of PGE or dibutyryl cyclic AMP to normal mononuclear cells in vitro can be shown to inhibit LPS-induced LAF production particularly at low cell concentrations (24).

However, we have made several observations which suggest that PGE may not be entirely responsible for macrophage mediated suppression or deficient LAF production: a) while certain patients exhibiting marked macrophage suppression of blastogenesis produced very high levels of prostaglandins, this finding was not invariable. Only 2 of 5 patients whose cultures showed suppressor macrophage activity had markedly elevated levels of PGE, and the remaining 3 had only slightly elevated levels. Conversely markedly elevated levels of PGE were found in the cultures of one of three patients who did not show suppressor macrophage activity; b) incubation of monocyte-rich mononuclear cells with indomethacin in our hands as usually been associated with a further fall in LAF production or no change; c) although indomethacin reduced the PGE concentration to very low levels, indomethacin treatment of unfractionated monocyte-rich cells was not as effective as monocyte-depletion in restoring T cell reactivity (Table V). These findings suggest that the effects of PGE on macrophage function are secondary, late events and that other mechanisms in addition to prostaglandin inhibition of lymphoproliferation may be involved in macrophage mediated suppression.

The role of deficient LAF production in the cultures of patients with monocyte suppressor activity probably also represents a secondary event. Suppression of blastogenesis by monocytes could conceivably result from deficient LAF production if, for example, baseline lymphocyte function has an absolute requirement for a minimum amount of LAF activity. However, the relationship between deficient LAF production and monocyte suppression of blastogenesis was not constant; therefore, it is more likely that

TABLE VI

Indomethacin vs Monocyte Depletion in PHA-Induced Lymphocyte Blastogenesis[a]

Subjects	Unfractionated Cells (MNL)	^{3}H-Thymidine Incorporation (DPS)	
		MNL + Indomethacin 10^{-5}M	Monocyte depleted MNL
Hodgkin's disease Untreated			
1. CD IV B	230	540 (+135%)[b]	770 (+235%)
2. LW IV A	1360	1940 (+42%)	2160 (+59%)
Relapsed or Stable			
3. BS IV A	480	470 (−2%)	1300 (+170%)
4. PS IV A	1290	1470 (+14%)	1880 (+46%)
Normal Controls			
1.	3110	5320 (+71%)	3950 (+27%)
2.	4950	3930 (−23%)	6760 (+36%)
3.	6490	6540 (+1%)	4000 (−26%)

[a]See footnotes to Table II.
[b]Figures in parenthesis represent percent increase.

the LAF deficiency was a result of impaired T cell function, rather than the cause.

IN VIVO SIGNIFICANCE OF SUPPRESSOR MONOCYTES

The relationship of in vitro macrophage suppressor activity to deficient immune reactivity in vivo is not clear. Although suppression has been noted predominantly in acquired immune deficiency states, a number of findings raise questions about its in vivo relevance. For example, although all of the patients with Hodgkin's disease and suppressor macrophage activity that we studied were also anergic, the patients with tuberculosis and in vitro suppressor activity all manifested normal delayed hypersensitivity in the form of positive skin test responses to PPD-tuberculin (8,23). Monocyte-mediated suppression of polyclonal immunoglobulin synthesis provides an attractive hypothesis to explain the antibody deficiency found in patients with multiple myeloma (3). However, similar suppression of polyclonal antibody synthesis has also been observed in patients with sarcoidosis who have hypergammaglobulinemia and increased levels of specific antibodies (11). Presumably, suppressor macrophages can contribute to in vivo anergy but until indomethacin treatment or another means of inhibiting suppressor macrophages also restores delayed hypersensitivity and/or immunoglobulin synthesis, the in vivo role of these cells must remain unresolved.

In experimental animals the macrophage has been shown to play an important role as an effector of tumor immunity (5). While evidence for this function in man is small at present, it is possible that the tumor cytostatic effect of macrophages from patients with Hodgkin's disease and non-lymphoid malignancies is inadvertently directed against T lymphocytes. It should be emphasized that all of the studies of suppressor macrophages in human beings have been done with peripheral blood mononuclear cells. No studies of splenic, lymph node, or more importantly tumor-associated macrophages have been performed. Of interest, in this regard, is the finding of Alexander et al. (1) that delayed hypersensitivity (skin test reactivity) was most severely impaired in tumor-bearing animals who had the largest numbers of macrophages in their tumors. Animals with few macrophages in tumors had less frequent impairment in delayed hypersensitivity, but had a greater incidence of metastases. In this context, it is possible to consider that suppressor macrophages in the host with malignancy may be important in antitumor defenses despite suppressive effects on immune function.

SUMMARY

Suppressor monocytes have been found in a number of human diseases most of which are associated with lymphopenia and deficiences in cell mediated immunity. In our studies both quantitative and qualitative differences in monocytes were detected in certain patients with advanced Hodgkin's disease or tuberculosis. In certain patients lymphocyte activating factor production by monocytes was severely depressed in part secondary to decreased activation by suppressed T cells, although at times primary impairment of macrophage function was also probably contributory. Mononuclear cell cultures from patients with advanced Hodgkin's disease also manifested excessive prostaglandin secretion; however, the association of this with monocyte suppression and deficient LAF production was inconstant. Furthermore, reversibility of monocyte suppression could not regularly be achieved by inhibition of prostaglandin synthetase with indomethacin suggesting that excessive production of prostaglandins is unlikely to be the sole mechanism of monocyte inhibition of lymphoproliferation. It also remains to be established whether the inhibition of lymphoproliferation in vitro is important to in vivo delayed hypersensitivity or whether the mechanism is related to other macrophage effects such as tumor cytostasis and cytolysis.

ACKNOWLEDGEMENT

We wish to acknowledge the excellent technical assistance of Frances Soehnlen, Suanne Dougherty and Charles Carter, Jr., and John E. Jones. G. P. Schechter is supported by Medical Research Service of the Veterans Administration (USA).

REFERENCES

1. Alexander, P., Eccles, S. A., Gauci, C. L. L., Annals of N. Y., Acad. of Sci., 276 91976) 124.
2. Berlinger, N. T., Lopez, C. and Good, R. A., Nature (Lond) 260 (1976) 145.
3. Broder, S., Humphrey, R., Durm, M., Blackman, M., Meade, B., Goldman, C., Strober, W. and Waldmann, T., New Engl. J. Med., 293 (1975) 887.
4. Cassileth, P. A., In: Hematology (Ed. W. J. Williams et al.), McGaw Hill, New York (1977) 972.
5. Evans, R., and Alexander, P., In: Immunobiology of the Macrophage (Ed. D. S. Nelson), Academic Press, New York (1976) 535.
6. Gery, I., Gershon, R. K., and Waksman, B. H., J. Exp. Med., 136 (1972) 128.
7. Gery, I., and Waksman, B. H., J. Exp. Med., 136 (1972) 143.
8. Goodwin, J. S., Messner, R. P., Bankhurst, A. D., Peake, G.

T., Saiki, J. H. and Williams, R. C., Jr., New Engl. J. Med., 297 (1977) 963.

9. Hersh, E. M., Oppenheim, J. J., New Engl. J. Med. 273 (1965) 1006.

10. Humes, J. L., Bonney, R. J., Pelus, L., Dahlgren, M. E., Sadowski, S. J., Kuehl, F. A., Jr., and Davies, P., Nature, 269 (1977) 149.

11. Katz, P., Fauci, A. S., Clin. Exp. Immunol., (1978) in press.

12. Keller, R., Cell Immunol., 17 (1975) 542.

13. Kirchner, H., Muchmore, A. V., Chused, T. M., Holden, H. T., and Herberman, R. B., J. Immunol. 114 (1975) 206.

14. Kurland, J. I., Bockman, R., J. Exp. Med., 147 (1978) 952.

15. Laughter, A. H. and Twomey, J. J., J. Immunol. 119 (1977) 173.

16. Markenson, J. A., Morgan, J. W., Lockshin, M. D., Joachim, C., and Winfield, J. B., Proc. Soc. Exp. Biol. Med. 158 (1978) 5.

17. Meltzer, M. S., Oppenheim, J. J., J. immunol., 118 91977) 77.

18. Nelson, D. S., In: Immunobiology of the Macrophage (Ed. D. S. Nelson), Academic Press, New York (1976) 235.

19. Opitz, H. G., Niethammer, D., Lemke, H., Flad, H. D., and Huget, R., Cell. Immunol., 16 (1975) 379.

20. Oppenheim, J. J., Unpublished observations.

21. Schechter, G. P. and McFarland, W., J. Immunol., 105 (1970) 661.

22. Schechter, G. P., and Soehnlen, F., Blood, 48 (1976) 988.

23. Schechter, G. P. and Soehnlen, F., Blood 52 (1978) 261.

24. Schechter, G. P., Wahl, L., Oppenheim, J. J., in preparation.

25. Scott, M. T., Cell Immunol., 5 (1972) 469.

26. Stobo, J. D., Paul, S., Vanscoy, R., Herman, P., J. C. I., 57 (1976) 319.

27. Stobo, J. D., J. Immunol., 119 (1977) 918.

28. Twomey, J. J., Laughter, A. H., Farrow, S., and Douglass, C. C., J.C.I., 56 (1975) 467.

29. Wahl, L. M., Olsen, C. E., Wahl, S. M., Sandberg, A. L., Mergenhagen, S. E., In: Mechanisms of Localized Bone Loss Calcium Tissue Abstracts (Special Supplement) Information Retrieval Co., Washington, D. C. (1978) 181.

30. Zembala, M., Mytar, B., Popiela, T. and Asherson, G. L., Int. J. Cancer, 19 (1977) 605.

SUPPRESSOR CELL DEFECT IN PSORIASIS

D. N. SAUDER, P. L. BAILIN, and S. KRAKAUER

Departments of Dermatology and Immunology
Cleveland Clinic Foundation
Cleveland, Ohio (USA)

Psoriasis is a common chronic, intractable skin disease affecting 1-3% of the world's population (15). In the United States it affects an estimated 6-8 million persons with an annual cost approaching one billion dollars (21). Psoriasis is a disorder of epidermal-cell proliferation. The histologic hallmark of this disease is a collection of neutrophils in the stratum corneum (12) or stratum malpigii known as a spongioform pustule of Kogoj. This influx of neutrophils may then stimulate the epidermal change (13). While the etiology of psoriasis is unknown, recent studies suggest that autoimmunity may be involved in its pathogenesis (1, 8). Autoantibodies have been identified in patients with psoriasis (2,3,6,11,14). Rimbaud et al. (14) for example have demonstrated anti-IgG activity on the surface membrane of peripheral lymphocytes in patients with psoriasis. Anti-stratum corneum antibodies deposited with C3 and C4 have been found in patients with psoriasis (11). These autoantibodies are present in the sera of normal individuals as well as psoriasis patients; however, they are not bound with stratum corneum antigen in either the skin of normal patients or in the uninvolved skin of psoriasis patients (10). It is possible that the stratum corneum antigens normally have no contact with the immune system and hence do not bind to circulating antibodies; it is also possible that altered antigenicity of stratum corneum antigen is necessary for antigen binding and immune complex binding. Rheumatoid-like factors have been identified in IgA and IgG classes of immunoglobulins in psoriasis patients (3,6). Other immune abnormalities identified as psoriasis include increased serum IgG and IgA (the latter correlating somewhat with the extent of the disease), and increase in salivary IgA and an increase in serum IgE has been found in a significant number of

patients (6). Using immunofluorescence techniques Cormane (2)
has identified antinuclear antibody which reacts with nuclei
of the basal cell layer of uninvolved skin in patients with psoriasis. T cell dysfunction has also been reported in psoriasis
patients (4,7). Guilhou (7) reported a decrease T cell number as
assessed by E-rossetes and antiheterologous anti-human T lymphocyte anti-serum, and a decreased mitogen response to concanavalin
A. This T cell defect was further substantiated by Glinski et
al.(4). Furthermore serum thymic factor levels were increased in
psoriasis (7). Gross et al.(5) found a significantly greater migration inhibition in psoriatic patients as compared to controls.

In view of the findings of autoantibodies and a possible T
cell defect, it is postulated that the immunologic deficit may
reside with T cell regulation of the immune system. It was therefore undertaken to determine if a suppressor cell defect was present in psoriasis that might account for the above findings.
While we postulated primarily a lack of T cell suppression on B
cell function, we in fact measured a T cell on T cell suppression.
However, there is precedence for this hypothesis in systemic lupus
erythematosus. Talal et al.(18) measured loss of T cell on T cell
suppression and then speculated that loss of T cell suppression of
B cell function existed. This was substantiated by Krakauer et al.
(9).

Suppression of a one way mixed lymphocyte culture (MLC) was
therefore measured. A single cell put in tissue culture will not
incorporate DNA or undergo blast formation. This cell, "RESPONDER"
cell, will however 'respond' or undergo blast formation if it is
stimulated by another cell, "STIMULATOR" cell. If DNA synthesis
is measured (by thymidine incorporation) in the above system, one
would be unable to tell whether the stimulator cell or responder
cell is undergoing blast transformation. The stimulator cell is
therefore irradiated. This still allows the cell to participate
in the MLC as a stimulator cell but the cell can no longer incorporate DNA or undergo blast formation. This reaction can be regulated by another cell, "REGULATOR" cell. Again the regulator
cell is irradiated. This still enables it to regulate the above
reaction but it will no longer be able to undergo blast formation.
When the regulator cell is placed in the above MLC no inhibition
takes place and the responder cell incorporates DNA. If, however,
the regulator cell is pretreated with concanavalin A - a known T
cell mitogen, this one way MLC inhibited and DNA synthesis is
decreased. However, when cells from psoriasis patients are used
as con A treatment regulator cells DNA synthesis and blast transformation occurs i.e. no suppression.

MATERIALS AND METHODS

Separation of Cells: Peripheral blood mononuclear cells from normal volunteers and patients with active psoriasis receiving no systemic therapy were separated by centrifugation through a Ficoll-Hypaque gradient.

Mixed Lymphocyte Culture: Stimulator cells (1×10^5 in 0.1 ml) were inactivated with 4000 Rads of X-irradiation and cultured with a like number of like volume of responding cells in RPMI-1640 with 15% heat inactivated pooled human plasma. (1×10^5) (0.1 ml) of irradiated (4000 Rads) "regulator" cells were added at initiation of this culture. After a five day culture period, cells were "pulsed" with triated Thymidine (1 microCurie) for 4 1/2 hr, harvested in a MASH II automated harvester and counted in an NCS Mark I Liquid scintillation counter peaked for tritium.

Regular Cells: Putative suppressor cells from normals or patients with active psoriasis receiving no systemic therapy were separated from whole blood as above. The cells were cultured at 3×10^6/cc in 1 ml of RPMI 1640 with penicillin, streptomycin, glutamine and 15% heat inactivated AB serum. Cultures were carried out for 48 hr at 37 C in a 5% CO_2 atmosphere. Suppressor cells were generated by the addition of 40 µg of Con A/cc. Control regulator cells were cultured in a like manner without Con A. At the termination of these cultures, the cells were washed three times and given 4000 Rads of irradiation (so they could not undergo blast transformation) before addition to the one way MLC described above. These regulator cells and both allogenic and autologous suppression were therefore studied.

RESULTS

The results are shown in Table I. It can be seen that patients with psoriasis possess lymphocytes that do not respond to concanavalin A stimulation by suppressing mixed lymphocyte reactions as compared to lymphocytes from normals. When the regulator cells are autologous to the responding cells, Con A pulsed cells from untreated psoriasis patients suppress 2.9 ± 18.7%. This difference is significant ($p<0.01$). When the responder cells are allogeneic to the regulator cells, Con A pulsed lymphocytes from patients with untreated psoriasis suppress the mixed lymphocyte reaction 6.2 ± 25.9%. Con A pulsed lymphocytes from normal individuals on the other hand suppress the same reaction 45.6 ± 16.4%. This difference is also significant ($p<0.025$). In both the patients and normals lymphocyte blast transformation as measured by ^{3}H-thymidine incorporation does occur to Con A and in unregulated one-way mixed lymphocyte cultures; however, in

the numbers of patients we studied the difference between these
two groups is not significant.

DISCUSSION

Normal lymphocytes differentiate along at least two cell
lines: those that develop along the thymic pathway. T cells,
and those that develop along the bursal equivalent pathway, B
cells. B cells further differentiate into plasma cells which
then secrete immunoglobulins. Although T cells do not secrete
immunoglobulin they control cell mediated immunity and play a
critical role in regulating the maturation and differentiation of
B cells and other T cells. There are at least two different
types of regulator T cells, helper cells and suppressor cells.
Excessive suppression can be a major factor in hypogammaglobuli-
nemia (20) while lack of suppression can lead to autoantibody
formation (9). Suppression can be nonspecific or idiotypic in
which situation suppression is only for certain antibody forming
cells (19).

Con A stimulated lymphocytes from patients with psoriasis
demonstrate a significant decrease in their ability to suppress
a mixed lymphocyte reaction as compared to normals (Table I).
The implication of this is unclear at the present time but the
following hypothesis is suggested. Since patients with psoriasis
do not manifest major clinical or laboratory evidence of autoimmunity such as immune complex nephritis, rheumatoid, arthritis,
autoimmune thyroiditis, pernicious anemia, serum antinuclear antibody, serum rheumatoid factor, etc., we postulate that an idiotypic suppression defect exists in patients with psoriasis. Such
lack of suppression on the humoral immune system could lead to
autoantibody production against skin antigens. This in turn
would lead to antigen-antibody complex formation, which would
stimulate the complement cascade leading to activation of C3a and
C5a. C3a and C5a being potent chemotactants, together with lyso-
mal enzyme release could lead to microabscess formation. Support
for this is gleaned from the fact that leukotactic factors have
been found in psoriatic scale (16,17). This in turn leads to
tissue damage, release of more antigen then further immune complex formation.

Lack of suppression on the cell-mediated immune system,
could increase lymphokine production, in particular migration inhibition which would enhance abscess formation. This in turn
could lead to the above tissue damage, release of more antigen,
then further immune complex formation and the cycle perpetuates
itself.

TABLE I

Con A Inducible Suppression in Peripheral Blood
Lymphocytes from Psoriasis Patients and Normal Controls

Control (C) / Patient (P)	C.P.M. in M.L.C. Reactions Incorporating Regulator Cell that were		% Suppression (1–Con A/ non–Con A) x100	Mean (±SD)
	Con A Pulsed	Non–Pulsed		
Autologous Regulators				
1-C	11,900	18,066	33.6	49.5
2-C	3,550	13,283	73.3	(18.7)
3-C	11,560	25,920	55.4	
4-C	731	1,137	33.4	
1-P	18,481	17,806	-3.8	
2-P	3,175	2,592	22.5	2.9
3-P	4,040	4,623	12.6	(21.3)
4-P	2,192	1,542	-42.2	
5-P	3,875	4,358	11.1	
6-P	11,917	12,975	8.9	
7-P	987	1100	10.9	
Allogeneic Regulators				
1-C	1,948	3,165	62.5	
2-C	4,137	9,482	56.4	45.6
3-C	7,917	11,042	28.3	(16.4)
4-C	660	1020	35.8	
1-P	25,023	29,064	13.9	
2-P	12,275	16,708	26.5	
3-P	9,117	13,325	31.6	6.2
4-P	4,780	4,871	1.8	(25.9)
5-P	25,950	17,610	-47.4	
6-P	5,653	6,078	7.0	
7-P	1237	1370	10.0	

CONCLUSION

We have demonstrated a significant lack of suppressor activity
in patients with psoriasis compared to normal controls and propose
a hypothesis to link this in a causal relationship with psoriasis.
While we have by no means demonstrated that this mechanism is
active in the pathogenesis of psoriasis, it nevertheless gives
support to the role of the immune system or immunoregulatory defects in psoriasis.

REFERENCES

1. Beutner, E. H., Chorzelski, T. P., Jablonska, S., Auto-
    immunity in Psoriasis (1) Studies on the possible signifi-
    cance of the universal stratum corneum antibodies in the
    pathogenesis of psoriasis. In: Psoriasis Proceedings of the
    Second International Symposium, (1976) 63.
2. Cormane, R. H., Asghar, S. S., J. Invest. Dermatol. 67 (1976)
    129.
3. Florin-Christensen, A., Maldonato Cocco, J. A., Arana, R.,
    Pomini, A., Mom, A., Garicia, Moreteo, O., Dermatologica 149
    (1974) 220.
4. Glinski, W., O'Balek, S., Langner, A., Jablonska, S., Haftek,
    M., J. Invest. Dermatol. 70 (1978) 105.
5. Gross, W. L., Packhauser, U., Hahn, G., et al, Br. J. Dermatol.
    97 (1977) 529.
6. Guilhou, J. J., Clot, J., Meynadier, J., Lapinski, H., Br. J.
    Dermatol, 94 (1976) 501.
7. Guilhou, J. J., Meynadier, J., Clot, J., Charmasson, E., Dar-
    denne, M., Brochier, J., Br. J. Bermatol. 95 (1976) 295.
8. Jablonska, S., Chorzelski, T. P., Beutner, E. H., Jarzabek-
    Chorzelska, M., Chowaniec, O., Maciejowska, E., Rzesa, G.,
    Autoimmunity in Psoriasis (11) Immunohistologic studies on
    various forms of psoriasis and the Koehner phenomenon, In:
    Psoriasis Proceedings of the Second International Symposium,
    (1976) 73.
9. Krakauer, R. S., Waldmann, T. A., Stroker, W., J. Exp. Med.
    144 (1976) 662.
10. Krogh, H. K., The significance of stratum corneum antibodies:
    An experimental model in guinea pigs, In: Psoriasis Proceed-
    ings of the Second International Symposium, Yorke Medical
    Books (1976) 55.
11. Krogh, H. K., Tonder, O., Scand. J. Immunol. 2 (1973) 42.
12. Lever, W. F., Schaumberg-Lever, G., Histopathology of the
    Skin, J. B. Lippincott Company, Toronto, (1975).
13. Pinkus, H., Mehregan, A. H., A Guide to Dermatohistopatho-
    pathology, Prentice-Hall, Inc., New York (1976).
14. Rimbaud, P., Meynadier, J., Guilhou, J. J., Clot, J., Arch.
    Dermatol. 108 (1973) 371.

15. Rook, A., Wilkinson, D. S., Ebling, F. J. G., Textbook of
     Dermatology, Blackwell Scientific Publishing, London,
     (1972) 1192.
16. Tagami, H., Ofuji, S., Br. J. Dermatol. 95 (1976) 1.
17. Tagmi, H., Ofuji, S., Br. J. Dermatol. 95 (1977) 509.
18. Talal, N., Steinberg, A. D., Curr. Top Microbiol. Immunol.
     64 (1974) 79.
19. Waldmann, T. A., Blaese, R. M., Broder, S., Krakauer, R. S.,
     Ann. Intern. Med. 88 (1978) 226.
20. Waldmann, T. A., Broder, S., Krakauer, R., et al., Fed. Proc.
     35 (1976) 2067.
21. Whedon, G. D. (Opening Remarks), Psoriasis Proceedings of
     the Second International Symposium, Yorke Medical Books,
     (1976) XXII.

STIMULATION OF THE RETICULOENDOTHELIAL SYSTEM AND AUTOIMMUNITY

J. I. MORTON and B. V. SIEGEL

University of Oregon Health Sciences Center
Portland, Oregon (USA)

The events leading to the development of autoimmune diseases in the New Zealand Black (NZB) strain mouse appear to have a genetic basis. Neonatally, these animals display an abnormally high level of production of nonspecific IgM (21), hyperresponsiveness to foreign antigenic stimuli (6), and excessive hemopoietic stem cell cycling activity in the spleen (16). By two weeks of age, antinuclear autoantibodies are already evident (25), thymocytotoxic autoantibodies appear by four weeks (24), and after three to four months, antierythrocyte autoantibodies (30) are detectable.

The transplantability of the lympho-hemopoietic abnormalities of the NZB mouse (17) by bone marrow cell grafts into H-2 histocompatible nonautoimmune mouse strains, and its prevention in the NZB model by marrow grafts from nonautoimmune strains (18) have led us to propose that the etiology of NZB disease may reside in a fundamental disorder of hemopoietic regulation innate to the stem cell and its lymphocytic progeny. In this regard, autoimmune disease may be a consequence of the altered steady-state equilibrium which we have observed to exist between the resting and cycling stem cell populations (14), the augmented cycling fraction spontaneously and randomly generating the increased numbers of antigen-reactive cells responsible for NZB immunologic hyperresponsiveness and increased autoantibody formation.

The observation that clinically normal humans and nonautoimmune strain mice produce significant autoantibody during the latter part of their life-spans suggests that the NZB model may reflect an early loss or absence of a regulatory system which becomes defective only during old age in normal individuals. It has been found that autoimmune phenomena may also be triggered by

environmental factors such as infections (23,29). Experimentally,
autoantibody formation can be induced by exposure to various antigens (8,20) and to polyclonal B-cell activators (9,11). The present report deals with the accelerated development of Coombs' positive hemolytic anemia in tumor-bearing (19) and in Freund's adju-
vant- and antigen-injected NZB mice (15,16), and the initiation of
transient antinuclear antibody (ANA) formation in nonautoimmune
strain animals treated with mitogens or non-cross reacting antigen.

   Coombs' positive hemolytic anemia. We have observed that
chronic stimulation of the reticuloendothelial system (RES) may
exacerbate autoimmune hemolytic disease in the NZB strain. For
example, the formation of antierythrocyte autoantibodies undergoes
an earlier onset and shows higher incidences in NZB mice bearing
primary, 3-methylcholanthrene (3-MC)-induced skin tumors (Fig. 1).
In these experiments, NZB mice were injected subcutaneously with
150 µg of carcinogen at 4 months of age. Those animals bearing
skin tumors, one cm in diameter or greater, showed enhanced Coombs'
positivity by 9 months of age compared to 3-MC-injected mice which
failed to develop skin tumors. Animals developing tumors after 9
months of age manifested less striking differences in Coombs'
reactivity, possibly due to the development of these tumors after
Coombs' conversion in the non-tumor-bearing NZB group was already
well underway.

   This adjuvant effect of tumor-bearing on antierythrocyte autoantibody formation may be associated with the profound nonspecific
stimulatory effects of the tumor on the host reticuloendothelial
system. In this connection, Smith and Konda (28) noted that the
presence of primary 3-MC-induced tumors markedly enhanced T- and
B-cell content and immune reactivity of mouse spleens, and also
increased transplantable stem cell numbers as assessed by the
colony-forming cell assay. Since stem cell and immunocyte hyper-
activity is characteristic of the NZB and linked with its autoimmune disorders, the augmentative effects of tumor bearing on
autoimmunity would not be unexpected. The mechanisms for tumor-
induced alterations in the RES are not well understood, but may
be antigen-driven (12), or due to the stimulatory effects of an
inflammatory process (2).

   Immunological adjuvants, such as complete Freund's adjuvant
(CFA) which possesses a mycobacterial component, also stimulate
T- and B-cell function (13) and activate hemopoietic stem cells
into proliferative cycle (26). As seen in Fig. 2, single and
multiple injections of Difco complete Freund's adjuvant-saline
emulsion, also accelerated Coombs' conversion in NZB mice.

   In another study (Fig. 3), soluble antigens were injected
into NZB mice twice weekly from 2 months of age (16). Some
augmentation of Coombs' conversion was observed in animals

injected with bovine serum albumin (BSA) or human gamma globulin
(HGG). Mice injected with phytohemagglutinin (PHA) showed diminished Coombs' conversion, possibly due to its failure to bring
about B-cell differentiation, while stimulating stem cell cycling
(27,21) and T-cell, including suppressor cell, activity (13).
These modalities of chronic RES stimulation, although exacerbating
autoimmune hemolytic anemia in the NZB model, failed to precipitate significant Coombs' conversion in conventional nonautoimmune
strains such as the DBA/2, BALB/c or C57Bl/6. It is possible that
a genetic factor necessary for Coombs' conversion may be absent
in these strains. Alternatively, it may be that extension of the
treatment or exposure period beyond that employed in the present
studies might have triggered autoreactivity.

     Antinuclear antibody formation. In contrast to the formation
of antierythrocyte autoantibodies, antibodies to nuclear antigens
such as DNA (antinuclear antibodies, ANA) are readily precipitated
in nonautoimmune strains by RES stimuli. ANA conversion was
transiently induced in the normally non-ANA-forming DBA/2 strain by
single injection of 1×10^9 or 2×10^7, but not by 5×10^5 saline-
washed sheep red blood cells (SRBC) (Fig. 4); 1×10^9 cells induced a higher incidence and longer-lasting response than 2×10^7
SRBC. The intensity and duration of this ANA response paralleled
the germinal center expansion and antigen-specific immune response
reported by Hanna et al. (10) following injection of comparable
doses of SRBC. In this connection, we have observed that three
absorptions of peak (6-day) antisera with one volume of SRBC each
did not abolish or diminish the induced ANA activity, indicating
that cross-reacting antibodies were not involved. Similar ANA
induction was elicited in a number of different nonautoimmune
mouse strains following injection of 1×10^9 SRBC (Fig. 5). These
increased ANA levels were observed to persist for as long as 30
days.

     In another experiment, intraperitoneal injection of 50 µg E.
coli lipopolysaccharide (LPS, Difco) was observed to induce transient ANA formation in DBA/2 mice (Fig. 6). By 17 days post-inject-
ion, ANA was no longer present. 1×10^9 rat erythrocytes (Fig. 6)
elicited an ANA response similar to that of 2×10^7 SRBC (Fig. 4)
suggesting that the magnitude of the nonspecific effect was dependent in part upon the immunogenicity of the antigen.

                         DISCUSSION

     It is well established that following a specific immune
stimulus there is induced nonspecific hyperimmunoglobulinemia of
a polyclonal nature. This has been observed to be dependent upon
specific antigen recognition, and cannot be induced by an antigen
to which the animal has been made tolerant, or in the absence of

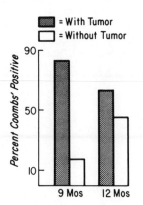

Fig. 1. Incidence of positive Coombs' tests for antierythrocyte autoantibody in tumor-bearing and non-tumor-bearing NZB mice injected subcutaneously with 150 μg of the carcinogen 3-methylcholanthrene at four months of age (19).

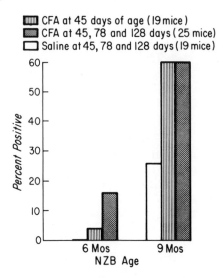

Fig. 2. Development of positive Coombs' test in NZB mice injected i.p. with complete Freund's adjuvant (CFA) (17).

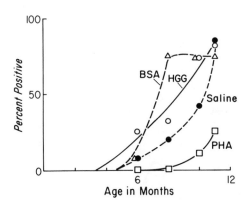

Fig. 3.   Effects of continuous twice weekly injections of BSA (2.5 mg), HGG (2.5 mg) or PHA (1 mg) from 2 months of age on Coombs' conversion in NZB mice (3).

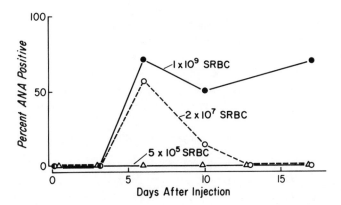

Fig. 4.   Antinuclear antibody ANA) formation in DBA/2 mice as a function of the sheep red blood cell (SRBC) immunization dose.

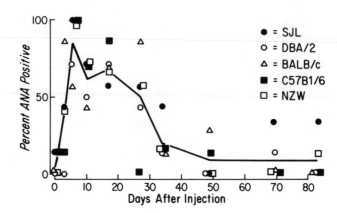

Fig. 5. Antinuclear antibody formation in several strains of mice following a single injection of 1 x 10^9 sheep red blood cells.

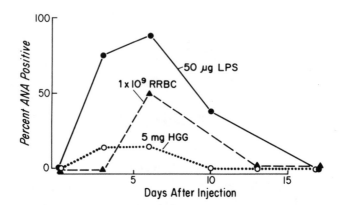

Fig. 6. Antinuclear antibody formation in 3-month-old DBA/2 mice following a single i.p. injection of E. coli lipopolysaccharide (LPS), human gamma globulin (HGG) or rat erythrocytes (RRBC).

a thymus (1,20). Interestingly, splenic hemopoietic stem cells are also triggered into proliferative cycle by nonspecific immune stimuli (3), which has been noted to be a thymus-dependent pheno- menon (7). One might thus speculate that lymphokines released by immunologicaly-activated T cells may act to stimulate stem cells into the cycling phase, thereby generating increased immunocyte populations including autoantibody-forming cells.

Antibodies to DNA (11) and to autologous red blood cells (9) are also observed following polyclonal B cell stimulation by B cell mitogens such as LPS. This appears to be a direct effect which is independent of the thymus and, in addition, is not enhanced by the removal of T suppressor cells (22). Infectious agents, acting either as antigens or mitogens, presumably trigger hyperglobulin- emia with concomitant autoantibody formation by these T cell de- pendent and independent mechanisms.

Recent reports suggest that autoantibodies, such as rheumatoid factor (5) and antibody to bromelain-treated autologous erythro- cytes (4) may comprise a significant fraction of secreted immuno- globulin. These observations reinforce the thesis that the capa- city for autoantibody formation is a normally expressed component of the immunoglobulin repertoire (17), and one which may even be necessary for certain physiological functions (5). Autoimmune disease ensues only when sustained excessive production of auto- antibody is stimulated, through either a genetically- or environ- mentally-determined disturbance in homeostasis. It would not be anticipated, as demonstrated in the present studies, that genera- ting transient autoreactivity following single injections of or exposures to antigen or polyclonal B cell activator would have pathogenetic consequences. However, chronic stimulation of the RES as through certain infectious, inflammatory or neoplastic states, could in some cases play a significant role in the initia- tion of autoimmune disorders.

This work was supported by USPHS Grant CA-18149 from The National Cancer Institute. Jane I. Morton is a Fellow of The Arthritis Foundation.

REFERENCES

1. Antoine, J. D., Petit, C., Bach, M. A., Bach, J. F., Salomon, J. C. and Avrameas, S., Eur. J. Immunol. 7 (1977) 336.
2. Baum, S. J., MacVittle, T. J., Brandenburg, R. T. and Levin, S. G., Exptl. Hematol. 6 (1978) 405.
3. Boggs, D. R., Marsh, J. C., Chervenick, P. A., Bishop, C. R., Cartwright, G. E. and Wintrobe, M. W., J. Exp. Med. 126 (1967) 850.

4. Cunningham, A. J., Nature 274 (1978) 483.
5. Dresser, D. W., Nature 274 (1978) 480.
6. Evans, M. M., Williamson, W. G. and Irvine, W. J., Clin. Exp. Immunol. 3 (1968) 375.
7. Frindel, E. and Croizat, H., Ann. N. Y. Acad. Sci. 249 (1975) 468.
8. Hamers, R., Hamers-Casterman, C., Van der Loo, W., Strosberg, A. D. and Baetselier, P. De., Z. Immun.-Forsch. 149 (1975) 187.
9. Hammarstrom, L., Smith, E., Primi, D. and Möller, G., Nature 263 (1976) 60.
10. Hanna, M. G., Jr., Congdon, C. C. and Wust, C. J., Proc. Soc. Exp. Biol. Med. 121 (1966) 286.
11. Izui, S., Kobayahawa, T., Zyrd, M. J., Louis, J. and Lambert, P. H., J. Immunol. 119 (1977) 2157.
12. Lala, P. K., In: Stem Cells of Renewing Cell Populations, (Eds. A. B. Cairnie, P. K. Lala, and D. G. Osmond), Academic Press, New York (1976) 343.
13. Moatamed, F., Karnovsky, M. J. and Unanue, E. R., Lab. Invest. 32 (1975) 303.
14. Morton, J. I., In: Microbial Infections and Autoimmunity, (Eds. H. Friedman and T. J. Linna) (1978) in press.
15. Morton, J. I. and Siegel, B. V., Immunology 18 (1970) 379.
16. Morton, J. I. and Siegel, B. V., In: Virus Tumorigenesis and Immunogenesis, (Eds. W. Ceglowski and H. Friedman), Academic Press, New York (1973) 91.
17. Morton, J. I. and Siegel, B. V., Immunology 34 (1978) 863.
18. Morton, J. I. and Siegel, B. V., Transplantation (1978) in press.
19. Morton, J. I., Siegel, B. V. and Moore, R. D., Amer. J. Pathol. 93 (1978) 469.
20. Moticka, E. J., Cell. Immunol. 19: 32, 1975, ibid. 36 (1978) 151.
21. Moutsopoulos, H. M., Boehm-Truitt, M., Kassan, S. and Chused, T., J. Immunol. 119 (1977) 1639.
22. Primi, D., Smith, C. I. E. and Hammarström, L., Scand. J. Immunol. 7 (1978) 121.
23. Rosenberg, Y. J., Nature 274 (1978) 170.
24. Shirai, T. and Mellors, R. C., Proc. Nat. Acad. Sci. USA, 68 (1971) 1412.
25. Siegel, B. V., Brown, M. and Morton, J. I., Immunology 22 (1972) 457.
26. Siegel, B. V. and Morton, J. I., J. Nat. Cancer Inst. 48 (1972) 1681.
27. Siegel, B. V. and Morton, J. I., J. Nat. Cancer Inst. 50 (1973) 539.
28. Smith, R. T. and Konda, S., Int. J. Cancer 12 (1973) 577.
29. Williams, R. C., In: Autoimmunity, Genetic, Immunologic, Virologic and Clinical Aspects, (Ed. N. Talal), Academic Press, New York (1977) 457.

30. Wilson, J. D., Warner, N. and Holmes, N. C., Nature 233 (1971) 80.
31. Wlodarski, K., Jakobisiak, M., Kossakowska, A. and Zelechowska, M., Folia Biol. (Praha) 20 (1974) 133.

MITIGATION OF EXPERIMENTAL ALLERGIC ENCEPHALOMYELITIS BY

CATHEPSIN D INHIBITION

D. H. BOEHME and N. MARKS

Laboratory Service, Veterans Administration Hospital
East Orange, New Jersey (USA)

Experimental allergic encephalomyelitis can be experimentally
induced by the intracutaneous administration of myelin or its antigenic subfraction, basic protein, into a great variety of animal
species. Our own investigations were conducted on the susceptible
BSVS mouse (the only mouse strain with predictable susceptibility
to the immunizing antigen), the highly susceptible Lewis rat and
Hartley strain guinea pigs. Numerous experimental attempts have
been made to prevent the development of this disease by induction
of tolerance and immunosuppressive agents (1,7,8,9,15). In the
present report, however, we employed a different approach using a
fungus derived enzyme inhibitor, pepstatin, which was previously
shown to inhibit the enzyme acid proteinase (cathepsin D). This
approach was based upon the rationale that EAE is attended by a
significant increase of lysosomal proteolytic activity in neural
tissue, notably acid proteinase (4,13,16). Previously, it had
been demonstrated that pepstatin is the most potent inhibitor of
acid proteinase of brain and other tissues (11,18). In this investigation, pepstatin was administered in various concentrations
intraperitoneally immediately following the administration of
antigenic mixture and conducted up to the day of sacrifice. In
some animal strains, these results were compared with proteolytic
inhibitors of cathepsin B1, i.e. leupetin, and an inhibitor of
arylamidase, i.e. benzothonium chloride.

MATERIALS AND METHODS

Experimental Procedures. Susceptible BSVS and resistant BRVR
mice were obtained from a colony maintained in our laboratory.
Lewis rats and Hartley strain guinea pigs were purchased from the

Charles River Breeding Lab. (Wilmington, Mass.).

  Sensitization Procedures. The principal source of antigen
was frozen guinea pig spinal cord from Dutchland Lab. (Denver,
PA). Bovine basic protein was prepared from both brain and spinal
cord according to Benuck, et al. (3). As an adjuvant, complete
Freund's adjuvant DIFCO (Detroit, MI) with H37Rv and, as an immunological stimulator, pertussis vaccine from Eli Lilly and Co.
(Indianapolis, IN) were employed. Pepstatin was supplied through
the Institute of Microbial Chemistry (Tokyo, Japan).

  Mice received four days prior to immunization pertussis
vaccine i.p., diluted 1:5. Lewis rats received 0.1 ml of undiluted pertussis vaccine into the dorsum of the foot on the day of
immunization. The antigen was administered to mice i.c. in the
skin of the back (3 times 0.1 ml) in complete Freund's adjuvant
on days +4 and +8 of the experiment; in Lewis rats, into the foot
pad, on day 0. The injection mixture in Lewis rats consisted of
20 mg guinea pig spinal cord in 0.5 ml NaCl v/v with an adjuvant
consisting of 8.5 parts Bayol F, 1.5 parts Arlacel A and 4 mg/ml
killed H37Rv. Pepstatin was given as an aqueous emulsion i.p.
(Tables I-III).

  The degree of EAE was evaluated on a score based on: hind
leg paralysis, weight loss and loss of sphincter control. Histological examination was conducted on formalin fixed brains after
paraffin processing. The histological score was ranging from –
to 4+.

                                RESULTS

  Lewis rats developed dependably EAE with a mean of 24.6 ±
5.2 days and showed severe clinical signs ranging up to 4+ histo-
pathologically (Table I). Administration of 2 mg pepstatin/day,
conducted from day 1-35, totally suppressed the onset of clinical
signs and significantly mitigated the histological signs of disease.
Histological examination of brain and spinal cord in one group
carried without sacrifice to day 35, exhibited a marked decrease
in severity in incidence of inflammatory lesions. The histological lesions encountered in the unprotected, fully immunized group
were absent from the pepstatin protected group listed in Table II
and greatly reduced in groups 3 and 4. A reduction of dose below
2 mg/day partly removed the clinical and histological modification
of the experimental disease but shortening of the administration
schedule of pepstatin to day 1-9 following immunization still reduced markedly clinical and histological incidence of the disease.

  For BSVS mice, the i.p. administration of 0.8 mg of pepstatin i.p. from day 5-14 was followed by a high significant reduc-

TABLE I

Extended Pepstatin Treatment in Lewis Rats

Group	Treatment (mg. pepstatin i.p.)	No. Sick/ No. Tested	Onset of Clinical Signs of EAE (%SD)	Histo- logical Signs
Control	none	5/5	24.6 ± 5.2	4+
Treated	2	0/2	none	0
Day 1-35	2	0/3	none	1+
	2	0/1	none	2+

Groups of Lewis rats were challenged with 14 mg guinea pig spinal cord emulsified with 0.5 ml complete Freund's adjuvant and injected into the foot pad. Treatment with 2 mg pepstatin began on day 1 and continued through day 35 following challenge. Saline suspensions of pepstatin were administered intraperitoneally. Animals were sacrificed 2 days following cessation of treatment.

tion of clinical and histological signs of EAE when the animals were sacrificed on days 14, 18 and 21 (Table II).

In the Hartley strain guinea pigs, pepstatin treatment at two different levels of concentration was compared with the cathespin Bl inhibitor leupetin and the arylamidase inhibitor benzothonium chloride (10). A dose regime from 1-5 mg of pepstatin beginning with day 4 and ending with day 14 following immunization reduced histological and clinical incidence of disease significantly (Table III). Histologically, the animals showed a more variable picture; two guinea pigs were devoid of lesions, one exhibited 3+ lesions without clinical signs of disease and one showed clinical lesions with the fully developed histological lesions. Increase of pepstatin to 4 mg and higher did not provide any additional effect.

Neither leupetin nor benzothonium chloride had any influence upon the outcome of EAE.

TABLE II

Pepstatin Treatment And its Effect on Development of EAE
in Lewis Rats and BSVS Mice

Group No.		Treatment (pepstatin, mg)	No. Sick/ No. Tested	Day Killed	Histologic Lesion
A	Lewis rats				
	1	saline	1/6	12	2+
	2	saline	3/6	15	2+
	3	saline	5/6	19	3+
	4	2	1/3	12	1+
	5	2	2/3	15	2+
	6	2	3/3	19	2+
B	BSVS mice				
	1	saline	0/4	14	0
	2	saline	1/8	18	4+
	3	saline	4/11	21	3+ − 4+
	4	0.8	0/5	14	0
	5	0.8	0/10	18	0
	6	0.8	2/14	21	1+

Groups of six Lewis rats, and of 6–14 BSVS mice were challenged with guinea
pig spinal cord emulsified in complete Freund's adjuvant. Treatment with pepstatin given intraperitoneally commenced on day 1 and continued for 9 days
Lewis rats) or at day 5 to day 14 (BSVS mice). Animals were killed at days
noted and CNS tissues examined histologically.

TABLE III

Comparison of Effects of Pepstatin with Leupetin and Benzothonium Chloride on EAE in Guinea Pigs

Group	Treatment	Dose	No. Sick/ No. Tested	Day of Onset (± SD)	Histologic Severity
Control	Saline		4/4	12.25 ± 1.2	4+
Treated					
Day 4-14	pepstatin	2 mg	3/4	18.5 ± 3.0	0 (2) 3+ (2) 4+ (1)
Day 3-15	pepstatin	4 mg	4/5	18.6 ± 4.0	0 (2) 2+ (1) 4+ (2)*
Day 4-14	Leupeptin	1 mg	4/4	11.75 ± 0.3	4+ (4)
Day 4-14	Genzothonium Chloride	1 mg	4/4	12.0 ± 1	4+ (4)

*One of the 4+ in this group did not develop hind leg paralysis. Groups of 4-5 Hartley-strain guinea pigs with 100 µg bovine myelin basic protein emulsified with 50 µg M. butyricium in 0.1 ml total volume and injected into the hind foot pad. Treatment with pepstatin started on the days indicated. All guinea pigs were terminated on day 30 following challenge; brain and spinal cord tissues were isolated for histology. The numbers in parentheses represent animals showing the histopathology indicated.

DISCUSSION

At present it is only possible to speculate on the mode of action of pepstatin which is chemically an N-acylated microbial pentapeptide. Its principal inhibitory activity affects the action of cathepsin D which splits myelin basic protein (the most potent antigen producing EAE) at its Phe-Phe linkages to release smaller toxic fragments (3). There are data showing infiltration of pepstatin into cells by pinocytosis and this mechanism could account for altering sensitive cells (circulating T-cells) known to mediate the hypersensitivity associated with EAE. Previously, pepstatin has been reported to affect protein turnover in cells (5), degradation of collagen (6), and in vivo to affect liver regeneration (14) and to delay degeneration of muscle in genetically dystrophic mice. Of particular interest is the fact that pepstatin possesses very low toxicity for the experimental animal organism which was born out of the present investigation. It appears that it has a far more benign effect than drugs which were previously employed to modify the autoimmune response leading to EAE as methotrexate, anti-lymphocyte serum, steroids or ACTH (2).

SUMMARY

Intraperitoneal treatment with the enzyme inhibitor, pepstatin, of BSVS mice, guinea pigs and Lewis rats which were sensitized with guinea pig spinal cord and pertussis vaccine resulted in complete or partial suppression of paralysis dependent on the species studied and alterations of histological signs of experimental allergic encephalomyelitis (EAE). The effect was dose-dependent but had no relationship to the age of the experimental animal at the time of the experiment.

REFERENCES

1. Alvord, E. C., et al., Ann. NY Acad. Sci, 122 (1965) 333.
2. Arnason, B. G. W., Immunosuppression in experimental demyelinating diseases. In: Multiple Sclerosis - Immunology, Virology and Ultrastructure, (Eds. R. Wolfgram, G. W. Ellison, V. G. Stevens and J. M. Andrews), Academic Press, New York, (1972) 487.
3. Benuck, M., et al., Eur. J. Biochem., 52 (1975) 615.
4. Boehme, D. H., et al., Brain Res., 75 (1974) 153.
5. Dean, R. T., Nature, 257 (1975) 414.
6. Dingle, J. T., et al., J. Biochem., 127 (1972) 443.
7. Driscoll, B. F., et al., J. of Immunology, 112 (1974) 392.
8. Hashim, G. A., et al., Arch. Biochem., 156 (1973) 287.
9. Levine, S., et al., Proc. Soc. Exp. Biol. and Med., 139 (1972) 506.

10. Marks, N., et al., Texas Reports on Biol. and Med., 31 (1973) 345.
11. Marks, N., et al., Science, 181 (1973) 949.
12. Marks, N., et al., Neurochem. Res., 1 (1976) 93.
13. Marks, N., et al., Brain Res., 123 (1977) 147.
14. Miyamoto, M., et al., Biochem. Biophys. Res. Commun., 55 (1973) 84.
15. Paterson, P. Y., et al., J. Immunol., 103 (1969) 795.
16. Smith, M., Neurochem. Res., 2 (1977) 233.
17. Stracher, A., et al., Science, 200 (1978) 50.
18. Umezawa, H., Univ. Park Press (1972).

LOCALIZATION AND CLEARANCE OF PASSIVELY ADMINISTERED IMMUNE

COMPLEXES AND AGGREGATED PROTEIN, IN THE CHOROID PLEXUS OF MICE

P. M. FORD

Department of Medicine of Queen's University
Kingston, Ontario (Canada)

The presence in the choroid plexus of immune complex material
has been observed both in human disease and a variety of experimental animal models. In human systemic lupus erythematosus (SLE)
such deposits were first noted by Atkins et al. (1) and he suggested that immune complex deposits in the choroid plexus might
contribute to the central nervous system disease seen in some
cases of SLE.

Similar deposits have been observed in the choroid plexus of
the NZW/NZB F1, hybrid mouse model of SLE (10), in mice chronically infected with lymphocytic choriomengitis virus (11) and in
both passive (14) and active serum sickness (9, 15) in rats and
mice.

The ultra-structure of the villi of the choroid plexus
suggests a filtration function with intermittently fenestrated
endothelium (12) of the type seen in the renal glomerular capillaries where, however, the fenestration is continuous. The epithelial surface of the choroid plexus resembles that of the pro-
ximal renal tubule in consisting of cuboidal cells with brush
borders. Between these two layers of cells may be found the pial
cell which probably covers about 85% of the endothelial basement
membrane (12). The function of the pial cell in the choroid is
not entirely clear, but a phagocytic role has been postulated (12).

In all the above mentioned situations where immune complexes
are found in the choroid plexus they are also deposited in the
renal glomerulus. In the study reported here using the passive
serum sickness model in the mouse, the object was to study the

effect of varying doses of immune complexes in terms of their deposition in the choroid, to compare immune complexes with an
aggregated protein of similar molecular size having presumably
less biological activity and to observe relative amounts of deposition in the choroid plexus and the renal glomerulus.

MATERIALS AND METHODS

Antiserum to bovine serum albumen (BSA) was produced in
rabbits. The equivalence point of antigen-antibody reactivity
was established by the method of Kabat and Meyer (8) and the antibody content determined. Immune complexes were prepared in 5X
antigen excess as previously described (3) and expressed as mg
antibody protein.

BSA was aggregated using the method of Ilo and Wagner (7).
This results in an aggregate size of approximately 780,000 daltons.

Reticuloendothelial system blockade was effected by I. V.
injection of 30 mg/100 g body weight colloidal carbon 24 hr before subsequent injections (3). Colloidal carbon was prepared by
dialysing Pelikan Ink C11/1431 (a) (Gunther Wagner) against phosphate buffered saline for 24 hr before use.

CBA mice of 3-6 months of age and weighing between 25 and
30 g were used. At the termination of the experiments the animals
were killed by cervical dislocation; both kidneys and the area of
brain containing the lateral ventricles were then removed, a part
being fixed in buffered formal saline and the remainder being
snap-frozen.

Immunofluorescence studies were carried out on 5 μ air-dried
cryostat cut sections using FITC anti-rabbit immunoglobulin
(Behring) to demonstrate rabbit immunoglobulin, and a "sandwich"
technique using FITC anti-rabbit immunoglobulin and rabbit anti-
BSA to localize BSA within tissues.

Both immune complexes· and aggregated BSA were injected I.V.
through a tail vein. Immune complex material was injected in a
dose of 28 mg antibody protein/100 g body weight of mouse. One
tenth of the dose was given initially followed 20 min later by
the remainder. This method has been found to minimize deaths
from anaphylaxis.

Aggregated albumen was given in either high (45 mg/100 g
body weight) or low dosage (15 mg/100 g body weight) as a single
dose.

RESULTS

Injection of Preformed Immune Complexes (Table I)

Group I. A single dose of 28 mg antibody protein/100 g body weight with death at 6 hr.

These animals showed ++ to +++ staining in a mesangio-capillary pattern in the renal glomerulus, but only a trace of material was seen in the choroid.

Group II. Daily injections of 28 mg antibody protein/100 g body weight for 5 days with death 6 hr after the last injection. Much enhanced deposition was noted in the kidney (Fig. 1) with some deposited material in the choroid with a focal pattern of deposition (Fig. 2).

Group III. Daily injections of immune complexes for 5 days with the animals being killed at 36 hr. The amount of material in the renal glomerulus, mainly in the mesangial region was comparable with that in group II at 6 hr. A clear decrease was noted in the choroid plexus with 5 out of 8 animals having no demonstrable deposits at 36 hr.

Group IV. These animals had a single injection of complexes 24 hr after RES blockade with particulate carbon. In comparison with group I a marked increase in glomerular deposition was observed with only a minimal increase in choroid plexus deposits.

No animals from any group showed any histological change on light microscopy when compared to uninjected controls.

Aggregated Albumen (Table 2)

Group I. Animals given a single low dose of aggregated BSA (15 mg/100 g body weight) and killed 6 hr after injection showed only a small amount of material in the renal glomerular mesangium with no detectable material in the choroid.

Group II. Animals receiving a single high dose injection (45 mg/100 g body weight) and killed 6 hr after injection showed an increase in renal deposition, but with only a slight amount of BSA being detected in the choroid of 2 out of 6 mice.

Group III. Animals given a single high dose injection of aggregated BSA and killed at 36 hr showed minimal renal retention, the most prominent staining being in the mesangial "stalk" region, and no deposits in the choroid.

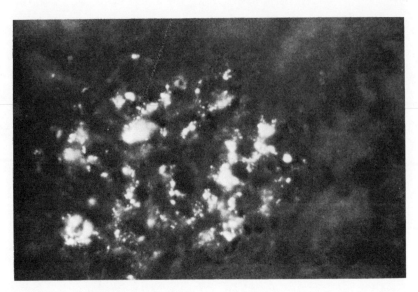

Fig. 1. Glomerulus from group II (immune complex) mouse showing +++ mesangio-capillary deposits. Stained with FITC anti-rabbit immunoglobulin X 200.

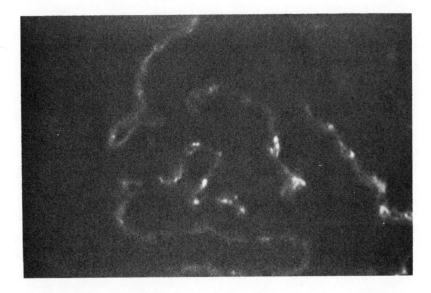

Fig. 2. Choroid plexus from group II (immune complex) mouse showing + focal deposition. Stained with FITC anti-rabbit immunoglobulin x 100.

TABLE I

Animals Injected with Immune Complexes

Staining Intensity[a]	Group I		Group II		Group III		Carbon Blocked	
	Kidney	Choroid Plexus	Kidney	Choroid Plexus	Kidney	Choroid Plexus	Kidney	Choroid Plexus
+ + + +			5		4		6	
+ + +	4		3		4		2	
+ +	3			2				1
+		5		5		3		7
none		2				5		

[a]Staining intensity observed in frozen sections stained with FITC anti-rabbit immunoglobulin. (See text for full explanation)

TABLE II

Animals Injected with Aggregated BSA

Staining Intensity[a]	Group I		Group II		Group III		Carbon Blocked	
	Kidney	Choroid Plexus	Kidney	Choroid Plexus	Kidney	Choroid Plexus	Kidney	Choroid Plexus
+ + + +							1	
+ + +			3				4	
+ +	4		3					2
+	3			2	2			4
none		6		4	4	6		

[a]Staining intensity observed in frozen sections stained with rabbit anti-BSA followed by FITC anti-rabbit immunoglobulin. (See text for full explanation)

Group IV. Carbon blockage of the RES followed 24 hr later by
I. V. aggregated BSA 15 mg/100 g body weight, resulted in a
marked increase in renal glomerular deposition as compared to the
unblocked group I and only a moderate increase in choroid plexus
deposits.

In group IV mice from both immune complex injected and BSA
injected mice rabbit immunoglobulin and BSA respectively were
shown in the CSF space in small amounts staining in a particulate
manner.

                              DISCUSSION

The results presented here confirm the observations of Peress
et al. (14) that following injection of passively prepared immune
complexes, immune material is deposited in the choroid plexus.
Such deposition as occurs however is small in amount and there
are a number of differences compared to renal glomerular mesangial
uptake and handling of the same material.

The scanty and focal nature of deposits may be partly explained by the observation (12) that the fenestrated endothelium
of the choroid capillaries is only intermittent, unlike that of
the renal glomerulus which is continuous, and therefore only a
reduced area in the chorid may be involved in filtration and the
trapping of micro-particulate material. Furthermore, the drop in
hydrostatic pressure across the capillary wall is much less in
the choroid plexus than in the renal glomerulus. Germuth (5) has
shown that reduction of the hydrostatic gradient across the glomerular capillary wall reduces immune complex deposition.

Michael et al. (13) using passively injected aggregated
gamma globulin showed mesangial uptake and retention of the
material for at least 48 hr. In the experiments reported here
the staining intensity of injected immune complexes did not diminish during the 36 hr following injection. In the case of
aggregated BSA while the pattern of mesangial uptake is similar
to that of immune complexes at 6 hr, at 36 hr very little retention is seen, but some staining in the mesangial stalk region
suggests removal via this route. Also in the case of the mesangial system, prolonging the circulation time and enhancing the
concentration of both immune complexes and aggregate protein by
RES blockade, results in a much increased uptake (3). The choroid
plexus on the other hand does not appear to have the capacity to
retain immune complex material for 36 hr and RES blockade has
little effect on choroidal deposits of either immune complexes
or of aggregated BSA. These differences would appear to be due
to the lack of a mesangial cell equivalent capable of phagocytosing such particles as get lodged on the endothelial fenestrations

or penetrate through the endothelial cell layer. That immune complex material deposited in the choroid is capable of causing local damage is suggested in experimental chronic serum sickness in the rats by the correlation of such deposits with an apparent increase in permeability of the choroid capillaries to a marker protein (15).

The similar intensity and pattern of deposition of immune complexes and of aggregated BSA as previously noted for the renal glomerulus would indicate that such deposition is a relatively passive process and independent of vasoactive amine release or of complement activation (3,4).

The observation of particulate immune material in the CSF space after RES blockade suggests that deposited material may cause sufficient damage to pass on through the epithelial layer. However, a similar finding with aggregated albumen, which is supposedly relatively inert in terms of vasoactive amine release and complement activation, might indicate that this observation is artefactual and perhaps related to damage caused by the injection of particulate carbon, preparations of which have been shown to contain potentially irritant substances (6).

The total absence of any light microscopic change in the choroid plexus in any of the groups injected with immune complexes is in keeping with similar observations by other workers (14). Cochrane comments upon the difficulty of producing histological change in the kidney using injection of preformed complexes (2). Even in the established disease in humans (1) or in animals (10) where definite evidence of immune material in the choroid plexus has been obtained by immunofluorescence, light microscopic change has been minimal or absent. Such lack of evidence of local histological response might suggest that any alterations in permeability might be due to structural change in the basement membrane and indeed the evidence in human SLE for activation of the complement system within the CSF (16) might be explained by the damaged capillary wall allowing complexes to pass into the CSF or alternatively allowing passage of activated components of the earlier part of the complement pathway.

ACKNOWLEDGEMENTS

    This study is supported by the Canadian Arthritis Society Grant #6-226. Dr. Ford is an Associate of the Canadian Arthritis Society.

REFERENCES

1. Atkins, C. J., Kondon, J. J., Quismorio, F. P. and Friou, G. J.
    Ann. Int. Med. 76 (1972) 65.
2. Cochrane, G. G. and Koffler, D., Advances in Immunology (Eds.
    F. J. Dixon and H. G. Kunkel), Academic Press, New York, 16
    (1973) 185.
3. Ford, P. M., Brit. J. Exp. Path., 56 (1975) 523.
4. Ford, P. M., Brit. J. Exp. Path. 57 (1976) 148.
5. Germuth, F. G., Keleman, W. A., and Pollack, A. D., Johns
    Hopkins Med. J. 120 (1976) 252.
6. Hopps, C. H. and Dent, T. E., Arch. Pathol. 74 (1962) 285.
7. Ilo, M. and Wagner, H. N., J. Clin. Invest. 42 (1963) 417.
8. Kabat, E. A. and Meyer, M. M. (Ed. C. C. Thomas), Springfield,
    Illinois, (1961) 2nd edition, chapter 2.
9. Koss, M. N., Chernack, W. J., Griswold, W. R. and McIntosh,
    R. M., Arch. Pathol. 96 (1973) 331.
10. Lampert, P. W. and Oldstone, M. B. A., Science 180 (1973)
    408.
11. Lampert, P. W. and Oldstone, M. B. A., Virchows Arch. A. Path.
    Anat. and Histol. 363 (1974) 21.
12. Maxwell, D. S. and Pease, D. C., J. Biophysic Biochem. Cytol.
    2 (1956) 467.
13. Michael, A. F., Fish, A. J. and Good, R. A., Lab. Invest. 17
    (1967) 14.
14. Peress, N. S., Miller, F. and Palu, W., J. Neuropath. Exp.
    Neurol. 36 (1977) 561.
15. Peress, N. S., Miller, F. and Palu, W., J. Neuropath. Exp.
    Neurol. 36 (1977) 726.
16. Petz, L. D., Sharp, G. C., Cooper, N. R. and Irvin, W. S.,
    Arthritis Rheum. 14 (1971) 180.

CARDIAC SPECIFIC ANTIGEN AND ANTIBODY IN IMMUNOPATHOGENESIS OF CARDIAC DISEASE

K. CHANG, H. FRIEDMAN and H. GOLDBERG

Deborah Heart and Lung Institute, Browns Mills, NJ
College of Medicine, University of South Florida
Tampa, FLA. and Albert Einstein Medical Center
Philadelphia, Pennsylvania (USA)

Antibody with specificity to myocardial antigens often develop in the serum of patients after myocardial infarction or cardiac surgery (1,8). Earlier studies in this laboratory showed a relatively rapid rise in antibody titer to heart extracts in patients after myocardial infarction (5). The kinetics of the antibody rise indicated that the cardiac antigen was the actual stimulator of the antibody response. The role of such cardiac antigen in immune responsiveness to myocardial tissue after heart surgery is generally unknown, although it has been postulated that the surgical procedure results in release of cardiac antigen which, in turn, stimulates an immune response which may be involved in an immunopathogenic sequelae (1,7). In the present study antibody titers to human cardiac extracts were detected in the serum of patients undergoing cardiac surgery and related to the appearance of cardiac myoglobulin antigen in the serum of the patients.

MATERIALS AND METHODS

Patients undergoing open heart surgery at Deborah Heart and Lung Institute were examined in this study. Sera were obtained prior to and at various time intervals after surgery. Antibody to cardiac tissue was determined by several serologic procedures. For these purposes a crude saline extract (10% v/v) of human heart tissue was prepared after autopsy of a patient who died for reasons unrelated to heart disease as well as hearts with massive myocardial infarcts (5). These extracts were used interchangeably without observable differences. The passive hemagglutination assay was utilized, in which heart antigen sensitized sheep or human erythro-

335

cytes were used for microtitration exactly as described elsewhere
(5). In brief a 10% saline extract of heart tissue was coated
onto washed 10% suspensions of tannic acid treated (1:20,000)
erythrocytes. These antigen sensitized red cells were then added
to serial dilutions of human sera in microtiter plates. Controls
consisted of addition of similarly treated erythrocytes without
antigen or others coated with similar 10% liver extracts. In
additional studies gel diffusion precipitin reactions, counter
current immunoelectrophoresis and microcomplement fixation procedures were utilized with the heart extract antigen. Myoglobulin
was determined by the conventional radioimmunoassay procedure.

RESULTS

Antibody with specificity to cardiac tissue was evident in
sera of patients at various times after open heart surgery. As
can be seen in Table I, very few of the 32 patients examined

TABLE I

Appearance of Cardiac Reactive Antibody in Sera of
Patients After Open Heart Surgery

Day After Surgery	No. of Specimens	Percent of Specimens with Anti-Heart Antibody[a]		
		H. A.	Ppt'n	CF
Before	32	6	5	<5
1-3 days	29	7	8	5
5-8	21	38	10	7
10-15	20	60	20	40
15-25	22	50	28	31

[a]Patient specimens with positive antibody

before surgery showed antibody either by the hemagglutination
technique, the gel precipitin assay or micro complement fixation
test. One to three days after surgery a small percentage of the
patients showed some evidence of antibody activity, usually with
a titer of 1:10 to 1:20. By the end of the first week after
surgery a larger percentage of patients showed antibody activity,
often at a level of 1:20 or greater. This was most evident by the
hemagglutination assay. By the second to third week after surgery
at least half of the patients showed titers of 1:40 or more by the
hemagglutination test and significant reactivity by the precipitin
and CF tests.

This response to cardiac tissue in the surgical patients was
generally similar to that observed in patients diagnosed as having
a myocardial infarction (Table II). Seventeen of 22 patients had

TABLE II

Antibody Appearance After Surgery or Myocardial Infarction

Patients Tested	Positive Immunofluorescence[a]		
	Cardiac Tissue	ANA	FTA
Before surgery	1/28[b]	0/20	0/20
After surgery	17/22	2/18	1/18
Post-myocardial infarct -			
early	15/38	3/17	2/17
late	24/43	2/18	4/18

[a]Indirect fluorescent antibody test performed with either human
cardiac tissue, liver tissue for ANA or treponemes for FTA
[b]Number of specimens positive/number tested.

titers of 1:20 or greater by the hemagglutination assay between
one and two weeks after the surgical procedures. Similarly 15
out of 38 patients after myocardial infarction (1 to 2 weeks)
showed titers of 1:20 or greater and even a higher percentage
had such titers by the second or third week after the infarction.
In control serologic tests anti-nuclear antibody assays were performed on the same specimens, as well as the treponema fluorescent
antibody test. Very few of these patients showed positive ANA or
FTA reactivity after surgery or after myocardial infarction,
although there was a somewhat greater positivity after an infarct
as compared to heart surgery.

Myoglobin antigen was readily detected for half the patients
undergoing cardiac surgery (Table III). Thirty-three percent of
the patients examined showed a 2-3 fold increase in serum myoglobin levels 1-3 days after surgery, while 25% of the patients
showed a 4-5 fold increase.

A good correlation was evident between appearance of peak
hemagglutinating antibody to cardiac extracts in the patients
and appearance of myoglobin in serum (Table IV). An increased
level of myoglobulin antigen 1-3 days after surgery was often
followed by appearance of anti-heart antibody in the patient's
sera.

TABLE III

Change in Serum Myoglobin Levels After Cardiac
Surgery

Serum Myoglobin Levels	No. of Patients	Percent
No change	15	45
Increase – moderate[a]	12	33
– marked[b]	9	25

[a]x 2–3 above normal
[b]x 4–5 above normal

TABLE IV

Correlation Between Antibody Titers and Appearance of
Serum Myoglobin After Surgery

Myoglobin Levels (μg)	Peak Antibody Titers After Surgery[a]				
	1:10	1:10 – 1:20	1:40 – 1:80	1:160 – 1:320	1:320
<2	6	1	0	0	0
2–20	2	5	0	0	0
20–40	1	0	2	0	0
40–80	1	1	0	2	0

[a]Antibody determined by hemagglutination assay

DISCUSSION AND CONCLUSION

In earlier studies antibody reactivity to cardiac extracts were detected in sera of patients after myocardial infarction (2,3,4,5,8). Lower titers and reactivity were observed in sera of patients with myocardial insufficiency and essentially no reactivity was evident in normal control patients (5). In the present study similar antibody activity was detected in the sera of patients undergoing open heart surgery. Peak titers occurred approximately 1-3 weeks after the surgical procedure. In addition, cardiac myoglobin antigen was also detected in the sera of many of the surgical patients, with peak levels varying between 1-3 days after the cardiotomy. It was also found that complexes of antibody and cardiac antigen could be detected, with peak levels approximately one week after the surgical procedure (unpublished data). These complexes were detected by radioimmunoassay and appeared to be composed of specific anticardiac antibody and either myoglobin or another unidentified antigen. No significant alterations in serum immunoglobin levels were evident (unpublished data).

As determined by the passive hemagglutination, gel precipitin and complement fixation assays, the appearance of anti-cardiac specific antibody seemed directly related to the surgical procedure. Thus it seems likely that some of the cardiac complications which occur after cardiac surgery may be related to development of a specific immune response to the circulating heart antigen. Antigen upon complexing with the antibody could have immunopathologic effects. The results of the present study thus lend support to the view that immunologic disease may be a complication of cardiac surgery (1,5,6,7,8).

SUMMARY

Antibody to human cardiac extracts was detected in the sera of many patients undergoing open heart surgery. A passive hemagglutination assay using cardiac extracts as antigen coated onto erythrocytes showed the development of cardiac antibody in the patients, with peak titers usually one to three weeks after the surgery. Radioimmunoassay revealed the presence of cardiac specific myoglobin antigen in the sera of many patients, with peak levels 1-3 days after the procedure. A correlation was observed between development of circulating serum antibody and appearance of cardiac myoglobin antigen. These results support the view that immunologic disease related to release of cardiac antigen in patients undergoing heart surgery may be a factor in post-cardiotomy disease.

REFERENCES

1. Das, S. K., Cassidy, J. T. and Petty, R. E. Amer. Heart J. 83 (1972) 159.
2. Davies, A. M. and Gery, I. Am. Heart J. 60 (1960) 1966.
3. Dressler, Am. J. Med. 18 (1955) 591
4. Elster, S. K., Wood, H. F. and Seely, R. D. Amer. J. Med. 17 (1954) 826.
5. Heine, W. H., Friedman, H., Mandell, M. S. and Goldberg, H., Am. J. Card. 17 (1966) 768.
6. Kaplan, M. H. and Fringley, D. Amer. J. Card. 24 (1969) 459.
7. Lessof, M. H. Hosp. Pract.   (1976) 81
8. Strausz, I. and Dubias, G. J. Clin. Path. 20 (1967) 161.
9. Talano, J. J. Arch. Inter. Med. 137 (1977) 570.

PHAGOCYTE FUNCTIONS IN FAMILIAL MEDITERRANEAN FEVER

M. BAR-ELI[1], M. LEVY[2], M. EHRENFELD[2], M. ELIAKIM[2],
and R. GALLILY[1]

[1]The Lautenberg Center for General and Tumor Immunology
The Hebrew University-Hadassah Medical School, Jerusalem
(Israel)
[2]Department of Medicine A, Hadassah University Hospital
Jerusalem (Israel)

Familial Mediterranean fever (F.M.F.) is a form of polysero-
sitis characterized by recurrent attacks of abdominal pain and
fever. Pleuritis and arthritis involving one or more joints
occurs in over 50% of the patients while erysipeloid rashes have
been less frequently described (8,17). This familial disorder
inherited as an autosomal recessive trait usually runs a benign
course, although amyloidosis may develop in as many as 25% of the
cases (10). Etiologic factors responsible for F.M.F. are still
unknown; several investigators have invoked inborn errors of
metabolism and hypersensitivity states as possible pathogenetic
mechanisms (8,10,17). Administration of colchicine to patients
with F.M.F. can prevent the frequency of painful episodes although
the mode of its action is not clear (7).

The purpose of this study was to examine monocyte and polymorphonuclear leukocyte (PMN) functions in patients with F.M.F.
prior to and during treatment with colchicine. The results obtained indicate that colchicine significantly decreased enhanced
chemokinesis detected in patient's PMNs. In addition, monocytes
from these patients were found to have decreased phagocytic and
bactericidal capacity which colchicine did not alter.

MATERIAL AND METHODS

Thirty-six patients with F.M.F. and 14 healthy individuals
were investigated. Sixteen patients were male and 20 were female. Their age ranged between 15 and 60 years. All patients
investigated had been affected by the typical symptoms of the

disease for variable number of years. Seventeen patients were
examined prior to and 19 during treatment with colchicine (0.5 to
1.5 mg daily). All the treated patients were free of painful
attacks unless stated otherwise.

Monocyte cultures. Mononuclear cells were obtained from
heparinized blood using a Ficoll-Hypaque gradient (3). Monolayer
cultures of monocytes were obtained by cultivating 3×10^5 mononuclear cells per well on tissue culture microplates (6 mm well,
Nunc, Denmark) in Dulbecco's modified Eagle's medium supplemented
with 10% heat inactivated fetal calf serum (FCS). The cells were
incubated for three hr at 37 C in a humidified atmosphere containing 5% CO_2. Nonadhering cells were removed by intense rinsing
with phosphate buffered saline (PBS) and fresh medium added. The
number of plastic-adhering cells was determined by a modification
of the Na_2 $^{51}CrO_4$ uptake method as described by More et al. (15).
Of the plastic-adhering cells (about 10^5 cells/well) 85% were
monocytes and less than 5% were granulocytes.

Phagocytic assay. Suspension of bacteria was fixed with
0.25% glutaraldehyde and iodinated with ^{125}I were used for the
labeling of 400 mg (wet weight) bacteria. The final intensity of
labeling was 400 bacteria per cpm and 200 bacteria per cpm for
Shigella flexneri and Staphylococcus albus, respectively. The
labeled bacteria were added to the monocyte cultures in a concentration of 2.4×10^7 bacteria (6×10^4 cpm) per 100 µl/well. The
cultures were incubated for various periods of time (usually for
one hr), and phagocytosis was assessed by counting every well of
a cut microtissue culture plate in a scintillation counter (Packard 5110) (16).

Suspensions of S. albus in the log phase of growth (100 Klett
units) were labeled with ^3H thymidine (20 Ci/m mol, New England
Nuclear) for 30 or 60 min at 37 C. These ^3H thymidine-labeled
bacteria were added to the monocyte cultures in a ratio of 100
bacteria per cell and incubated for 30 to 120 min at 37 C. The
monocytes were rinsed with PBS and lysed with 1% sodium dodecyl
sulphate (SDS). The trichloroacetic acid (final concentration
10%) precipitable material was collected on filters (GF/C glass
filters, Whatman, England) which were then dried, immersed in
scintillation fluid, and the radioactivity was determined in a
Tri-Carb Spectrometer.

Enzyme assay. Monocyte monolayers were cultured in 30 x 10
mm plastic petri dishes (Nunc, Denmark) at 37 C for three hr,
rinsed with PBS, counted, and then added 1 ml distilled water to
each plate. The cell lysates were assayed for acid phosphase
and β-glucuronidase activities as previously described (11).

Bactericidal assay. Saline suspensions of S. albus in the

log phase of growth were added to the monocyte culture in a ratio
of 100 bacteria to one cell. After incubation for 30 min at 37 C,
the nonphagocytosed bacteria were removed by intensive rinsing
and the monocyte monolayers were incubated for an additional 30
and 60 min. The cells were then washed and lysed for three min
with 0.1% Trition X-100. The number of viable staphylococci was
determined by plating appropriate dilutions of the lysate in brain-
heart agar. The colonies were counted after 24 hr incubation of
the agar plates at 37 C.

Polymorphonuclear leukocyte (PWM) chemotaxis. Thirty-two
F.M.F. patients and nine healthy volunteers were studied. Sixteen
of the patients were male and 16 were female, and their ages
ranged between 15 and 60 years. Six patients were examined prior
to and 20 during treatment with colchicine. Six of the patients
were examined during attacks.

The chemotactic assay was performed by a modification of the
Boyden chamber technique (2), PMN were obtained by sedimentation
of heparinized human peripheral blood followed by ammonium chloride
lysis of erythrocytes. The PMN were washed twice with phosphate-
buffered saline (PBS) resuspended in RPMI-1640 medium and brought
to a concentration of 2.5×10^6 cells/ml for use in the upper
compartment.

The chemotactic attractant was prepared by incubating normal
human serum with 1.5 mg/ml Shigella flexneri lipopolysaccharide
W (Difco Laboratories, Detroit, Michigan) at 37 C for 90 min.
The endotoxin serum mixture was then heated at 56 C for 30 min
and centrifuged at 3000 x g for 30 min at 4 C. Aliquots of the
attractant were stored at -20 C. The chemotactic attractant was
diluted fourfold in RPMI-1640 before application to the lower well
of Lucite chambers (0.2 ml/well). Polycarbonate membrane filters
(5 μm pore size, Nucleopore Corporation, Pleasanton, California)
were placed over the lower wells. A volume of 0.2 ml of the cell
suspension in medium was added to the upper well (8 mm diameter).
The chambers were incubated at 37 C for one hr in humidified 5%
CO_2 in air. The filters were then air dried, fixed in methanol,
and stained with Giemsa. Ten high-power fields (HPF) were counted
using a microgrid, and the mean number of PMN per high-power field
which migrated through the filter was determined. The results of
each patient were then compared to the control and expressed as
percent control value.

RESULTS

Phagocytosis of Shigella flexneri. Fig. 1 compares the
phagocytic capacity of treated or untreated patients to that of
normal control. As shown, patients' phagocytic capacity was

lower than that of control during the two hr incubation. In subsequent experiments, 16 patients were evaluated while on treatment, two prior and six both prior and during treatment with colchicine. Monocytes from all F.M.F. patients demonstrated significantly less phagocytic capacity than those of healthy individuals (mean uptake about 40% of the normal, p<0.001). Fig. 2
summarizes the results obtained when all patients and controls
are evaluated together.

    Phagocytosis of Staphylococcus albus. Phagocytosis of ^{125}I-
labeled S. albus (killed bacteria) and ^{3}H–thymidine–labeled S.
albus (live bacteria) had no effect on the phagocytic capacity,
of F.M.F. patients' monocytes after one hour of incubation
(Table I).

    Bactericidal activity of monocytes. Intracellular survival
of phagocytosed S. albus was assessed 30 and 60 min following
their engulfment by monocytes from 13 F.M.F. patients and eight
control subjects. It was found (Table II) that the bactericidal
capacity of monocytes from F.M.F. patients was significantly
lowered after 30 and 60 min incubation so that the number of live
intracellular bacteria was up to eight times higher than that in
the control subjects. No significant effect (p<0.1) of colchicine treatment on the bactericidal effect of monocytes from F.M.F.
patients could be demonstrated.

    Monocyte enzyme activity. The activity of acid phosphatase
and β–glucuronidase (two lysosomal enzymes) in six untreated and
14 treated F.M.F. patients and in seven control subjects was not
significantly different (p<0.1) (Table III).

    Chemotactic response to LPS–activated serum. PMN from 32
patients and nine healthy subjects were assayed for their chemotactic responsiveness. Six patients were tested prior to and 20
during treatment with colchicine. It was found (Table IV) that
PMN from untreated patients exhibited a slight but significantly
higher chemotactic response than control (p<0.001). On the other
hand, PMN derived from patients during colchicine treatment
showed significantly decreased chemokinesis when compared to
either PMN from untreated or normal individuals (p<0.001).

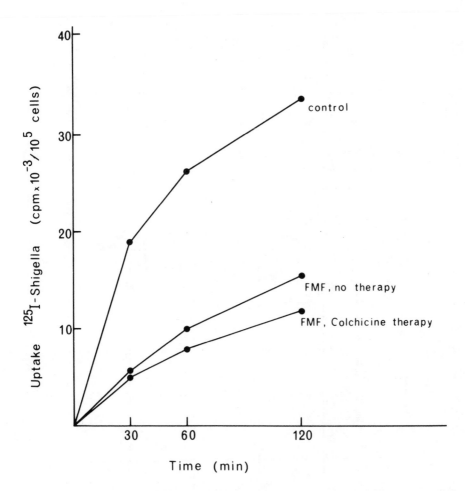

Fig. 1. Pagocytosis of <u>Shigella flexneri</u> by monocytes from one untreated and one treated F.M.F. patients and from one control subject. Each point represents the mean of 6 determinations (1).

TABLE I

Phagocytosis of ^{125}I-Labeled and ^{3}H-Thymidine
Labeled Staphylococcus albus by Monocytes
Derived from Patients with F.M.F. (1)

		Phagocytosis ± S.D.		
Patients	No. of Patients	%Uptake ± S.D. of ^{125}I.S.albus	No. of Patients	%Uptake ± S.D. of ^{3}H-S albus
F.M.F. (treated)	4	48.9 ± 1.0	4	5.4 ± 1.9
F.M.F. (untreated)	8	47.8 ± 3.8	9	5.8 ± 1.2
Healthy subjects	5	47.2 ± 3.2	8	6.2 ± 1.3

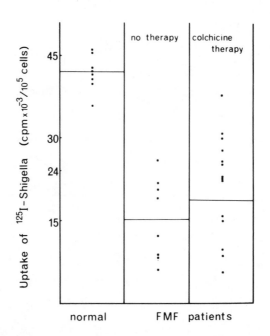

Fig. 2.   Phagocytosis of <u>Shigella flexneri</u> by monocytes from
F.M.F. patients and healthy subjects. Note decreased phagocytosis
in F.M.F. patients (p<0.001) and lack of significant effect of
colchicine (p>0.1).   Each dot represents one subject.   The mean
for each group is shown as a solid line (1).

TABLE II

Killing of Staphyloccus Albus by Monocytes Derived from Patient with FMF

Ex. No.	Subjects Normal	Subjects FMF	Colchicine Treatment	No.Bacteria per Monocyte after 30 min	Relative Bactericidal Activity %a	No. Bacteria per Monocyte after 60 min	Relative Bactericidal Activity %a
1		D.M	+	13.8	21	25.5	40
		S.D	+	23.6	12	32.9	31
	S.U			2.9	100	10.3	100
2		M.D	–	9.9	20	22.9	24
		N.S	–	4.8	41	8.6	63
	P.I			2.0	100	5.5	100
3		A.Z	+	6.6	21	58.1	22
	C.E			1.4	100	13.0	100
4		O.B	–	8.3	57	11.9	50
	O.M			4.8	100	5.9	100
5b		O.H	–	14.3	20	12.7	28
		O.J	–	14.3	20	12.2	29
		P.J	+	10.6	27	20.2	17
		W.R	–	6.8	43	14.7	24
		O.M	–	9.3	31	11.5	30
		M.L	–	4.9	59	16.3	22
		T.R	+	N.D	N.D	12.6	27
	G.S			2.5		2.7	
	G.R			2.7	100	1.1	100
	B.M			3.5		6.7	
Mean±S.D			+		20.3± 5.3		27.4± 7.8
			–		35.3±15.1		33.7±13.7
			normal		100		100

a% of normal monocytes.   bAll the patients in this group belong to the same family (1).

TABLE III

Acid Phosphatase and β-Glucuronidase activities in
Monocytes from F.M.F. Patients and Healthy Subjects

Subjects	No. of Subjects	$M.D.U/10^6$ Monocytes ± S.D. Acid Phosphatase	β-Glucuronidase
F.M.F.(treated)	14	3.7 ± 1.0	0.50 ± 0.11
F.M.F. (untreated)	6	4.0 ± 0.4	0.42 ± 0.10
Healthy subjects	7	3.5 ± 1.0	0.52 ± 0.10

TABLE IV

Chemotactic Activity of PMN Derived
From F.M.F. Patients and Healthy Subjects

Subjects	No. of Subjects	Chemotaxis Mean Count[a]	P-value	Mean Response[b]
F.M.F (untreated)	6	118±8	p<0.02	117±10
F.M.F. (treated)	20	46±26	p<0.001	43±23
F.M.F. (during attack)	6	140±29	p<0.001	148±17
Healthy subjects	9	96±17		100

[a]Number of cells per high-power field (HPF)± standard deviation.
[b]% of control ± standard deviation.

DISCUSSION

The etiology and pathogenesis of F.M.F. is still unclear. During disease activity the fundamental lesion encountered is a nonspecific, nonbacterial inflammation which affects primarily serous membranes. During painful episodes, fever, leukocytosis, increased erythrocyte sedimentation rate, and serum levels of acute phase reactants have been reported. Cell-mediated immune responses in patients with F.M.F. have not been thoroughly examined. In a few studied cases leukocytes from patients receiving small doses of colchicine have shown an intact ability to ingest S. albus and to migrate in chemotactic chambers as well as normal production of pyrogen (6). In addition, these patients exhibited normal numbers of circulating T and B as well as an intact blastogenic response to polyclonal mitogen.

This study demonstrates that monocytes from untreated patients show decreased phagocytosis of labeled Shigella bacilli as well as diminishing bacterial activity against engulfed S. albus. In concordance to the data reported by Dinarello et al. (6), phagocytosis of S. albus was normal. These functional derangements could reflect an in vivo failure to eliminate inflammatory stimuli which might have pathogenetic significance. Administration of colchicine can prevent attacks in the majority of F.M.F. patients. This drug arrests cell division in metaphase (4), interferes with phagocytosis by PMN (14), and prevents appearance of immature lymphocytes in peripheral blood (13). In addition, it can also decrease fibrinogen output by fibroblasts (9) and increase collagen degradation in vitro (12). Dinarello et al. (6) showed that the "skin-window" response in untreated F.M.F. patients is normal and that colchicine inhibits this response (2). Our study shows that colchicine has no significant effect on monocyte phagocytosis and bactericidal activity. In contrast, colchicine decreased significantly chemokinesis of PMN obtained from F.M.F. patients. It is suggested therefore, that this might represent the mechanism whereby colchicine exerts its anti-inflammatory effects.

SUMMARY

Monocytes derived from peripheral blood of patients with familial Mediterranean fever (F.M.F.) demonstrated lower phagocytic capacity for Shigella flexneri and depressed bactericidal activity against S. albus when compared to monocytes from healthy individuals. Treatment of patients with colchicine did not alter these functions. On the other hand, chemokinesis of PMN of F.M.F. patients was enhanced especially during attacks. Colchicine treatment decreased significantly the PMN chemotactic migration.

REFERENCES

1. Bar-Eli, M., Gallily, R., Levy, M., and Eliakim, M. Amer.
    J. Med. Sci. 274 (1977) 265.
2. Boyden, S. J. Exp. Med. 115 (1962) 454.
3. Boyum, A. Scan. J. Clin. Lab. Invest. 21 (1968) 77.
4. Brues, A. M., and Cohen, A. Bioch. J. 30 (1936) 1363.
5. Carpenter, R. R. J. Immunol. 96 (1966) 992.
6. Dinarello, C. A., Chusid, M. J., Fauci, A. S., Gallin, J. I.,
    Dale, D. C., and Wolff, S. M. Arthr. & Rheum. 19 (1976) 618.
7. Editorial. Brit. Med. J. 3 (1975) 60.
8. Ehrenfeld, E. N., Eliakim, M., and Rachmilewitz, M. Amer.
    J. Med. 31 (1961) 107.
9. Ehrlich, H. P., and Bornstein, P. Nature, New Biol. 238
    (1972) 257.
10. Eliakim, M. Israel J. Med. Sci. 6 (1970) 2.
11. Gallily, R., and Eliahu, H. Immunol. 26 (1974) 603.
12. Harris, E. D., and Krane, S. M. Arthr. & Rheum. 14 (1971)
    669.
13. Killen, D. A. J. Surg. Oncol. 2 (1970) 125.
14. Malawista, S. E. Arthr. & Rheum. 11 (1968) 191.
15. More, R., Yron, I., Ben Sasson, S., and Weiss, David W.
    Cell. Immunol. 15 (1975) 382.
16. Schroit, A. J., and Gallily, R. Immunol. 33 (1977) 121.
17. Sohar, E., Gafin, J., Pras, M., and Heller, M. Amer. J. Med.
    43 (1967) 227.

Part IV
The Reticuloendothelial System and Immunomodulation in Cancer

Recent work in many laboratories has focused attention on the important role of macrophages in tumor immunity and immuno-modulation in cancer. This section includes several papers which deal specifically with macrophages as regulators of immune responses against tumors, and tumor immunity in general, as well as the generation of tumor cytotoxic factors and activities. Modulation of tumoricidal activity of activated macrophages also is described, as well as the effects of endotoxin on tumor resistance. Furthermore, the complexity of the interactions of tumors and macrophages is evident by discussion of the possible enhancement of tumor growth by macrophages in normal and tumor-bearing mice. Macrophage involvement in leukemia virus-induced tumorigenesis and in other lymphoid tumors is also presented. It is apparent from these papers that there is much activity at present concerning the role of macrophages in anti-tumor immunity, both in a positive and negative manner. Undoubtedly, additional studies in many laboratories concerning the nature and mechanism of macrophage involvement in tumor resistance and immunity will provide new and fundamental information in the future which could eventually lead to prevention, diagnosis and immunotherapy in cancer.

MACROPHAGES IN TUMOR IMMUNITY

M. G. HANNA, JR.

Cancer Biology Program
NCI Frederick Cancer Research Center
Frederick, Maryland   (USA)

As a result of the fact that experimentally induced animal tumors evoke a specific anti-tumor response in a syngeneic host, much effort has been devoted to defining the role of T and B lymphocytes as effector cells in anti-tumor immunity. This immune reactivity is presumably induced by and directed against tumor-specific transplantation antigens (TSTA) and may be manifested as humoral antibodies and/or cytotoxic lymphoid cells. The latter effector mechanism has been exhaustively studied by _in vitro_ techniques, and it is now recognized that this approach may only be of potential relevance _in vivo_. Important differences between immune-mediated tumor regression _in vivo_ and tumor cell destruction _in vitro_ involve the complexities of the former. Clearly, tumor regression _in vivo_ is limited by the ability of effector cells to search and find the tumor, and then to destroy it. In contrast, in an _in vitro_ assay the need to search for the tumor cell is eliminated. The only measurable phenomenon involves the capacity of various effector cells at appropriate ratios to destroy relatively few tumor cells confined to an _in vitro_ environment.

Although there is ample biological evidence both _in vitro_ and _in vivo_ for acquired immunity to specific antigens in the newly transformed cells, it is of limited relevance since it generally does not operate optimally and the tumor ultimately overwhelms the syngeneic host. For specific tumor immunity to operate effectively under natural conditions, it would probably be necessary for the tumor cells to be highly antigenic and to appear in sufficient quantity in order to produce a fully immunogenic stimulus. Anything less would result in little or no immunity, which would lag behind the growth potential of the tumor and

be ineffective. An analogy can be made with immunity to microorganisms, which tend to be highly antigenic, and yet still require a substantial antigenic stimulus to produce a measurable
immunologic effect. In brucellosis, for example, the infection
is cyclic (undulant fever) because the immunologic stimulus from a
declining bacterial population allows resistance to diminish and
permits the microorganism to grow again until the antigenic stimulus is high enough to reactivate the host defense (16). If indeed defense against highly antigenic infectious agents demands
such a strong immunogenic stimulus, it seems unlikely that a
small clone of transformed cells could provoke a specific immune
response that would be protective.

Analogies between resistance to infectious disease and resistance to tumors have been made in several earlier reviews (14,18,
19) and today are even more fundamental to any concept of host-
tumor relationship (15). A major component of host defense against
infectious microorganisms is a native form of immunity, which is
called "innate resistance." The cell types responsible for innate
resistance are of the macrophage-histiocyte series. Cells of this
series have three important qualities which qualify them as effector cells of innate resistance: they possess a primitive mechanism
for distinguishing foreigness, are actively phagocytic, and can
destroy ingested material by a series of endocytic molecular
events. The effectiveness of phagocytic cells in innate resistance to infections depends upon several important variables,
such as rate of influx of phagocytic cells to an infectious focus,
rate of phagocytosis relative to the rate of target microbial replication, and capacity of phagocytes to kill ingested organisms.
Thus, it is clear that microorganisms must be able to survive
their encounter with host phagocytes.

It now seems that tumor cells may be subject to the same
host defense mechanism. North and associates (23-25) present
evidence that mice possess an innate defense mechanism which
operates against both allogeneic and syngeneic tumor cells in the
apparent absence of any known specific immunologic mechanism.
Their data also suggest that this mechanism of resistance is
counteracted by the tumor itself, thus providing a means of
escape from the body's innate defenses. This aggressive quality
in tumor cells is analogous to the antiphagocytic properties
that characterize many infectious agents. Although these are the
first studies which have implied an innate resistance through
macrophages as a component of host defense against tumors, numerous experiments in the past have provided inferential evidence
for the involvement of macrophages in tumor immunity. Early
evidence for the involvement of macrophages in tumor cell destruction in vivo was mainly from histopathologic studies of regressing tumors. Several investigators observed that macrophages

were consistently seen in regressing tumors, but more importantly, they also observed that macrophages invaded the tumor before any degenerative changes in the tumor could be detected.

Possibly a basis for the previous lack of acceptance of the macrophage as a major participant in host immunity to malignant tumor cells is the fact that phagocytosis, which is an essential property of macrophages, is usually not a conspicuous feature of resistance to tumors; because macrophages undoubtedly have a scavenger role, their presence in regressing tumors does not imply that they are playing an active or primary role in the process. Also, as mentioned above, other cell types have been shown to be capable of killing tumor cells in vitro, so that an absolute requirement for macrophages would be difficult to prove. It was thus reasonable to conclude that the macrophage did not play a primary role in host defense against malignancy.

This attitude, however, is chanigng as a result of a large amount of evidence demonstrating that some increased resistance to transplantable tumors may be obtained from nonspecific stimulation of the reticuloendothelial system by a variety of unrelated agents {chronic infection with certain microorganisms (2,7,9,11), endotoxin and double-stranded RNA (1), complete Freund's adjuvant (12), allogeneic and syngeneic tumor cells (5), and pyran copolymer (13)}, and in vitro major effector cells shown to be cytotoxic to tumor cells are macrophages. The induction of a sterile inflammatory exudate in the peritoneal cavity of mice, for example, is not a sufficient stimulus to transform macrophages into tumor-cytotoxic effector cells (4,8); in most cases, a "mediator" produced in response to the inducing agent is needed. Evans and Alexander (5) and Piessens et al. (26) have demonstrated that a product of a reactive lymphocyte (lymphokine) induces macrophage-mediated tumor cytotoxicity. Fidler (6) has shown that normal macrophages as well as macrophages from tumor-bearing mice can be converted to effector cells in vitro by incubating the macrophages with mediators released from sensitized syngeneic, allogeneic, or xenogeneic lymphocytes.

Hibbs et al. (8,10) made the observation that the cytotoxic effect of activated macrophages was selective. Neoplastic cells are destroyed by cytotoxic activated macrophages under in vitro conditions in which nonneoplastic target cells are spared and grow to confluency. Activated peritoneal macrophages from mice with chronic toxoplasma, chlamydia, listeria, or BCG infection did not destroy contact-inhibited allogeneic fibroblast or kidney cell strains that have surfaces of high immunogenic potential, but were markedly cytotoxic to both syngeneic and allogeneic tumorigenic cell lines. These experiments suggest that normal cells may acquire a property similar to neoplastic transformation

that elicits nonimmunologic recognition and subsequent destruction
by activated macrophages.

The observation that activated macrophages had a selective
cytotoxic effect against neoplastic target cells has been confirmed
by others (26). In addition, using a mixture of neoplastic and
nonneoplastic cell lines prelabelled with ^{3}H-thymidine, Meltzer
et al. (17) demonstrated that BCG-activated macrophages selectively
destroyed neoplastic cells. The nonneoplastic cells were not
affected as "innocent bystanders".

A more fundamental question is: what is the mechanism by
which activated macrophages first recognize the subtle differences
between malignant and normal cells, and then kill the former in
deference to the latter? This question has recently been approached
in the different experimental models with some success.

Neoenzymatic agents that accumulate and are stored in the
vacuolar system of macrophages were used to study the nonphago-
cytic contact-dependent mechanism or mechanisms of target cell
destruction by activated mouse peritoneal macrophages and murine
tumor target cells (9). Normal and activated macrophages readily
take up dextran sulfate, which is concentrated in secondary lysosomes. Dextran sulfate is indigestible and nontoxic, and it
stains metachromatically with toluidine blue. Normal and activated macrophages were labelled with dextran sulfate and Hibbs
(9) demonstrated that the transfer of the dextran sulfate secondary lysosome marker to target cells paralleled their susceptibility to destruction by activated macrophages. For example,
after a 24-hr incubation period, 68 ± 8% of BALB/3T12 cells BCG-
activated macrophages had metachromatic cytoplasmic vacuoles.
Similar results were obtained with the same target cells with
the use of C3H macrophages activated by chronic toxoplasma infection. These results indirectly support the idea that activated macrophages transfer the contents of secondary lysosomes
into susceptible target cells.

A morphologic study performed in my laboratory using BCG-
activated peritoneal macrophages from guinea pigs and syngeneic
hepatocarcinoma target cells yielded direct evidence that the
transfer of lysosomal oranelles is a necessary and essential step
in the tumoricidal mechanism of activated macrophages (3). Strain
2 guinea pigs cured of a transplanted hepatocarcinoma by intralesional BCG injection were used as the source of PEC.

The morphological data were obtained by a sequential time
lapse, immunofluorescence, scanning electron microscopy (SEM),
and transmission electron microscopy (TEM) study of single
macrophage-tumor cell interactions. Observations of adherent
macrophage-tumor cell interaction, which by time lapse cinemato-

graphy were judged just to precede tumor cell degeneration, were followed by determination of the identity of the effector cells by immunofluorescence using specific goat anti-guinea pig macrophage serum. Then the identified macrophage-tumor cell interaction was examined by SEM and TEM. This approach eliminated the uncertainties of: (a) the identity of the effector cell, and (b) the relevance of static morphological observations to functional aspects of identified cellular interactions.

Two important observations characterized the interaction of activated macrophages with tumor cell surfaces. There was active extension and contraction of cytoplasmic processes of the macrophages on and into the tumor cell surface. This "probing" was sustained for long periods of time without much lateral movement of the activated macrophage. This activity resulted in considerable clasmatosis of the macrophage at the tumor cell surface. Furthermore, exocytosis of osmiophilic organelles from the macrophage was observed. These organelles have the morphological and histochemical characteristics of primary and/or secondary lysosomes. By TEM it was clear that some of the lysosomal organelles were still within pieces of macrophage cytoplasm that had detached at the tumor cell surface. These lysosomal organelles probably had been intracellular in macrophage cytoplasmic extensions. This is supported by the fact that the intracellular blebs morphologically identified in the cytoplasmic processes of macrophages had the approximate size of the lysosomal organelles. Clasmatosis of macrophage processes with intracellular organelles would result in these structures remaining attached at the tumor cell surface. Other lysosomal products were identified as intercellular entities. These released lysosomal products would not be limited by the single-unit membrane, since fusion of the lysosome membrane with the cell surface would be required for release of the lysosomal products into the intercellular space. Such a mechanism of extracellular localization of lysosomal products has been suggested in other experimental systems (20,21).

Uptake of exocytosed lysosomes of macrophage origin at the intercellular space between macrophages and line 10 tumor cells could be achieved through endocytosis. The endocytic capacity of tumor cell surfaces has been described (21,22) and may be requisite to the translocation of lysosomes from macrophages to tumor cells.

Both normal and activated macrophages contain phosphatase-positive granules (lysosomes). However, the extracellular release of these organelles or their products was not detected by TEM when activated macrophages were mixed with normal guinea pig embryo cells or when normal macrophages were mixed with line 10 tumor cells. Thus, although there were certain qualitative similarities, there

were distinct differences in these systems. These results are in
agreement with the findings that cytotoxic macrophages discriminate between neoplastic and nonneoplastic cells (9,26). Since
the macrophages were isolated from tumor-immune animals, they may
also be "armed" as well as "activated," as described by Evans and
Alexander (5). The question of whether we were dealing with specific tumor cytotoxicity, however, was not approached in this
study. Nevertheless, our results suggest that the cytotoxic
reaction has both an effector cell recognition and a target cell
susceptibility component. The macrophage-tumor cell interaction
initiating the recognition phase may result in the extracellular
release of lysosomes, the exocytosis phase of this cytotoxic reaction. Target cell susceptibility of neoplastic cells to effector
cell events appears to be a result of an active or passive uptake
of lysosomes and, consequently, cytolysis. Basically, the macrophage should, at least, be considered as an important accessory
cell and, in some particular instances, a major effector cell in
host resistance to neoplasia.

REFERENCES

1. Alexander, P. and Evans, R., Nature New Biol, 232 (1971) 76.
2. Bašic, K., Milas, L., Gardina, D. C. and Wither, H. R., J.
   Natl. Cancer Inst. 52 (1974) 1839.
3. Bucana, C., Hoyer, L. C., Hobbs, B., Breesman, S., McDaniel,
   M. and Hanna, M. G., Jr., Cancer Res. 36 (1976) 4444.
4. Cleveland, R. P., Meltzer, M. S. and Zbar, B., J. Natl. Cancer
   Inst. 52 (1974) 1887.
5. Evans, R., and Alexander, P., Nature, 236 (1972) 168.
6. Fidler, I. J., J. Natl. Cancer Inst. 55 (1975) 1159.
7. Hibbs, J. B., Jr., Science, 180 (1973) 868.
8. Hibbs, J. B., Jr., J. Natl. Cancer Inst. 53 (1974) 1487.
9. Hibbs, J. B., Jr., Science, 184 (1974) 468.
10. Hibbs, J. B., Jr., In: The Macrophage in Neoplasia, (Ed. Mary
    Fink) Academic Press, New York, New York (1976) 83.
11. Hibbs, J. B., Jr., Lambert, L. H., Jr. and Remington, J. S.,
    J. Infect. Diseases, 124 (1971) 587.
12. Hibbs, J. B., Jr., Lambert, L. H., Jr. and Remington, J.,
    Proc. Soc. Exptl. Biol. Med., 139 (1972) 1049.
13. Kaplan, A. M., Morahan, P. S. and Regelson, W., J. Natl.
    Cancer Inst., 52 (1974) 1919.
14. Mackaness, G. B., J. Exp. Med., 129 (1969) 973.
15. Mackaness, G. B., In: The Macrophages in Neoplasia, (Ed.
    Mary Fink) Academic Press, New York, New York (1976) 3.
16. Mackaness, G. B. and Blanden, R. V., Progr. Allergy, 11 (1967)
    89.
17. Meltzer, M. S., Tucker, R. W., Sanford, K. K. and Leonard,
    E. J., J. Natl. Cancer Inst. 54 (1975) 1177.
18. Nelson, D. S., CRC Crit. Rev. Microbiol., 1 (1972) 353.

19. Nelson, D. S., Transplant. Rev., 19 (1974) 226.
20. Nichols, B. A. and Bainton, D. F., Lab. Invest. 29 (1973) 27.
21. Nicolson, G. L., Biochim. Biophys. Acta, 458 (1976) 1.
22. Nicolson, G. L., Lacorbiere, M. and Hunter, I. R., Cancer Res.,
    35 (1975) 144.
23. North, R. J. and Kirsten, D. P., J. Exp. Med., 145 (1977) 275.
24. North, R. J., Kirsten, D. P. and Tuttle, R. L., J. Exp. Med.,
    143 (1976) 559.
25. North, R. J., Kirsten, D. P. and Tuttle, R. L., J. Exp. Med.,
    143 (1976) 574.
26. Piessens, W. F., Churchill, W. H., Jr and David, J. R., J.
    Immunol., 114 (1975) 293.

MACROPHAGES AS REGULATORS OF IMMUNE RESPONSES AGAINST TUMORS

R. B. HERBERMAN, H. T. HOLDEN, J. Y. DJEU[*], T. R.
JERRELLS[*], L. VARESIO, A. TAGLIABUE, S. L. WHITE,
J. R. OEHLER and J. H. DEAN[*]

Laboratory of Immunodiagnosis, National Cancer Institute,
Bethesda, Maryland; and [*]Department of Immunology, Litton
Bionetics, Inc., Kensington, Maryland (USA)

There is an increasing body of in vitro and in vivo evidence
that macrophages play an important role in regulating or modulating a wide variety of immune responses. This is being found to
have particular relevance in studies of immune responses against
tumors. Not only are they effector cells against tumors, they
have major positive and negative regulatory effects on the immune
responses against tumors by other types of lymphoid cells.

The positive effects of macrophages in immune responses
against tumors can be summarized as follows:

Direct anti-tumor effects of macrophages. Many studies in
mice and rats have demonstrated that macrophages, after various
activating procedures, have cytotoxic effects against tumor cells.
Both cytolytic (46, 48) as well as cytostatic or growth inhibitory effects (29,30) have been associated with activated macrophages. Most studies on cytotoxic effects of macrophages have
utilized macrophages activated by immune adjuvants or other agents.
However, macrophages harvested from the spleen and peritoneal
cavity of tumor-bearing mice (29,30,46) and from the actual site
of tumor growth (22,46,48) have also been shown to be highly cytotoxic against tumor cells. There have been very few comparable
studies on macrophages or monocytes from patients with cancer,
but a recent study in our laboratory has demonstrated that peripheral blood monocytes of a substantial proportion of patients
with carcinomas, particularly those with advanced disease, have
cytostatic activity against cultured cell lines (24).

Macrophages have been shown to be required as accessory cells
for various types of T cell-mediated immune responses against
tumors. a) in tumor systems in mice (33) and rats (50), histocompatible macrophages have been shown to be required for production of migration inhibitory factor (MIF) in response to some
tumor antigens. b) furthermore, for expression of the biological
effects of MIF, functional macrophages are required to respond to
this lymphokine and be slowed in their migration. c) there have
been some recent indications, mainly in studies of the lymphoproliferative response of cancer patients to extracts of autologous
tumor, that macrophages are required for response (7). d) similarly, in studies in mice, macrophages have appeared to be required for in vitro generation of secondary cytotoxic responses
to tumor cells (53).

Requirement for macrophages for activation of natural killer
(NK) cells and of K cells mediating antibody-dependent cell-
mediated cytotoxicity (ADCC) by production of interferon. Recent
studies have indicated that macrophages may play an important
role in activating these effector cells, and in maintaining their
activities in vivo, by means of their central involvement in
interferon production (11).

In the past several years, it has also become apparent that
macrophages can mediate negative or inhibitory effects on various
immune responses to tumors. Although the initial findings of
suppression by macrophages involved lymphocyte proliferative
responses, more recently macrophages have been found to mediate
suppression of several other types of cell-mediated immune
reactions. These include suppression of: a) in vitro generation
of primary or secondary cytotoxic responses; b) production of
MIF and other lymphokines; and c) responses of macrophages to
MIF. In this report, we will concentrate on the various suppressor activities of macrophages, but will also discuss some
recent information on the role of macrophages in activating
mouse NK cells.

Before summarizing in any detail the data on suppression of
immune responses by macrophages, it is important to discuss the
methods used to incriminate macrophages as the suppressor cells.
Similar steps, looking for effects in the opposite direction,
have usually been taken to document the role of macrophages as
helper or accessory cells. Two main approaches have been employed:

Demonstration of restoration or augmentation of immune
responses by removal or inactivation of macrophages. The most
frequent and useful methods for eliminating most macrophages are:
a) adherence to nylon or rayon fiber or Sephadex G-10 columns or
to glass or plastic dishes. Our experience has been that rayon
and G-10 columns are quite efficient in removing suppressor cells

and tend to be somewhat more selective for macrophages than nylon columns, which in addition deplete a higher proportion of B cells. A particular problem that we have encountered in depletion experiments is that some suppressor macrophages are only loosely adherent and therefore the usual procedures to remove strongly adherent cells on petri dishes usually fail to adequately deplete suppressor macrophage activity. b) phagocytosis of carbonyl iron with subsequent removal of macrophages by a magnet or by centrifugation on a Ficoll-Hypaque gradient. This method has been quite useful but, depending on the actual technique used, may suffer from non-specific losses of non-phagocytic cells. c) treatment with macrophage-toxic agents, silica or carrageenan. These agents appear to be fairly selective in their effects on macrophages (1), but we must be aware of the possibility of more general toxic effects by some preparations. It is clear that none of these depletion procedures are ideal and it is therefore desirable to obtain evidence of restoration of immune reactivity when more than one type of treatment is used. Furthermore, merely restoring or augmenting responsiveness by depletion procedures cannot be taken as definitive evidence for suppressor activity. Some of the same results could be produced by enriching for reactive cells, by removal of many inactive but non-suppressive cells. This has led to extensive use of the second approach.

Suppression of normal responses by addition of either a) small numbers of purified macrophages or b) macrophage-containing populations of cells. With the latter approach, it has been necessary to show that the addition of equal numbers of cells, after depletion of macrophages, no longer inhibits the immune reaction. With all of these procedures to prepare macrophage-depleted or enriched cell populations, it has been important to document the purity of the resultant population. We have relied on the ingestion of latex particles to identify phagocytic cells and on nonspecific esterase stains.

Our laboratory has investigated a number of cases of suppressed immune responses in vitro and, in most instances, we have identified the macrophage as the cell responsible for the effects. Many of the original observations were made by Kirchner et al. (26,27,28,30). It was initially observed that spleen cells from C57BL/6 mice-bearing tumors induced by murine sarcoma virus (MSV) responded poorly if at all to T cell mitogens such as PHA and Con A and frequently had a depressed response to the B cell mitogen endotoxin (LPS) (26,27). After removal of adherent or phagocytic cells, it was shown that cells capable of lymphoproliferative responses were present in the spleens. Furthermore, mixture of spleen cells from MSV-tumor-bearing mice with normal spleen cells resulted in a depressed response. This suppressor activity was depleted by removal of adherent or phagocytic cells or by treatment with anti-Thy 1 plus complement. There has been a number

of subsequent studies of tumor-bearing mice (42,44) and rats (15,
32,55) in which the depressed responses to mitogens have been
attributed to the presence of suppressor macrophages. We have
recently documented that not only are the effector cells independent of T cells, the generation of suppressor cells in tumor-
bearing mice is independent of thymic function since nude mice
bearing MSV-induced tumors develop comparable levels of suppressor
cells as do conventional mice of the same strain. In addition to
the suppression of mitogen responses, macrophage-mediated suppressive effects have been demonstrated for lymphoproliferative
responses of mice and rats to alloantigens in mixed lymphocyte
cultures (MLC) (12,13,38,56) and to tumor antigens in mixed lymphocyte tumor interactions (MLTI) (15,30,37).

TABLE I

Suppressor Cell Activity in Lung and Breast Cancer Patients

Patient Group	No. Tested	% with Suppressor Cell Activity	% with Adherent Suppressor Cells	% with Nonadherent Suppressor Cells
Lung cancer	21	52% (11/21)	64% (7/11)	27% 3/11)[a]
Breast cancer	20	35% (7/20)	29% (2/7)	57% (4/7)[a]

[a]One patient in each group had detectable suppressor cell activity
which was not further characterized.

        In addition to suppression of lymphoproliferative responses
by macrophages in tumor-bearers, some bacterial immune adjuvants
have been paradoxically associated with the induction of suppressor macrophages. Both Corynebacterium parvum (28,49) and BCG
(35) have been shown to produce such effects.

        In mice, suppressor macrophages have usually been detected
only after induction of tumors or after some other treatment. In
contrast, suppressor macrophages have been found in the spleens
of most normal rats. Addition of normal rat spleen cells to MLC
or MLTI cultures as third part cells led to suppression, although
not as marked as that seen with cells from tumor-bearing donors

(38,40,56). Furthermore, removal of most macrophages from the spleen cells of normal rats substantially improved their lymphoproliferative responses in MLC (38,56) and the same procedure with rats immune to a syngeneic tumor allowed us to more consistently demonstrate reactivity in MLTI (40). These findings indicate that the suppressive nature of macrophages may not necessarily represent a pathologic state but rather reflect a normal regulatory mechanism which is intensified in some pathological conditions.

Recently it has been shown that the depressed lymphoproliferative responses to mitogens or in MLC or many patients with cancer were due to suppression by monocytes (2,4,17,23,61). We have recently performed a study of patients with carcinoma of the breast or lung who had depressed lymphoproliferative responses (23), and our overall experience is summarized in Table I. Approximately one-half of the lung cancer patients with depressed reactivity had demonstrable suppressor cell activity which at least partially accounted for the low responses. The suppressor cell in two-thirds of these patients were adherent to Sephadex G-10 and in some instances were also shown to be phagocytic. With a few other lung cancer patients, the suppressor cells were nonadherent and their nature (? suppressor T cells) remains to be determined. With the breast cancer patients with depressed responses, a lower proportion had evidence of suppressor cells and more of these were not monocytic in nature. We have also found that the lack of lymphoproliferative response of some lung or breast cancer patients to autologous tumor extracts (8,9) could be attributed to the presence of suppressor monocytes in the peripheral blood. The results of experiments with two such patients are summarized in Fig. 1. The peripheral blood mononuclear leukocytes (PBL) of these patients, obtained by centrifugation on a Ficoll-Hypaque gradient, failed to give a significant response to autologous tumor membrane extracts. To look for a role of suppressor monocytes, the PBL were passaged over Sephadex G-10 columns. Since we have found that the lymphoproliferative responses to these extracts require the presence of some monocytes, a small number (1%) of the autologous monocytes were added back. These cultures then showed quite substantial reactivity. In addition, with the first patient, addition of higher numbers of autologous monocytes resulted in complete abrogation of the response. As a further interesting point in this experiment, addition of indomethacin reversed some of the suppression.

The use of indomethacin in this and similar experiments was prompted by the report of Goodwin et al. (17) that the suppression by monocytes of lymphoproliferative responses in patients with Hodgkin's disease was due to their production of prostaglandins. Addition to the cultures of indomethacin, a prostaglandin synthetase inhibitor, caused a significant increase in reactivity. As illustrated in Fig. 1, we have also observed that indomethacin

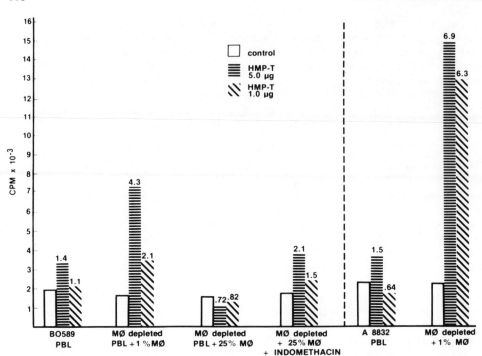

Fig. 1.   The peripheral blood mononuclear leukocytes (PBL) of
patient B 0589 (lung cancer) and of patient A 8832 (breast
cancer) were tested for their lymphoproliferative response to
hypotonic membrane preparations (HMP) of their own tumors.   For
some groups, the monocytes were depleted from the PBL by passage
over Sephadex G-10 columns.   Enriched populations of monocytes,
obtained by elution from the columns by 0.25% lidocaine, were
added back to these cultures.   In one set of cultures, indomethacin (1 μg/ml) was also added.

can at least partially reverse the suppression in some patients.
We have studied this in somewhat more detail in mice bearing
MSV-induced tumors (Table II).   When small numbers of suppressor
spleen cells were added to cultures of normal spleen cells, partial
suppression of reactivity to PHA or LPS was seen, and this was reversed rather well by indomethacin.   However, the stronger inhibition by larger numbers of added suppressor cells was usually un-
affected by the presence of indomethacin.   Even higher doses of
drug, up to 10 μg/ml, were unable to reverse some of the suppression.   This suggests that macrophages may be able to suppress by
other mechanisms in addition to prostaglandin production or that
indomethacin, under the in vitro conditions of our experiments,

TABLE II

Effect of Indomethacin on Suppression of Mitogenic Responses
by Spleen Cells from MSV-Tumor-Bearing Mice

Expt.	Mitogen	Indomethacin (1μg/ml)	cpm ^{3}HTdR Incorporation (% Suppression)[a]		
			.67:1	33:1	.17:1
1	PHA (165,977 cpm)[b]	–	50,175 (70)	78,926 (52	119,422 (28)
		+	35,289 (79)	87,638 (47)	164,138 (1)
	LPS (18,584 cpm)	–	13,966 (25)	17,706 (5)	20,299 (0)
		+	20,225 (0)	21,656 (0)	23,001 (0)
2	PHA (70,488 cpm)	–	17,197 (81)	52,513 (30)	64,865 (10)
		+	28,042 (70)	90,621 (0)	68,501 (4)
	LPS (22,019 cpm)	–	9,216 (58)	14,137 (36)	18,461 (16)
		+	10,899 (51)	21,025 (5)	23,013 (0)

[a] Spleen cells from C57BL/6 mice 13-15 days after intramuscular injection of MSV, added at various ratios, to normal spleen cells.

[b] cpm ^{3}H-TdR incorporated into spleen cells of normal C57BL/6 after incubation with mitogen for three days.

was unable to completely block prostaglandin synthesis.

In constrast to the inhibitory effects of suppressor macrophages on lymphoproliferative responses, cytotoxicity by previously generated effector cells seems not to be affected. T
cell-mediated cytotoxicity to tumor-associated antigens (27), PHA-
induced T cell-mediated cytotoxicity (28) and ADCC (45) were un-
affected by suppressor macrophages. In contrast, the generation
of cytotoxic T cells in MLC (31,38,56) or in MLTI (16,40) has
been suppressed by the presence of suppressor macrophages. Since
the generation of cytotoxic lymphocytes in primary MLC (5,43)
and in secondary MLTI (3,51) requires some proliferation, it was
postulated that the primary effect of suppressor macrophages was
on proliferation of lymphocytes (39).

However, we have recently obtained evidence that some proliferation-independent immune responses can also be inhibited by
suppressor macrophages. This has come from studies of the production of MIF in response to tumor cells by T cells from immune
mice (54). Although spleen cells from mice bearing MSV-induced
tumors produce MIF upon culture with intact tumor cells, T cells
isolated from the tumors have been unreactive. Since high levels
of suppressor macrophage activity have been found in these tumors
(22), it was of interest to determine whether such cells could
cause suppression of MIF production. Addition of adherent cells
from MSV tumors to cultures of immune spleen cells and RBL-5
tumors resulted in abrogation of detectable MIF production
(Table III). In contrast, normal mouse peritoneal macrophages
had no suppressor activity. This suppressor activity, however,
is not restricted to tumor-bearing mice, since peritoneal cells
from mice inoculated with BCG had strong suppressor activity.
As with the suppression of lymphoproliferative responses by macrophages, the suppression of MIF production has not been antigen
specific. Suppressor macrophages from MSV tumors have also been
able to suppress MIF production of alloimmune spleen cells in
response to allogeneic cells, and of normal spleen cells in
response to the mitogen Con A (Table IV). The production of MIF
by lymphocytes has been shown to be independent of proliferation,
with mitomycin C blocked cells being fully capable of response.
These results indicate that macrophages are able to suppress
immune phenomena independent of proliferation. It seems likely
that the primary effect of suppressor macrophages is on an early
phase of the metabolic activity of lymphocytes which is induced
by stimulation, and that the inhibition of proliferation is a
secondary manifestation. The indications for a role of prostaglandins in the suppression by macrophages would be consistent
with this hypothesis, since some of the primary effects of prostaglandins are on metabolic pathways separate from DNA synthesis
or cell division (18).

TABLE III

Suppressive Effect of Macrophages from MSV-Induced Tumors or
from BCG-Induced PEC on MIF Production by MSV-Immune
Macrophage-Depleted Spleen Cells in Response to RBL-5 Tumor

Macrophages Added (10%)	% Migration Inhibition
-	55
PEC[a]	45
-	40
SV tumor[b]	2
-	47
CG-induced PEC[c]	-8

[a]Uninduced peritoneal exudate cells.

[b]Adherent cells from MSV tumor at 14 days after induction.

[c]15-21 days after i.p. inoculation of viable BCG.

TABLE IV

Suppressive Effect of Macrophages from MSV-Induced
Tumors of MIF Production by Macrophage-Depleted C57BL/6 Spleen
Cells

Immunization of Responder	Stimulus	Suppressor Cells[a]	% Migration Inhibition
MSV	RBL-5 tumor cells	-	41
		+	-1
K36(H-2^k)	K36 tumor cells	-	57
		+	-4
none	Con A	-	36
		+	-2

[a]10% adherent cells from MSV tumors added to incubation mixture.

As noted earlier, the biologic effects of MIF are dependent on the response of macrophages to the lymphokine, with slowing of their migration. We have recently studied the response to MIF of macrophages from C3H/HeJ mice since these cells were found not to become cytotoxic in response to macrophage activating factor (47). In addition of the genetic defect for response of their B cells to LPS, these mice appear to have deficient macrophage functions. Peritoneal macrophages from most normal C3H/HeJ mice were not inhibited in their migration upon exposure to a super- natant fluid containing a high titer of MIF (52) (Fig. 2). In contrast, peritoneal cells from the related C3H/HeN strain, which lacks the genetic defect in LPS responsiveness, responded well to the lymphokine. Although the lack of response to MIF of C3H/HeJ macrophages might be taken as another form of intrinsic defect in the lymphoid cells of this strain, the finding of responsiveness to MIF by some normal C3H/HeJ mice (Fig. 2), and by macrophages from BCG-inoculated C3H/HeJ mice, suggested some other explana- tion. Among the peritoneal cells of C3H/HeJ mice, there appear to be cells capable of suppressing the migration responses of macro- phages to MIF. Addition of 10% peritoneal cells from normal C3H/HeJ mice to C3H/HeN cells resulted in suppression of the in- hibition of migration by MIF (Fig. 3). Preliminary data indicate that adherent cells, probably macrophages, of normal C3H/HeJ are the suppressor cells in this system. If so, this would indicate another type of proliferation-independent suppressive effect of macrophages.

Having summarized much of the available information on sup- pression by macrophages, we will now turn to a discussion of the relationship of macrophages to natural killer (NK) cells. Natu- ral cell-mediated cytotoxicity against tumors has been found to be mediated by a particular subpopulation of lymphocytes which have been termed NK cells (19). Considerable circumstancial evi- dence also suggests that radioresistant rejection of bone marrow allografts is mediated by NK cells (19,25). Neither NK activity nor bone marrow resistance are mediated by macrophages, but there have been some indications of an important role of macrophages in these functions. The most direct evidence has been that ad- ministration of silica or carrageenan to mice resulted in a de- crease in NK activity (25) and bone marrow resistance (6,60). Data from a representative experiment, showing the inhibitory effects of silica and carrageenan on NK activity, are summarized in Table V. The apparent link between these functional activi- ties and macrophages was quite puzzling, but some recent find- ings on factors regulating the activation of NK cells have pro- vided some important clues. These have allowed us to formulate the model shown in Fig. 4. It has been possible to rapidly and substantially augment the levels of NK activity in mice and rats by inoculation of tumor cells, viruses and some bacterial immune

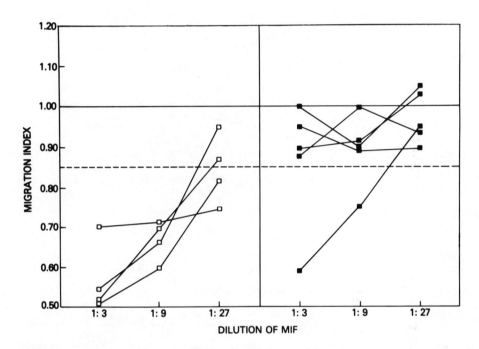

Fig. 2. Effect of MIF on migration of PEC from C3H/HeN (□) and C3H/HeJ (■) mice. Each line represents the results obtained when simultaneously testing PEC from several groups of mice (pools of PEC from 3 mice/group).

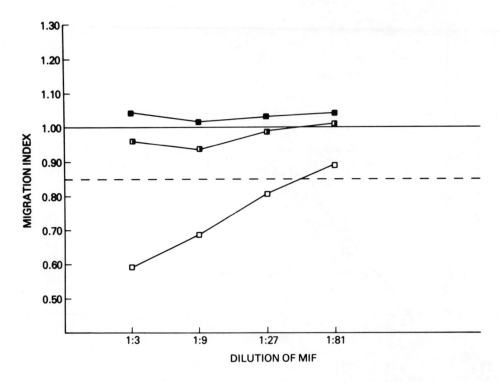

Fig. 3.   Effect of MIF on migration of PEC from C3H/HeN (□) and
C3H/HeJ (■) mice or on mixture of 90% PEC from C3H/HeN mice plus
10% PEC from C3H/HeJ mice (◨).

TABLE V

Effect of In Vivo Administration of Silica and
Carrageenan on NK Activity in 6-8 Week Old Mice

Treatment[b]	% Cytotoxicity[a]	
	CBA/J	Swiss Nude
BSS	31.9	33.5
Silica (750 mg/kg i.p.)	5.6	17.2
Carrageenan (100 mg/kg i.v.)	8.1	20.1

[a]Effector: target cell ratio of 100:1 against RLδ1 target cells.
[b]Administered 1 day before testing.

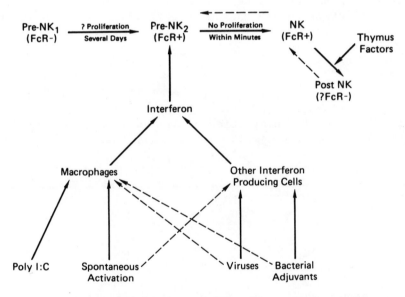

Fig. 4. Model for activation of NK cells and the important roles
of interferon and macrophages.

adjuvants (21,34,41,57,58,59). When it was found that poly
I:C, a potent inducer of interferon, could also augment NK activity in rats (41), it seemed likely that interferon might play an
important role in boosting NK activity. In studies in mice, inoculation of interferon, as well as poly I:C and other interferon
inducers, could strongly augment NK activity (10,14) and this
could be blocked by anti-interferon (14). It was also possible
to incubate mouse spleen cells with poly I:C or interferon and
produce rapid augmentation of NK reactivity (10). A similar
stimulatory role of interferon for human NK and K cell (20) activities has been demonstrated. The initial indications for a role
of macrophages in boosting of NK activity came from experiments
in which rats (36) or mice (11) were treated with silica or
carrageenan prior to inoculation with poly I:C. As shown in
Table VI, these agents at least partially interfered with the
augmentation of cytotoxic reactivity. In contrast, when poly
I:C was given first and the mice were treated with silica or
carrageenan just a few hr before testing, no inhibitory effect
was seen. To further examine the role of macrophages in boosting
of NK activity, a series of experiments were performed in vitro.
After pretreatment of spleen cells with silica or carrageenan,
their NK activity no longer could be boosted by poly I:C (Table
VII). However, if the sequence were reversed, with carrageenan
or silica being added after poly I:C, strong augmentation was seen.
The pattern of boosting in these experiments correlated well with
the levels of interferon in the culture fluids, with much lower
amounts being detectable in those of cells treated with the

TABLE VI

Effect of In Vivo Administration of Silica and Carrageenan on
Boosting of NK Activity of 12 Week Old CBA/J Mice by Poly I:C

Treatment[a]	% Cytotoxicity[b]
BSS	2.1
Poly I:C	16.6
Poly I:C + silica, 15 mg i.p.	7.0
Poly I:C + carrageenan, 1 mg i.v.	3.4

[a]Poly I:C was administered 4 hr after silica or carrageenan and
 NK activity was tested 18 hr later.
[b]Attacker: target cell ratio of 200:1, against RL♂1 target cells.

TABLE VII

Effect of Macrophage Removal on the In Vitro Augmentation
of NK Activity by Poly I:C

Treatment In Vitro[a]			% Cytotoxicity[b]	
-3 hr	0 hr	+18 hr	CBA/J	Swiss Nude
−	−	−	2.8	2.0
−	Poly I:C	−	15.8	24.3
Silica	Poly I:C	−	4.9	5.0
Carrageenan	Poly I:C	−	4.5	3.1
Nylon column	Poly I:C	−		3.4
−	−	−	9.2	1.2
−	Poly I:C	−	22.6	22.0
−	Poly I:C	Silica	28.0	17.0
−	Poly I:C	Carrageenan	24.2	17.9

[a]Spleen cells incubated with 10 µg/ml of silica or carrageenan
for 3 hr at 37 C, 3 hr before, or 18 hr after, addition of
Poly I:C (100 µg/ml).
[b]Attacker: target cell ratio 200:1, RL∂1 target cells.

macrophage-toxic agents prior to poly I:C. These results
suggested that the interference with boosting by poly I:C was
due to a block in the production of interferon, either by the
macrophages themselves or due to the requirement for macrophages
for interferon production by other cells. However, macrophages
did not appear to be required for some other accessory role in
boosting. This was supported by the findings that spontaneous
levels of NK activity (Table VII) or in vitro boosting by interferon (Table IX) were not affected by treatment with silica or
carrageenan. Studies are now in progress to clarify the role of
macrophages in the spontaneous appearance and maintenance of
levels of NK activity in vivo.

TABLE VIII

Effect on NK Activity of In Vitro Incubation of Spleen Cells
with Silica or Carrageenan

Treatment[a]	% Cytotoxicity	
	CBA/J	Swiss Nude
Medium	25.4	21.6
Silica	24.2	19.6
Carrageenan	24.9	20.2

[a]Spleen cells preincubated with 10 µg/ml of agent for 3 hr at
37 C and then tested, without washing, for NK activity against
RL♂1 target cells, at 200:1 attacker:target cell ratio.

TABLE IX

Effect of Macrophage Removal on In Vitro Augmentation by
Interferon of NK Activity of Spleen Cells from CBA/J Mice

Treatment[a]	% Cytotoxicity[b]
Medium	8.6
Interferon	17.1
" + silica	18.6
" + carrageenan	24.3
" + rayon column	24.9

[a]Spleen cells preincubated with silica or carrageenan (10 µg/ml)
for 3 hr at 37 C or column passed before exposure to interferon (10^4 U/ml) for 1 hr.
[b]Attacker:target cell ratio 200:1, RL♂1 target cells.

As illustrated by the studies described above, there is now abundant evidence for a major regulatory role of macrophages in a variety of cell-mediated immune reactions against tumors. It is no longer appropriate to restrict one's attention to T cells and other lymphocytes in considering the host defenses against neoplasia. On the one hand, macrophages may be essential for the development of effective immune responses; and, on the other hand, these cells may interfere with the development of immunity and with the expression of immunity by sensitized lymphocytes. Since these various functions of macrophages are strongly affected by BCG, C. parvum and other immunotherapeutic agents, the positive and negative effects by the activated macrophages need to be carefully considered.

REFERENCES

1. Allison, A. C., Hammington, J. S. and Birbeck, M., J. Exp. Med., 124 (1966) 141.
2. Berlinger, N. T., Lopez, C. and Good, R. A., Nature, 260 (1976) 145.
3. Bernstein, I. D., Cohen, E. F. and Wright, P. W., J. Immunol. 118 (1977) 1090.
4. Broder, S., Humphrey, R., Durm, M., Blackman, M., Meade, B., Goldman, C., Strober, W. and Waldmann, T., N. Eng. J. Med., 293 (1975) 887.
5. Cantor, H. and Jandinski, J., J. Exp. Med., 140 (1974) 1712.
6. Cudowicz, G. and Yung, Y. P., J. Immunol. 119 (1977) 483.
7. Dean, J. H., Jerrells, T. and Herberman, R. B., (1978) unpublished observations.
8. Dean, J. H., Jerrells, T. R., Cannon, G. B., Kibrite, A., Baumgardner, B., Weese, J. L., Silva, J. and Herberman, R. B., (1978), submitted for publication.
9. Dean, J. H., McCoy, J. L., Cannon, G. B., Leonard, C. M., perlin, E., Kreutner, A., Oldham, R. K. and Herberman, R. B., J. Nat. Cancer Inst., 58 (1977) 549.
10. Djeu, J. Y., Heinbaugh, J. A., Holden, H. T. and Herberman, R. B., (1978),submitted for publication.
11. Djeu, J. Y., Heinbaugh, J. A., Holden, H. T. and Herberman, R. B., (1978), submitted for publication
12. Fernbach, B. R., Kirchner, H., Bonnard, G. D. and Herberman, R. B., Transplantation, 21 (1976) 381.
13. Fernbach, B. R., Kirchner, H. and Herberman, R. B., Cell. Immunol. 22 (1976) 399.
14. Gidlund, M., Orn, A., Wigzell, H., Senik, A. and Gresser, I., Nature (1978), in press.
15. Glaser, M., Kirchner, H. and Herberman, R. B., Int. J. Cancer, 16 (1975) 384.
16. Glaser, M., Kirchner, H., Holden, H. T. and Herberman, R. B., J. Nat. Cancer Inst., 56 (1976) 865.

17. Goodwin, J. S., Messner, R. P., Bankhurst, A. D., Peake, G. T., Saiki, J. H. and Williams, R. C., Jr., N. Eng. J. Med., 297 (1977) 963.
18. Henney, C. S., Bourne, H. R. and Lichtenstein, L. M., J. Immunol. 108 (1972) 1526.
19. Herberman, R. B. and Holden, H. T., Advances in Cancer Research (Ed. G. Klein and S. Weinhouse). Academic Press, New York (1978) in press.
20. Herberman, R. B., Djeu, J. Y., Ortaldo, J. R., Holden, H. T., West, W. H. and Bonnard, G. D., Cancer Treatment Reports, (1978) in press.
21. Herberman, R. B., Nunn, M. E., Holden, H. t., Staal, S. and Djeu, J. Y., Int. J. Cancer, 19 (1977) 555.
22. Holden, H. T., Haskill, J. S., Kirchner, H. and Herberman, R. B., J. Immunol. 117 (1976) 440.
23. Jerrells, T. R., Cannon, G. B., McCoy, J. L. and Herberman, R. B., J. Nat. Cancer Inst. (1978) in press.
24. Jerrells, T., Dean, J. H. and Herberman, R. B., (1978) unpublished observations.
25. Kiessling, R., Hochman, P. S., Haller, O., Shearer, G. M., Wigzell, H. and Cudkowicz, G., Eur. J. Immunol. 7 (1977) 655.
26. Kirchner, H., Chused, T. M., Herberman, R. B., Holden, H. T. and Larvin, D. H., J. Exp. Med., 139 (1974) 1473.
27. Kirchner, H., Herberman, R. B., Glaser, M. and Larvin, D. H., Cell. Immunol. 13 (1974) 32.
28. Kirchner, H., Holden, H. T. and Herberman, R. B., J. Immunol., 115 (1975) 1212.
29. Kirchner, H., Holden, H. T. and Herberman, R. B., J. Nat. Cancer Inst., 55 (1975) 971.
30. Kirchner, H., Muchmore, A. V., Chused, T. M., Holden, H. T. and Herberman, R.B., J. Immunol. 144 (1975) 206.
31. Klimpel, G. R. and Henney, C. S., J. Immunol., 120 (1978) 563.
32. Kruisbeek, A. M. and Van Hess, M., J. Nat. Cancer Inst., 58 (1977) 1653.
33. Landolfo, S., Herberman, R. B. and Holden, H. T., J. Immunol., 118 (1977) 1244.
34. MacFarlan, R. I., Burns, W. H. and White, D. O., J. Immunol., 119 (1977) 1569.
35. Mitchell, M. S., Kirkpatrick, D., Mokyr, M. B. and Gery, I., Nature New Biol., 243 (1973) 216.
36. Oehler, J. R. and Herberman, R. B., Int. J. Cancer, 21 (1978) 221.
37. Oehler, J. R., Campbell, D. A., Jr. and Herberman, R. B., Cell. Immunol., 28 (1977) 355.
38. Oehler, J. R., Herberman, R. B., Campbell, D. A., Jr. and Djeu, J. Y., Cell, Immunol., 29 (1977) 238.
39. Oehler, J. R., Herberman, R. B. and Holden, H. T., J. Pharmacol. Ther., 2 (1978) 551.

40. Oehler, J. R., Landolfo, S. and Herberman, R. B., (1978) submitted for publication.
41. Oehler, J. R., Lindsay, L. R., Nunn, M. E., Holden, H. T. and Herberman, R. B., Int. J. Cancer, 21 (1978) 210.
42. Padarathsingh, M. L., Dean, J. H., Jerrells, T. R., McCoy, J. L., Lewis, D. D. and Northing, J. W. (1978) submitted for publication.
43. Peavy, D. L. and Pierce, C. W., J. Immunol., 115 (1975) 1521.
44. Pope, B. L., Whitney, R. B., Levy, J. G. and Kilburn, D. G., J. Immunol., 116 (1976) 1342.
45. Poplack, D. G., Bonnard, G. D., Holiman, B. J. and Blaese, R. M., Blood, 48 (1976) 809.
46. Puccetti, P. and Holden, H. T., J. Immunol, (1978) in press.
47. Ruco, L. P. and Meltzer, M. S., J. Immunol., 120 (1978) 329.
48. Russell, S. W., Gillespie, G. Y. and McIntosh, A. T., J. Immunol., 118 (1977) 1574.
49. Scott, M. T., Cell, Immunol., 5 (1972) 459.
50. Sharma, J. and Herberman, R. B. (1978) unpublished observations.
51. Stiller, R. A. and Holden, H. T. (1978) submitted for publication.
52. Tagliabue, A., McCoy, J. L. and Herberman, R. B., J. Immunol. (1978) in press.
53. Taniyama, T. and Holden, H. T., (1978) unpublished observations.
54. Varesio, L., Herberman, R. B. and Holden, H. T., (1978) submitted for publication.
55. Veit, B. C. and Feldman, J. D., J. Immunol., 117 (1976) 655.
56. Weiss, A. and Fitch, F. W., J. Immunol., 119 (1977) 510.
57. Welsh, R. M., Jr. and Zinkernagel, R. M., Nature, 268 (1977) 646.
58. Wolfe, S. A., Tracey, D. E. and Henney, C. S., Nature, 262 (1976) 584.
59. Wolfe, S. A., Tracey, D. E. and Henney, C. S., J. Immunol., 119 (1977) 1152.
60. Yung, Y. P. and Cudkowicz, G., J. Immunol., 119 (1977) 1310.
61. Zembala, M., Mytar, B., Popiela, T. and Asherson, G. L., Int. J. Cancer, 19 (1977) 605.

MACROPHAGE ACTIVATION FOR TUMOR CYTOTOXICITY:

MECHANISMS OF MACROPHAGE ACTIVATION BY LYMPHOKINES

M. S. MELTZER, L. P. RUCO and E. J. LEONARD

Immunopathology Section, Laboratory of Immunobiology
National Cancer Institute, Bethesda, Maryland (USA)

Animals infected with certain intracellular parasites such as
Mycobacterium bovis, strain BCG, Toxoplasma gondii or Listeria
monocytogenes develop macrophages localized to the site of infection
that are cytotoxic to tumor cells (3,1). Nonspecifically tumoricidal macrophages, defined as "activated", also occur at reaction sites
of allograft and tumor rejection and of specific antigen or mitogen-
induced immune responses (4,8). Development of activated macrophages during each of these reactions requires the simultaneous
presence of effective activation signals and mononuclear phagocytes able to respond. We have analyzed interactions between
mononuclear phagocytes and activation stimuli using an in vitro
cytotoxicity assay based on release of nuclear label from prelabeled
tumor cells (5) (Fig. 1). Release of ^{3}HTdR showed good correlation
with tumor cell death estimated by morphologic changes on cinemicroscopy (6) (Fig. 2). Cytotoxicity curves for tumor cell
death by both criteria were superimposable except for a time factor: death estimated by ^{3}HTdR release occurred about 2-fold
later than death defined by morphologic changes.

Using this assay, we have begun to characterize macrophage
activation factors in supernatants of antigen or mitogen-stimulated
leukocyte cultures (Fig. 3). By Sephadex G-100 chromatography,
MAF elutes as a single peak with a molecular weight of about
55,000 daltons. This elution pattern, however, is too broad for
a single entity and suggests a limited heterogeneity within the
MAF species (7,4). MAF activity is heat labile (80% loss of
activity at 56 C for 30 mins), destroyed at pH 4 or 10 (90% loss
after 16 hrs) and susceptible to proteolytic enzymes (Fig. 4).

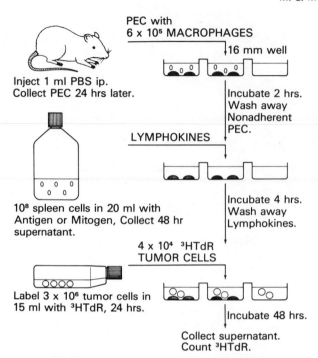

PEC with
6 x 10⁵ MACROPHAGES

16 mm well

Inject 1 ml PBS ip.
Collect PEC 24 hrs later.

Incubate 2 hrs.
Wash away
Nonadherent
PEC.

LYMPHOKINES

10⁸ spleen cells in 20 ml with
Antigen or Mitogen, Collect 48 hr
supernatant.

Incubate 4 hrs.
Wash away
Lymphokines.

4 x 10⁴ ³HTdR
TUMOR CELLS

Label 3 x 10⁶ tumor cells in
15 ml with ³HTdR, 24 hrs.

Incubate 48 hrs.

Collect supernatant.
Count ³HTdR.

Fig. 1.   Tumor cytotoxicity by lymphokine–activated macrophages:
quantification of the cytotoxic reaction by release of tritiated
thymidine from prelabeled target cells.

The time course for lymphokine activation of peritoneal macrophages in vitro is shown in Fig. 5. Cytotoxic activity was evident
after 4 hrs of incubation in lymphokines, increased to maximal
levels by 8–12 hrs, then progressively decreased to untreated levels by 24–36 hrs. Loss of tumoricidal activity was not due to macrophage death in cultures: no changes in vital dye uptake or in
phagocytic capacity was observed over this time period. Loss of
tumoricidal activity was also not due to depletion or destruction
of active lymphokines: replacement of lymphokine supernatants at
16 hr did not alter this decay (9). Thus, tumoricidal activity
of lymphokine-activated macrophages was short-lived in vitro.
This loss of activity, although not due to cell death or lymphokine depletion was irreversible. Identical decay of tumoricidal
activity in vitro was observed with macrophages activated in vivo
by BCG infection (3,1). Capacity of macrophages to be activated
by lymphokines in vitro for tumor cytotoxicity was short-lived as
well (Fig. 6). Macrophages cultures in medium for various times
prior to the addition of lymphokines gradually lost capacity to be
activated for tumor cytotoxicity. This loss of lymphokine responsiveness with time in culture was also irreversible and not due
to cell death (9,10).

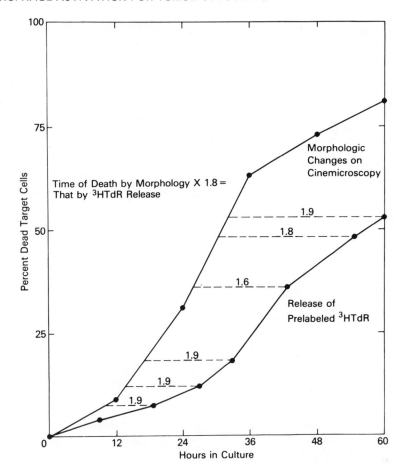

Fig. 2. Macrophage-mediated tumor cytotoxicity: correlation of morphologic changes on cinemicroscopy (loss of nuclear rotation) with release of [3]HTdR from target cells as indices of tumor cell death. Dashed line shows factor that arithmetically superimposes the [3]HTdR release point upon the morphologic change curve.

The tumoricidal activity of lymphokine-activated macrophages, even under optimal in vitro conditions, was consistently less than that of equal numbers of macrophages activated in vivo during any of several immune reactions (9). To gain insight into this difference, we analyzed the cellular changes which occurred during macrophage activation in vivo (Fig. 7). BCG-immune mice were inoculated intraperitoneally with PPD. Within 8 hrs of antigen injection, activated tumoricidal macrophages were recovered from the peritoneal cavity. Cytotoxic macrophages were present through 24 hrs, then progressively decreased to untreated levels by 48-60 hrs.

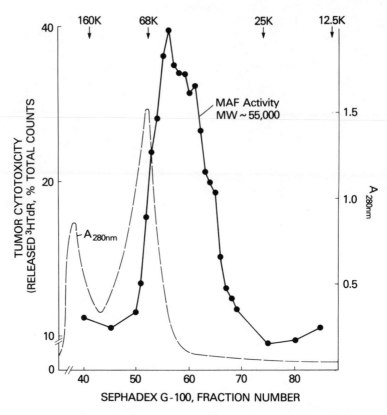

Fig. 3.   Sephadex G-100 gel chromatography of macrophage activation factor activity present in Con A-induced lymphokine supernatants.

This decrease may have been related to antigen clearance and could be prevented by another injection of PPD at 24 hrs (8).   The percentage of peroxidase-positive macrophages in these cell populations closely followed the onset and loss of cytotoxic activity.   Changes in peroxidase cytochemistry, however, were entirely nonspecific sequela of inflammation and not of the immune response per se: identical changes occurred in control mice injected with PPD without development of activated tumoricidal macrophages (8,10).

In vivo, inflammation and the influx of immature, peroxidase-positive mononuclear phagocytes were coincident with development of cytotoxic macrophages during immune reactions.   Indeed, macrophages from peritoneal exudates induced by sterile irritants were more responsive to lymphokines in vitro than equal numbers of more differentiated, peroxidase-negative resident macrophages (Fig. 8). Peritoneal macrophages were harvested at various times after injection of a sterile irritant (fetal calf serum) and assayed for

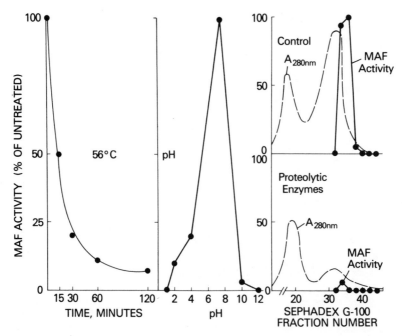

Fig. 4.   Susceptibility of macrophage activation factor activity to temperature, pH and proteolytic enzymes.

peroxidase cytochemistry, phagocytic capacity and lymphokine activation for tumor cytotoxicity. Changes in peroxidase cytochemistry and lymphokine responsiveness were closely correlated throughout this time period and suggest that the lymphokine responsive cell was associated with peroxidase-positive blood-derived mononuclear phagocytes. Comparison of dose and time-responses by peritoneal exudate and resident cell populations to dilutions of lymphokines demonstrated that differences in lymphokine responses were quantitative: increased responsiveness of peritoneal exudate macrophages was not due to qualitative changes in macrophage-lymphokine interaction but rather to quantitative changes in the number of macrophages able to respond (Fig. 9). Cytotoxicity curves for exudate and resident macrophages were superimposable after multiplication by a constant factor. This factor, about 10, represents the relative difference in numbers of lymphokine responsive cells between the two populations (10). The lymphokine responsive cell, however, was the same for each population. This 10-fold difference in lymphokine-responsive cells was similar in magnitude to differences in macrophage turnover during steady-state (resident) and acute inflammation (exudate) described by Van Furth et al. (15) and suggests that the macrophages able to be activated by lymphokines in resident cell populations were not the well differentiated resident cells but rather the immature, peroxidase-

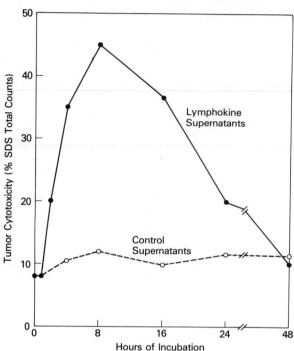

Fig. 5. Tumor cytotoxicity by lymphokine-activated macrophages:
time course of lymphokine activation. Adherent PC were incubated
in lymphokines for various times, washed and cultures with ^{3}HTdR-
labeled target cells for 48 hrs. Cytotoxicity was estimated at
48 hrs by measurement of ^{3}HTdR release.

positive mononuclear phagocytes responsible for steady-state turnover. This conclusion was supported by results of experiments on
the effect of X-irradiation on lymphokine responsiveness (Fig. 10).
Mice were irradiated 1 day prior to injection of a sterile irritant.
Peritoneal cells were collected 1 day later. Bone marrow precursors
of macrophages are radiosensitive. Peripheral blood monocytes have
a turnover time of about 30 hrs and resident macrophages are radioresistant. Whole body X-irradiation prevented the influx of young
mononuclear phagocytes into the peritoneal cavity; percent peroxidase-positive cells during inflammation decreased from 40% to 3%.
The ability of macrophages to respond to lymphokines showed a
corresponding decrease. These data suggest that the lymphokine
responsive cell, the mononuclear phagocyte precursor to activated
tumoricidal macrophages in steady-state and inflammation is the
immature, peroxidase-positive macrophage.

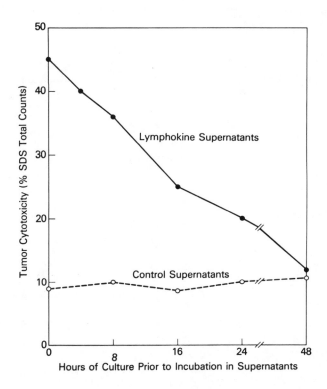

Fig. 6. Tumor cytotoxicity by lymphokine-activated macrophages:
effect of time in culture prior to lymphokine activation. Adherent
PC were cultured in medium for 0-48 hrs, then incubated in lymphokines for 4 hrs. Cultures were washed and incubated with ^{3}HTdR-
labeled target cells for 48 hrs. Cytotoxicity was estimated at
48 hrs by measurement of ^{3}HTdR release.

     In certain instances, a normally adequate activation stimulus
and mononuclear phagocytes able to respond to this stimulus were
not sufficient for development of macrophage cytotoxic activity.
Macrophages from endotoxin-unresponsive C_3H/HeJ mice infected i.p.
with viable BCG were not cytotoxic to tumor cells in vitro (Fig. 11).
Varying time of macrophage collection after BCG infection, numbers
of BCG organisms in the infectious inoculum or numbers of macrophages from BCG infected mice added to tumor cells did not evoke
cytotoxic activity (11). Macrophage tumoricidal activity also did
not develop after in vitro treatment of C_3H/HeJ cells with lymphokines (Fig. 12). Increasing time of macrophage incubation in
lymphokines, concentration of lymphokines or numbers of lympho-
kine-treated macrophages added to tumor cells also did not evoke
tumoricidal activity (11).

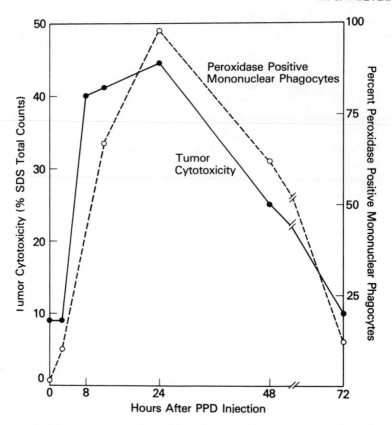

Fig. 7. Tumor cytotoxicity by macrophages from PPD-injected BCG-immune mice: time course of macrophage activation. Mice immunized with BCG intradermally were injected i.p. with PPD. Peritoneal macrophages were assayed for tumoricidal capacity and peroxidase cytochemistry at various times after PPD injection.

The tumoricidal defect of macrophages from C_3H/HeJ mice was highly selective: inflammatory responses to BCG infection in C_3H/HeN and C_3H/HeJ mice were indistinguishable; macrophage responses to chemotactic lymphokines in vitro were also normal (11,12). Moreover, production of macrophage activation factors by spleen cells from C_3H/HeJ mice was entirely normal (12) (Fig. 13). Thus, endotoxin-unresponsive C_3H/HeJ macrophages possess a profound and selective defect in tumoricidal capacity following in vivo and in vitro treatments not directly dependent upon bacterial endotoxins. By backcross linkage analysis we have determined that the gene for control of macrophage tumoricidal capacity in several mouse strains by both LPS-dependent and LPS-independent

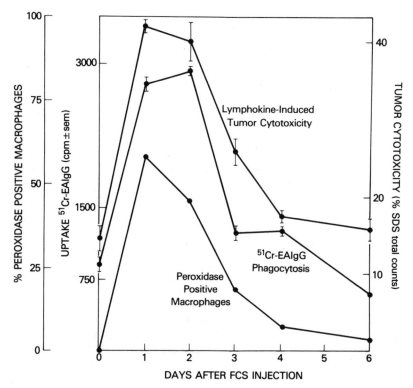

Fig. 8.   Peritoneal macrophage function during acute inflammation.
PC were collected from mice treated i.p. with 1 ml fetal calf serum
0-6 days previously and assayed for phagocytosis of ^{51}Cr-labeled
antibody-coated sheep erythrocytes, peroxidase cytochemistry and
response to lymphokine-induced macrophage activation.

stimuli is either closely linked or identical to the LPS gene
on chromosome 4 (12).

    We have shown that despite extensive manipulation of single
activation stimuli in vivo (BCG) or in vitro (lymphokines) macrophages from C$_3$H/HeJ mice fail to develop cytotoxic activity.
Under certain conditions, however, macrophages from C$_3$H/HeJ mice
could become tumoricidal (Table I). Macrophages from in vivo
immune reactions (BCG infection, Con A injection) but not from
irritant-induced peritoneal exudates, developed full cytotoxic
capability after further exposure in vitro to additional activation stimuli.   These stimuli include mcg/ml concentrations of LPS
and certain factors in lymphokine supernatants (13).   The effect
of LPS but not that of lymphokines was abrogated by polymyxin B,
an antibiotic that binds to lipid A (13).   This polymyxin B effect
suggests that at least two factors can provide the second activa-

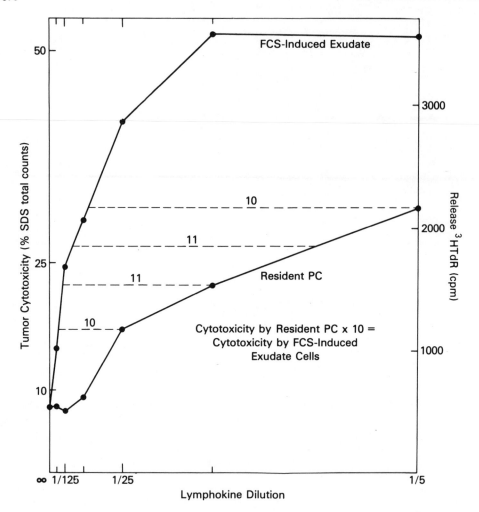

Fig. 9. Tumor cytotoxicity by lymphokine-activated macrophages: lymphokine responsiveness of resident and inflammatory macrophages. PC were collected from untreated mice and from mice treated i.p. with fetal calf serum 1 day previously. Cells were adjusted to an equal macrophage concentration and assayed for lymphokine-induced tumoricidal capacity. Dashed line shows factor that arithmetically superimposes the resident PC point upon the FCS-induced exudate curve.

tion stimulus for macrophage activation. Thus, cytotoxic activity by C₃H/HeJ macrophages required a progression of activation signals: preparative stimuli from in vivo immune reactions followed by a second and qualitatively different signal for expression of tumoricidal activity. This multistage activation sequence could also be completed entirely in vitro: preparative signals from in vivo immune

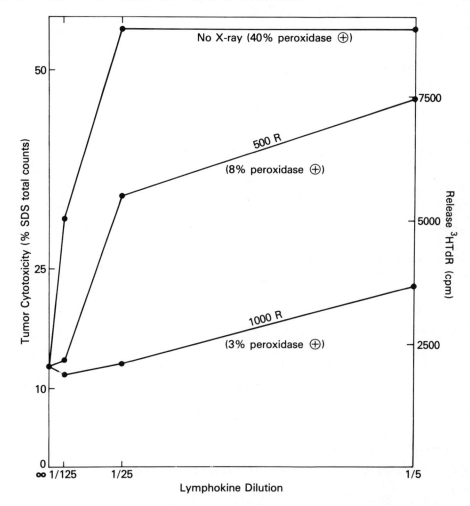

Fig. 10. Tumor cytotoxicity by lymphokine-activated macrophages: effect of X-irradiation on lymphokine-induced macrophage activation.

reactions were supplied by factors in lymphokine supernatants (Table II). C_3H/HeJ macrophages cultured in lymphokines and LPS were fully cytotoxic; macrophages cultured in either stimulus alone had no cytotoxic activity.

A similar multistage reaction sequence for macrophage activation can be demonstrated with LPS-responsive C_3H/HeN mice as well (Fig. 14). Tumoricidal activity by C_3H/HeN macrophages incubated in lymphokines plus 25 ng/ml LPS was significantly greater than that of cells cultured in lymphokines alone at each lymphokine dilution. Macrophages cultured in 25 ng/ml LPS alone were minimally cytotoxic. If this minimal cytotoxicity is subtracted from that of lymphokines plus LPS, the remaining cytotoxicity is still

TABLE I

Tumor Cytotoxicity by Macrophages from BCG-Infected C₃H/HeJ
Mice Treated In Vitro with LPS or Lymphokines

Tumor Cytotoxicity By Macrophages Treated With:	Macrophages From C₃H/HeJ Mice Treated With:		
	Saline	BCG	Con A
Medium	6%	8%	5%
LPS, 2 ug/ml	6%	46%[a]	35%[a]
+Polymyxin B	8%	10%[a]	7%[a]
Lymphokines	6%	52%[a]	26%[a]
+Polymyxin B	7%	54%[a]	29%[a]

[a]Morphologically evident tumor cell destruction.

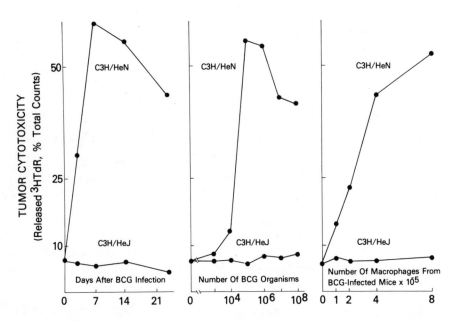

Fig. 11. Tumor cytotoxicity by macrophages from BCG-infected C₃H/
HeJ and C₃H/HeN mice: effect of varying time of macrophages collection after BCG infection, numbers of BCG organisms in the infectious
inoculum of numbers of macrophages added to tumor target cells.

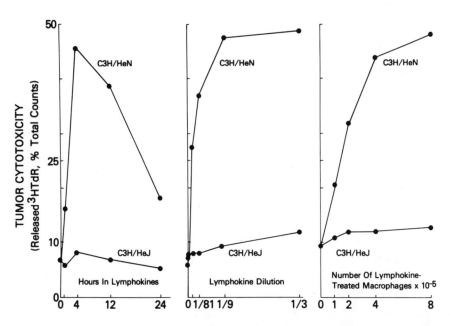

Fig. 12. Tumor cytotoxicity by lymphokine-activated macrophages from C_3H/HeJ and C_3H/HeN mice: effect of varying time of incubation in lymphokines, concentration of lymphokines or numbers of lympho-kine-treated macrophages added to tumor target cells.

TABLE II

Tumor Cytotoxicity by Macrophages from C_3H/HeJ Mice Treated
In Vitro with Lymphokines and LPS

C_3H/HeJ Macrophages Treated With:	Tumor Cytotoxicity By Treated Macrophages Incubated With:		
	No LPS	5 ug/ml LPS	50 ug/ml LPS
Medium	5%	6%	7%
Lymphokines	8%	22%[a]	34%[a]

[a]Morphologically evident tumor cell destruction.

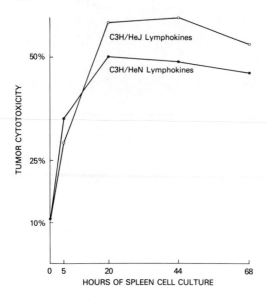

Fig. 13. Tumor cytotoxicity
by C3H/HeN macrophages treated
with lymphokines from Con A-
stimulated C3H/HeJ and C3H/HeN
spleen cell cultures.

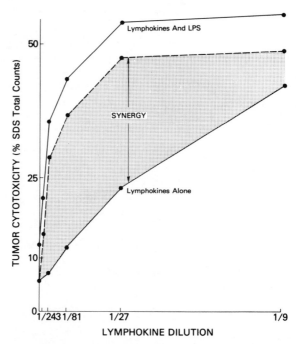

Fig. 14. Synergistic action of LPS on tumor cytotoxicity by lymphokine-activated macrophages. Adherent PC were incubated in lymphokines
with and without 25 ng/ml LPS for 4 hrs. Cultures were washed and
incubated with 3HTdR-labeled target cells for 48 hrs. Shaded area
(synergy) represents cytotoxic responses of cells treated with lymphokines and LPS minus responses of cells treated with LPS alone.

significantly greater than that by lymphokines alone. LPS therefore had a synergistic effect on the cytotoxic activity of lymphokine-activated macrophages. This synergistic effect was critically
dependent upon treatment sequence (Fig. 15). LPS was active only
if added simultaneously with or following lymphokine treatment;
LPS treatment prior to lymphokine exposure was ineffective. The
synergistic effect of LPS was also dependent upon treatment interval (Fig. 16). The capacity of macrophages pretreated with lympho-

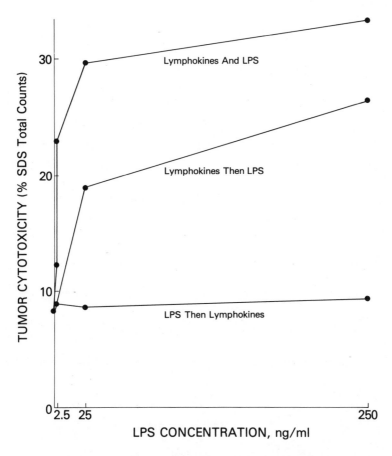

Fig. 15. Synergistic action of LPS on tumor cytotoxicity by
lymphokine-activated macrophages: effect of treatment sequence.
Adherent PC were incubated with lymphokines and LPS for 4 hrs or
with lymphokines for 3.5 hrs followed by LPS for 0.5 hrs or with
LPS for 0.5 hrs followed by lymphokines for 3.5 hrs. Cultures were
washed and incubated with ^{3}HTdR-labeled target cells for 48 hrs.

kines to develop tumoricidal activity after addition of LPS was short-lived and gradually decayed over 24 hrs in vitro. Thus, in both C_3H/HeN and C_3H/HeJ mice macrophage activation required mul-tiple stimuli in a defined sequence (14). Lymphokine-derived preparative signals must be followed by other, qualitatively different stimuli for expression of cytotoxicity (Fig. 17).

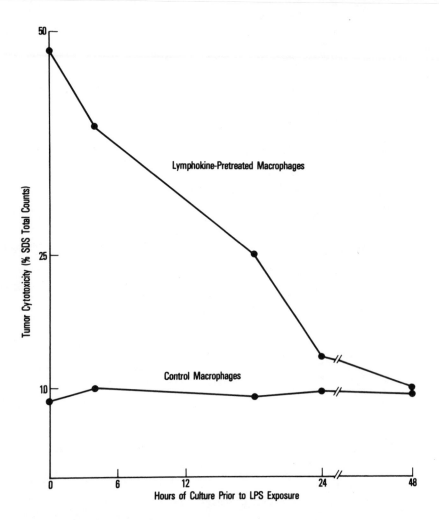

Fig. 16. Synergistic action of LPS on tumor cytotoxicity by lymphokine-activated macrophages: effect of treatment interval. Adherent PC were incubated in lymphokines for 0-48 hrs, washed and exposed to LPS for 0.5 hrs. Cultures were washed and incubated with [3]HTdR-labeled target cells for 48 hrs. Cyto-toxicity was estimated at 48 hrs by measurement of [3]HTdR release.

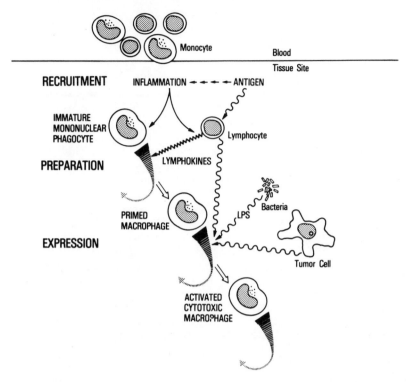

Fig. 17. Macrophage activation for tumor cytotoxicity: development of macrophage cytotoxic activity requires completion of a sequence of short-lived intermediary reactions.

We believe that macrophage activation for tumor cytotoxicity is the final result of a cascade of short-lived intermediary reactions. Tumoricidal activity of fully activated cells and responsiveness of noncytotoxic intermediates to activation stimuli were all short-lived macrophage functions. Analysis of each stage of macrophage activation suggests that none of the intermediary reactions was reversible. Each stage of macrophage activation was completely dependent upon the simultaneous presence of localized activation signals and precursor cells responsive to those signals. The nature of the activation signal and the responsive cell was different from stage to stage. These interactions provide a basic framework for macrophage activation which can be and almost certainly are affected by second level control systems: factors at the reaction site or in serum or from tumors which can modify activation signals or responsive precursors to affect alterations in macrophage function.

REFERENCES

1. Cleveland, R. P., Meltzer, M. S. and Zbar, B. J. Natl. Canc. Inst. 52 (1974) 1887.
2. Evans, R. and Alexander, P. Nature 236 (1972) 168.
3. Hibbs, J. B., Jr. In: The Macrophage in Neoplasia (Ed. M. A. Fink) Academic Press, New York (1976) 83.
4. Leonard, E. J., Ruco, L. P. and Meltzer, M. S. Cell Immunol. (1978) in press.
5. Meltzer, M. S., Tucker, R. W., Sanford, K. K. and Leonard, E. J. J. Natl. Canc. Inst. 54 (1975) 1177.
6. Meltzer, M. S., Tucker, R. W. and Breuer, A. C. Cell. Immunol. 17 (1975) 30.
7. Meltzer, M. S. Clin. Immunol. Immunopath. 6 (1976) 638.
8. Ruco, L. P. and Meltzer, M. S. Cell. Immunol. 32 (1977) 203.
9. Ruco, L. P. and Meltzer, M. S. J. Immunol. 119 (1977) 889.
10. Ruco, L. P. and Meltzer, M. S. J. Immunol. 120 (1978) 1054.
11. Ruco, L. P. and Meltzer, M. S. J. Immunol. 120 (1978) 329.
12. Ruco, L. P., Meltzer, M. S. and Rosenstreich, D. L. J. Immunol. (1978) in press.
13. Ruco, L. P. and Meltzer, M. S. Cell. Immunol. (1978) in press.
14. Ruco, L. P. and Meltzer, M. S. J. Immunol. (1978) submitted.
15. Van Furth, R., Diesselhoff-Den Dulk, M. M. C. and Mattie, H. J. Exp. Med. 138 (1973) 6.

THE TREATMENT OF ESTABLISHED MICROMETASTASES WITH SYNGENEIC MACROPHAGES

I. J. FIDLER, W. E. FOGLER, Z. BARNES and K. FISHER

Cancer Biology Program
NCI-Frederick Cancer Research Center
Frederick, Maryland (USA)

The establishment and growth of cancer metastases is a complex biological process which can be conveniently divided into several sequential steps. The phenomenon begins with the invasion of host stroma, blood vessels and/or lymphatics by cells from the primary tumor. Single tumor cells or clumps of cells can then detach from the primary tumor mass, circulate as emboli and reach a distant microvasculature of an organ. Following arrest, tumor cells must infiltrate the parenchyma, followed by multiplication and growth of a vascularized stroma into the new tumor foci. The processes of invasion, embolization arrest and cell multiplication can reoccur, leading to secondary metastasis (11, 17). The process of metastasis is highly selective and represents the end point of many destructive events from which only a few tumor cells can survive. Thus, only some tumor cells in a primary malignant neoplasm are invasive and of those even fewer can survive in the circulation. Similarly, not every metastasizing tumor cell can evade host defense mechanisms, which could destroy malignant cells during any of the steps described above.

One host factor which profoundly influences metastasis is the immune system. The interaction of host immunity with malignant tumor cells may lead to two conflicting end results. In some tumor systems, immune cells can inhibit tumor spread; whereas in other systems, syngeneic lymphocytes may actually enhance metastasis (10,15,19,33). Host immunity to metastatic cells involves the interaction of both lymphocytes and macrophages. It is postulated that lymphocytes which are specifically sensitized to tumor-associated antigens can interact with tumor target cells to either lyse them (15) and/or to release soluble mediators, i.e., lymphokines. Lymphokines are also released by lymphocytes in response

to a variety of antigens (3,29) or mitogens (16). The soluble
lymphocyte mediator responsible for inducing macrophage activation
is referred to as "macrophage-activating factor" (MAF) and MAF-
treated macrophages (tumoricidal macrophages) acquire the ability
to recognize and destroy neoplastic cells both in vitro and in vivo
while leaving non-neoplastic cells unharmed. MAF is able to act
across species barriers (3,12,16), and tumoridical macrophages
activated by MAF induce destruction of a wide range of target tumor
cells from a variety of species via a nonimmunologic mechanism
which requires cell-to-cell contact (21). MAF-induced activation
can thus be distinguished from the so-called "arming" of macrophages by a specific MAF (SMAF) (7,25) which renders macrophages
cytotoxic to specific tumor cells. The remarkable discrimination
in vitro by tumoricidal macrophages between tumorigenic and normal
cells has been studied in a variety of systems. These include
syngeneic and allogeneic tumors of mice (8,16,20,22,34), syngeneic
rat tumor systems (14,23), and syngeneic guinea pig tumor systems
(2,29). Collectively, the data indicate that the ability of tumoricidal macrophages to discriminate in vitro between non-neoplastic
and neoplastic cells is independent of transplantation, species-
specific and tumor-associated antigens expressed on the surface
of neoplastic target cells. This is in complete contrast to the
immunologic specificity associated with tumor cell destruction
by sensitized lymphocytes.

Several studies have suggested that in rodents bearing a
progressively growing tumor, the interaction between lymphocytes
and macrophages fails to occur (1,4,7,12,25). We have previously
reported (12,25) that macrophages collected from normal or tumor-
bearing mice were not cytotoxic against a syngeneic tumor in vitro.
On the other hand, macrophages obtained from immunized mice were
cytotoxic to the tumor cells. Unreactive macrophages from normal
and tumor-bearing mice became cytotoxic after their in vitro incubation with supernatants from cultures containing lymphocytes
from immunized syngeneic mice, sensitized allogeneic mice, or
sensitized xenogeneic rats and tumor targets. At the same time,
macrophages incubated with supernatants from cultures of normal
nonsensitized allogeneic or xenogeneic lymphocytes did not exhibit tumor cytotoxicity. These observations suggested that
macrophages from tumor-bearing animals were potentially cytotoxic
to the syngeneic tumors and could be activated by mediators released from reactive, sensitized lymphocytes in vitro.

As stated above, the establishment and growth of cancer
metastases is determined by the outcome of two conflicting factors:
the rate of tumor cell division exceeds tumor cell destruction.
The present report concerns our studies of the treatment of ex-
tablished micrometastases by the intraveneous (i.v.) injection of
syngeneic macrophages activated either in vitro or in vivo (in
syngeneic mice which do not bear a progressive tumor). We primarily

wished to determine whether the i.v. injection of specific or
nonspecific cytotoxic macrophages could increase the rate of
tumor cell destruction in vivo and thus lead to beneficial therapeutic effects against disseminated disease.

MATERIALS AND METHODS

Mice. Specific-pathogen-free C3H/HeN(MTV⁻) mice were obtained from the Animal Production Area of the Frederick Cancer
Research Center. They were usually 8 weeks old at the beginning
of the experiment; within a single experiment all mice were age-
and sex-matched. The mice were given drinking water that contained 10 ppm of chlorine (13).

Tumors. The UV-2237 is a fibrosarcoma that was induced by
chronic UV irradiation in a female C3H⁻ mouse according to the
procedure detailed previously (24). Trocar implants of the
primary tumor were transplanted to syngeneic mice immunosuppressed
by adult thymectomy and sublethal (450 R) whole-body X-irradiation.
Four weeks after transplantation, two implants were removed, minced
and trypsinized to prepare a tissue culture line (18). Cell cultures were maintained in plastic flasks in CMEM (see below) Antibiotics were not included in the medium for routine maintenance
of cell lines. The B16 melanoma, syngeneic to the C57BL/6 mouse,
has been adapted to culture as described previously (12,25). The
tumor cultures were screened and found free of mycoplasma and
pathogenic murine viruses including lactate dehydrogenase virus
(Microbiological Associates, Bethesda, Maryland, USA).

Tissue culture conditions. All cultures were maintained on
plastic flasks in Eagle's minimum essential medium (MEM) supplemented with 10% fetal calf serum, sodium pyruvate, nonessential
amino acids, penicillin-streptomycin, L-glutamine and two-fold
vitamins. The medium, designated complete MEM (CMEM), and supple-
ments were obtained from Flow Laboratories, Rockville, Maryland,
USA. All cultures were kept in a humidified incubator containing
5% CO_2 atmosphere at 37 C.

Immunization of mice against UV-2237 fibrosarcoma. C3H mice
were injected subcutaneously (s.c.) with 1×10^6 tumor cells which
were pretreated with mitomycin C. Two weeks later the mice were
challenged with a lethal dose of viable UV-2237 cells. Only those
mice which rejected the tumor challenge were considered immune
and used for the subsequent studies.

Sensitization of mice to BCG. C3H mice were injected intraperitoneally (i.p.) with 1×10^7 viable organisms (Trudeau
Institute, Saranac Lake, New York). Ten days later, they were
injected i.p. with thioglycollate (see below) and their peritoneal

exudate cells (PEC) were harvested and used for the in vitro and in vivo studies.

Preparation and purification of normal macrophage cultures.
Homogeneous C3H mouse macrophage cultures were prepared as
described previously (12,25). Briefly, mice were injected i.p.
with 2 ml of thioglycollate, killed after 5 days, and their PEC
were harvested by washing with Hanks' balanced salt solution (HBSS)
containing 5 units of heparin/ml. The PEC were centrifuged, resuspended in CMEM, and plated into 60 x 15 mm plastic dishes (Falcon
Plastics, Oxnard, California) at a concentration of 2 x 10^6 PEC
per dish. Forty min after incubation at 37 C, all nonadherent
cells were removed and the adherent cells were then incubated for
one additional day. By culture day 2 all the adherent cells (50%
of originally plated cells) had the typical macrophage morphology
and phagocytized carbon particles. These cells were used in all
of the subsequent in vitro cytotoxicity assays.

In vitro activation of normal mouse macrophages by rat lym-
phycyte supernatants. Concanavalin A (Con-A-MAF) was obtained
from cultures of normal F344 rat lymphocytes incubated in vitro
with insoluble Con-A (Pharmacia, Piscataway, N. J.) using the
methods described in detail elsewhere (16). C3H macrophages were
incubated with the rat lymphocyte supernatants (Con-A-MAF) for 24
hr at 37 C. All macrophage cultures were then washed twice with
CMEM prior to the in vitro cytotoxicity assay.

Harvest and preparation of immune or BCG-sensitized
macrophages. Immune mice or those injected i.p. with BCG organisms were injected i.p. with thioglycollate and PEC were harvested as described above. the PEC were plated into dishes and
the cultures were washed 40 min later. At this time labeled
target cells were added to the dishes (see below).

Assay for macrophage-mediated cytotoxicity in vitro. Macrophage-mediated cytotoxicity in vitro was studied by a radioactive
release assay as detailed previously (14,28). Target cells in an
exponential growth phase were labeled in vitro for 24 hr with 0.3
μCi of ^{125}I-5 iodo-2'-deoxyuridine (^{125}IUdR; 200 mCi/μmol) per ml
medium. Radioisotopes were obtained from the New England Nuclear
Corporation, Boston, Massachusetts. After the labeling period
and before the assays, the cultures were washed several times
with HBSS to remove all unbound radioactive label. Following a
1-min trypsinization (0.25% trypsin-0.02% EDTA) the labeled cells
were washed and suspended in CMEM. Ten thousand labeled target
cells were added to each 60 x 15 mm culture dish containing the
previously plated macrophages, yielding an initial ratio of
macrophages to target cells of 100:1. At this ratio, normal (non-
activated) macrophages are not cytotoxic to neoplastic cells,
while activated macrophages are (12,25,28). Target cells were

also plated alone, as an additional control group. Twenty-four
hr after plating, the cultures were washed and refed with CMEM to
remove target cells which did not plate. On day 4, the cultures
were washed twice with HBSS to remove all nonadherent cells. The
remaining adherent, viable cells were lysed with 1 ml 0.5 N NaOH,
and the lysate and HBSS washes were combined and placed directly
into tubes to determine the amount of cell-associated radioactivity
as monitored in a gamma counter. Maximal in vitro macrophage-
mediated cytotoxicity in this assay is obtained after 4 days of
incubation with target cells and macrophages do not reincorporate
^{125}IUdR released from dead target cells (28).

Calculations of percentage of significant cytotoxicity.
Percentage of significant cytotoxicity was computed by the following formula:

$$\% \text{ Significant Cytotoxicity} = 100 \times \frac{\text{cpm } ^{125}\text{IUdR in target cells with normal macrophages} - \text{cpm } ^{125}\text{IUdR in target cells with test macrophages}}{\text{cpm} ^{125}\text{IUdR in target cells with normal macrophages}}$$

The percentage of significant cytotoxicity was analyzed for statistical significance by the Student's t-test (2-tailed).

Procedures for study of experimental metastasis and the in
vivo effects of syngeneic macrophages. UV-2237 fibrosarcoma
cells grown in vitro were harvested during their exponential
growth phase by a 1 min treatment with 0.25% trypsin. The cells
were washed twice with CMEM and resuspended in HBSS. The number
of single viable tumor cells (95% viability as determined by the
trypan blue exclusion test) was adjusted to 100,000/ml. Tumor
cells were injected i.v. into the tail vein of normal C3H mice.
The inoculum dose was 0.2 ml containing 20,000 cells. Three days
later, when micrometastases are known to be firmly established
(6), treatment with macrophages commenced. Each treatment consisted of the i.v. injection of 3×10^6 viable macrophages in
0.3 ml HBSS. The treatment schedule consisted of mice injected
either once (3 days after i.v. tumor cell injection), twice (3,
5 and 7 days after i.v. tumor cell injection). The mice were
divided in five major treatment groups of 30 mice each: 1) control mice injected with tumor cells alone; 2) mice injected i.v.
with normal macrophages; 3) mice injected i.v. with normal MAF-
treated macrophages. 4) mice injected i.v. with macrophages
collected from BCG-stimulated mice; and 5) mice injected i.v.
with macrophages collected from mice immune to the UV-2237 fibrosarcoma. Thus, the major treatment groups of 30 mice consisted of
3 sub-groups of 10 mice each.

The groups were coded and 6 weeks after tumor cell injection
all the mice were killed. The number of subsequent pulmonary and
extrapulmonary metastases was determined with the aid of a dis-
secting microscope by 2 independent observers. The differences
in the number of metastases among the group were analyzed with
the two-tailed t-test.

RESULTS

Normal and activated C3H macrophages were incubated in vitro
with the syngeneic UV-2237 fibrosarcoma and the allogeneic B16
melanoma. Tumoricidal macrophages (nonspecific) are characterized
by their ability to discriminate between tumorigenic and normal
cells (14). On the other hand, specifically activated macrophages
destroy in vitro only tumor target cells against which they were
sensitized (7). The data shown in Table I demonstrated the following: a) normal (thioglycollate-induced) peritoneal macrophages
were not cytotoxic against either of the targets, which agreed
with our earlier results (12,14) and those of others (1,2,4,6,8,
13,18,20-24,28,29,34);   b) macrophages obtained from BCG-
stimulated mice were tumoricidal in vitro and destroyed 60% of
UV-2237 targets and 36% of the B16 melanoma cells (p<0.01);
c) normal C3H macrophages treated in vitro with rat Con-A-MAF
were rendered tumoricidal (9) and destroyed 40% of the UV-2237
cells and 47% of the B16 melanoma cells (p<0.01); and   d) in
contrast, macrophages collected from C3H mice immunized against
the syngeneic UV-2237 fibrosarcoma were specifically cytotoxic
in vitro. The immune macrophages destroyed 75% of UV-2237
fibrosarcoma target cells but were not cytotoxic against the B16
melanoma. The specific spectrum of cytotoxicity seen with immune
macrophages agrees closely with our recent work (25) and that of
Evans and Alexander (7).

The in vitro data can be summarized as follows. Macrophage
stimulation with BCG in vivo and incubation of macrophages with
MAF in vitro led to nonspecific activation, and these activated
macrophages were tumoricidal in vitro. In contrast, the immunization of mice with an antigenic tumor led to the generation of
highly cytotoxic but specific macrophages.

The in vitro experiments were performed simultaneously with
the in vivo studies. For the latter, C3H mice were injected i.v.
with 20,000 viable UV-2237 fibrosarcoma cells. Three days later,
treatment of the mice with the i.v. injection of various groups
of syngeneic macrophages began. Mice were treated with 3×10^6
viable macrophages (per injection) either once, twice or three
times at two-day intervals. Six weeks after the i.v. injection of
tumor cells, all mice were killed and the number of lung metastases was determined.

TABLE I

Specificity of In Vitro Cytotoxicity Mediated by C3H Macrophages

Source of C3H Macrophages	Macrophage Mediated Cytotoxicity[a] Against			
	UV-2237 Fibrosarcoma		B16 Melanoma	
	day 1	day 4	day 1	day 4
None, tumor cell control	21214 ± 301[b]	10138 ± 381	13489 ± 280	10228 ± 256
Normal, thioglycollate-induced	20348 ± 221	10400 ± 550	14132 ± 283	10020 ± 250
BCG-stimulated in vivo	20872 ± 262	4088 ± 201(60)[c]	14847 ± 189	6343 ± 401(36)[d]
MAF-treated in vitro	21567 ± 191	6178 ± 340(40)[d]	13572 ± 494	5242 ± 443(47)[d]
Immune, in vivo	20049 ± 301	2572 ± 105(75)[c]	12978 ± 250	9303 ± 225

[a] In vitro cytotoxicity mediated by C3H⁻ macrophages.

[b] Mean cmp ± standard deviation of triplicate cultures. Residual cpm of ^{125}IUdR prelabeled target cells 4 days after plating. Initial ratio of macrophages to tumor cells was 100:1.

[c] Percent cytotoxicity as compared with control macrophages at corresponding ratio to tumor cells ($p < 0.001$).

[d] Percent cytotoxicity as compared with control macrophages at corresponding ratio to tumor cells ($p < 0.01$).

The data are shown in Table II and demonstrated the following: a) injection(s) of normal (thioglycollated) peritoneal
macrophages did not influence the incidence of metastasis;
b) two and three treatments with BCG-stimulated macrophages significantly decreased metastasis (p<0.004 and <0.05, respectively);
c) two and three treatments with in vitro MAF-treated macrophages
significantly reduced the number of metastases (p<0.003 and <0.0001,
respectively); and d)   one, two and three treatments with specifically immune macrophages significantly reduced the incidence of
metastasis (p<0.006, <0.0001, <0.0001, respectively). In the
group receiving three courses of treatment, 4 of 10 mice, were
tumor free, indicating that cure of metastatic deposits could
have actually occurred. In all the treatment groups, except
those receiving normal macrophages, we observed a trend: three
treatments with macrophages were more effective in reducing metastasis than two treatments, which, in turn were more effective
than one treatment.

                              DISCUSSION

     The successful immune response against neoplasia, in gen-
eral and metastasis, in particular, involves the interaction of
lymphocytes and macrophages. Our recent studies with mice bearing
a progressively growing B16 melanoma demonstrated that the interaction of lymphocytes and macrophages failed to occur (12).
Lymphocytes of mice bearing the B16 melanoma did not release MAF
following their in vitro incubation with the B16 cells. Whether
this was a specific failure of MAF production, limited to antigens of the growing tumor, or a generalized inability of tumor-
bearing animals to produce MAF against other antigens was unclear.
In subsequent studies, we tested whether the lack of MAF production
by lymphocytes from tumor-bearing mice represented an eclipsed
response. Both MAF production and lymphocyte-mediated growth
inhibition were present during the early stages of tumor growth
and disappeared when the tumors reached an advanced stage. This
implied that the failure of lymphocytes from mice bearing large
tumors to produce MAF was not due to a lack of sensitization,
but rather, it appeared to be brought about by the presence of a
large tumor mass (25). The eclipsed reactivity in tumor-bearing
mice was specific for the growing tumor and did not include reactivity against an unrelated tumor. Lymphocytes from mice
bearing one tumor were able to produce MAF in response to a second tumor to which they had been preimmunized. This demonstrated
that the tumor-bearing mice are not generally immunosuppressed,
since they could still respond to a recall antigen. Macrophages
from rodents bearing progressively growing tumors are not cytotoxic to the tumor (12,25,31) and may also have a reduced chemotactic response (27,32). However, these unreactive macrophages

TABLE II

Number of Pulmonary Metastases in Control and Macrophage-Treated
C3H Mice Injected with Syngeneic UV-2237 Fibrosarcoma

Group[a]	Number of Treatments[b,c]	Median (Range) Pulmonary Metastases[d]		P[e]
Untreated	–	24	(6–50)	
Normal Macrophages	1	22	(8–30)	
	2	17.5	(6–56)	
	3	27	(4–44)	
BCG-stimulated Macrophages	1	22	(17–60)	
(In vivo)	2	14.5	(3–20)	<0.004
	3	9	(1–28)	<0.05
MAF-treated Macrophages	1	19.5	(8–25)	
(In vitro)	2	10	(3–16)	<0.003
	3	4	(2–17)	<0.0001
Immune Macrophages	1	10	(3–28)	<0.006
(In vivo)	2	7	(0–10)	<0.0001
	3	2	(0–10)	<0.0001

[a] Ten mice per group, except the untreated group which consisted of 30 mice.

[b] Each macrophage treatment consisted of i.v. injection of 3×10^6 viable cells.

[c] First treatment occurred 3 days post i.v. injection of tumor cells; second treatment was on day 5; and third treatment was on day 7.

[d] Pulmonary metastases were counted 6 weeks after the i.v. injection of 20,000 viable UV-2237 fibrosarcoma cells.

[e] Two-tailed pairwise comparisons (t-test).

could be rendered cytotoxic with either specific or nonspecific
MAF.

The in vivo inhibitory effects of specifically (immune) and
nonspecifically (BCG, MAF) activated macrophages on established
micrometastases were investigated. Mice with established pulmonary metastases, which if left untreated would progress to kill
the host, were injected i.v. with various syngeneic macrophages.
Six weeks later, the mice were killed and the fate of their pulmonary metastases was determined. The data clearly demonstrated
that multitreatment with syngeneic macrophages was of significant
benefit to the tumor-bearing mice. Immune macrophages (specific)
were the most efficient in reducing pulmonary metastasis and
multiple macrophage treatments were more beneficial than a single
treatment. In order of decreasing efficacy the macrophage treatment groups were: immune, MAF-treated (in vitro) and BCG-stimulated (in vivo). Normal macrophages were neither cytotoxic in
vitro nor effective in vivo. Clearly, both specifically and nonspecifically activated macrophages (whose cytotoxic specificity
was monitored by in vitro assays - Table I) were capable of inhibiting established micrometastases.

There are previously published reports regarding the efficacy of injected macrophages to reduce tumor burden and metastases. Activated syngeneic macrophages injected i.v. reduced
the formation of B16 melanoma pulmonary tumor colonies (10) and
the injection of nonspecifically activated macrophages (BCG-
stimulated) was recently shown to inhibit and prevent the formation of spontaneous metastases (26). In the latter studies
circulating activated macrophages were shown to reduce metastasis
by the prevention of tumor cell invasion into blood vessel and
implantation at distant microvasculature (26). Activated macrophages were also shown to inhibit the growth of tumors at primary
sites (4). Whether or not the i.v. injection of activated macrophages can be used successfully in treatment of extrapulmonary
metastases has been questioned (4,26). Intravenously injected
macrophages are arrested in the capillary bed of the first organ
encountered, i.e., the lungs. However, injected macrophages may
be released later and have been shown to accumulate at the site
of an inflammatory reaction (30). In the present studies, the
UV-2237 fibrosarcoma was injected i.v. and thus mostly pulmonary
metastases were produced. For treatment of metastases at other
organs such as liver or lymph nodes it is postulated that tar-
geting of macrophages could be determined by the route of injection. Liver metastases, for example, could be treated by the
injection of macrophages into a mesentery vein which empties into
the portal circulation.

SUMMARY

We demonstrated that macrophages injected systemically can profoundly inhibit the incidence of experimentally induced metastasis. In our system mice bearing established micro-metastases were treated with one, two or three i.v. injections of activated macrophages. Specifically activated (immune) macrophages were most efficient in reducing the number of metastases, but non-specifically activated macrophages were also effective in reducing the metastatic incidence. Macrophages play a major role in host defense against neoplasia (9,22) and have been shown to influence the outcome of spontaneous metastasis (9). Rat sarcomas whose macrophage content was found to be high were also shown to be non-metastatic. Conversly, rat sarcomas with low macrophage content were found to be metastatic (9). Our current data demonstrate that the systemic injection of syngeneic activated (exogenous) macrophages can bring about a significant reduction of lethal cancer metastases. Apparently, treatment with activated macrophages can increase the rate of tumor cell destruction as compared to the rate of tumor cell proliferation which ultimately leads to inhibition of clinical metastasis.

ACKNOWLEDGEMENTS

This research was sponsored by the National Cancer Institute under Contract No. NO1-CO-75380 with Litton Bionetics, Inc.

REFERENCES

1. Alexander, P., Evans, R., and Grant, C. K., Ann. Inst. Pasteur., 122 (1972) 645.
2. Churchill, W. H., Piessens, W. F., Sulis, C. A. and David, J. R., J. Immunol., 115 (1975) 781.
3. David, J. R., Fed. Proc., 34 (1975) 1730.
4. Den Otter, E., Dullens Hub, F. J., Van Lovern, H., and Pels, E., The Macrophage and Cancer (Ed. K. James, B. McBride and A. Stuart) Econoprint, Edinburgh (1977) 119.
5. Eccles, A. S., and Alexander, P., Nature 250 (1974) 667.
6. Evans, R., Brit. J. Cancer, 28 (1973) 19.
7. Evans, R., and Alexander, P. L., Transplantation, 12 (1971) 227.
8. Evans, R., and Alexander, P., Nature, 236 (1972) 168.
9. Evans, R. and Alexander P., In: Immunology of the Macrophage. (Ed. D. S. Nelson) Academic Press, New York (1976) 210.
10. Fidler, I. J., Cancer Res., 34 (1974) 491.
11. Fidler, I. J., In Cancer: A Comprehensive Treatise (Ed. F. F. Becker) Plenum Press, New York (1975) 101.

12. Fidler, I. J., J. Nat. Cancer. Inst., 55 (1975) 1159.
13. Fidler, I. J., Nature 270 (1977) 735.
14. Fidler, I. J., Isr. J. Med. Sci., 14 (1978) 177.
15. Fidler, I. J. and Bucana, C., Cancer Res., 37 (1977) 3945.
16. Fidler, I. J., Darnell, J. H. and Budmen, M. B., Cancer Res., 36 (1977) 3610.
17. Fidler, I. J. and Kripke, M. L., Science, 197 (1977) 893.
18. Fortner, G. W. and Kripke, M. L., J. Immunol. 118 (1977) 1483.
19. Hager, J. C., Griswold, D. E. and Heppner, G. H., Proc. AACR, 19 (1978) 61.
20. Hibbs, J. B., Jr., Nature, New Biol., 235 (1972) 48.
21. Hibbs, J. C., Jr., Science, 180 (1973) 868.
22. Hibbs, J. B., Jr., J. Natl. Cancer Inst., 53 (1974) 1487.
23. Keller, R. J., Natl. Cancer Inst., 56 (1976) 369.
24. Kripke, M. L., Cancer Res., 37 (1977) 1395.
25. Kripke, M. L., Budmen, M. B., and Fidler, I. J., Cell. Immunol., 30 (1977) 341.
26. Liotta, L. A., Gattozzi, C., Kleinerman, J. and Saidel, G., Br. J. Cancer, 36 (1977) 639.
27. Meltzer, M. S. and Stevenson, M. M., Cell. Immunol., 35 (1978) 99.
28. Norbury, K. C. and Fidler, I. J., J. Immunol. Method, 7 (1975) 109.
29. Piessens, W. F., Churchill, W. H., Jr. and David, J. R., J. Immunol., 114 (1975) 293.
30. Roser, B., In: Mononuclear Phagocytes (Ed. Van Furth), B. H. Blackwell, Oxford (1970) 166.
31. Russell, S. E., and McIntosh, A. T., Nature 268 (1977) 69.
32. Synderman, R., Pike, M. C., McCarley, D. and Lang, L., Infect. Immun., 11 (1975) 488.
33. Vaage, J., Cancer Res., 38 (1977) 331.
34. Zwilling, B. S., Meltzer, M. S. and Evans, C. H., J. Natl. Cancer Inst., 54 (1975) 743.

INFLUENCE OF TUMOR BURDEN, TUMOR REMOVAL, IMMUNE STIMULATION,

PLASMAPHERESIS ON MONOCYTE MOBILIZATION IN CANCER PATIENTS

R. SAMAK, L. ISRAEL and R. EDELSTEIN

Unité de Chimio-Immunothérapie. Université Paris XIII.
Centre Hospitalier Universitaire, Bobigny (France)

The cells of the monocyte-macrophage line probably represent
one of the most important means used by the body to prevent or at
least restrain the growth of a malignant tumor. The arguments in
favor of this theory are quite clear: (a) The cytoplasm of macro-
pages contains microfibrillary and microtubular structures (2,6,
23) which appear to represent a locomotor apparatus endowing these
cells with a major property, that of migration. In the majority
of cases this migration takes place in a directed fashion, that
of a chemical stimulus which may be of various types: components
of activated complement, immune complexes, cytoplasmic constituents
liberated by cell lysis (5), bacterial constituents (66) or dena-
tured proteins (68), chemotactic factor (CF). (b) The mechanisms
by which the macrophage is able to recognize these contituents or
cell structures would involve the use of Fc receptors and of receptors for complement components which by means of recognition
of immune complexes, offer a specificity of action. Other mechanisms are probably involved, such as differences in the electri-
cal charge of the membrane (68,69) or opsonization which also may
be specific, via cytophilic antibodies elaborated by sensitized
lymphocytes (39,48) and even C3b (7,56,62,63,67), but also nonspecific, via proteins such as C-reactive protein, and α-2-S.B.
glycoprotein (8) which would appear to play a fundamental role in
the phagocytosis of malignant cells (13,49,53,57); (c) Macrophages activated by different substances are selectively cytotoxic
against malignant cells (1,22,26,29,31,42,52); (d) The means by
which this activation in vivo takes place might also be either
specific via the secretion of certain factors by sensitized
lymphocytes: specific macrophage arming factor (SMAF) (17),
macrophage activating factor (MAF), monocyte migration inhibitory
factor (MIF), CF (55), or nonspecific, as a result of irritants,

BCG (19), Corynebacterium parvum, bacterial endotoxin, in vitro or
in vivo (17), endowing the animal with an increased resistance to
malignant disease (21,34);   (e) There is almost invariably a cytotoxic expression of macrophages at the inflammatory site, whether
a delayed hypersensitivity reaction (4) or a nonspecific reaction
caused for instance by irritants, by mediators of inflammation (44,
51,71) or even by a simple skin abrasion such as that of Rebuck
(54).   It has thus been possible to demonstrate their presence
within tumors in amounts which are all the higher when the tumors
have less of a tendency to metastasize and when their prognosis is
better (12,15,16,70);   (f) Changes in their function by an anti-
macrophage serum or by trypan blue decreases the inhibition of cell
growth in the mouse (28,32);   (g) In man, injection of BCG or of
glucan into metastatic skin tumor nodules causes a very localized
inflammatory reaction, containing an essentially monocytic infiltrate and rapidly followed by tumor necrosis (33,37,47); and (h)
Various authors have shown that the chemotaxis of macrophages in
vitro is altered in patients suffering from malignant disease,
regardless of the stage of extension and the site of the primary
tumor (10,25,41,46,59,61).

    These data have led various authors to seek such deficiences
in vivo in tumor-bearing animals.   It has been demonstrated that
in an artificially created inflammatory reaction, the animal with
malignant disease produces an exudate in which the macrophage
component is markedly decreased in comparison with that of normal
controls (4,50,58,60).   Synderman and Pike (60) incriminated a
factor produced by the tumor comparable with the Fauve's peptide
(18), responsible for inhibition of the in vivo accumulation of
macrophages and their in vitro chemotaxis.   Bernstein and Zbar (4)
noted that tumor-bearing guinea pigs had altered delayed hypersensitivity to PPD, while in vitro, the lymphocytes had a normal
response to this antigen and suggested that the dysfunction of
cellular immunity, responsible for the absence of tumor rejection,
was not located at the site of antigen-lymphocyte interaction but
in the nonspecific end-stage of the inflammatory response, i.e.
the accumulation of macrophages at the inflammatory site.

    Numerous hypotheses have since long been suggested regarding
the causes of this block.   While certain factors produced by the
tumor would appear to play an important role (18,60), it would
also seem that factors belonging to the host himself may intervene in this sense.

    Israël and Edelstein (36) have shown that serum glycoproteins
present in high levels in patients with malignant disease depressed
the in vitro lymphocytic response to PHA.   The same applies to
monocyte chemotaxis (personal unpublished data).   Surprising
clinical results have been obtained by eliminating these proteins
by repeated plasmapheresis (35).

Finally, the role of suppressive sub-populations would appear to be more and more worthy of being taken into account in the context of immune depression in the cancer patient.

On the basis of these various findings, we felt that it would be of interest to evaluate the macrophage mobilization in response to a nonspecific inflammatory stimulus (e.g., abrasion of a small skin area on the forearm) in order to: (a) determine whether data from animal experiments could be confirmed in man, with regard to the change in monocyte response at an inflammatory site in patients with malignant disease; (b) assess the nonspecific inflammatory response within the context of an evaluation of immune status in the cancer patient; and (c) determine the effects of certain types of treatment on this cell migration.

MATERIALS AND METHODS

The inflammatory stimulus. It was carried out according to the principles of Rebuck and Crowley (54), involving the following phases: (1) cleansing of the anterior aspect of the forearm with ether, (2) a skin abrasion was made using a small battery drill (Stichling) (usually used by make-up artists) fitted with a rounded head 2.4 mm in diameter. The abrasion was continued until micropoints of bleeding occurred, indicating that the connective tissue had been reached. The wound was left exposed to the air for a few seconds, in order to confirm that no bleeding appeared. It was then covered with a small glass coverslip, (3) this glass plate was covered by a gauze square folded in four, the whole dressing being fixed using a strip of elastoplast completely surrounding the limb, (4) the glass plates were removed and immediately replaced at pre-determined intervals which were: 3, 6, 12, 24 and 48 hr after initiation of the inflammatory stimulus, (5) the glass plates were dried, mounted on slides and stained with May-Grunwald-Giemsa. They were examined under the microscope at a magnification of 40X by two different individuals. All cells were counted individually, except when the smear contained more than 10,000 cells, in which cases only an approximation was recorded.

Subjects tested. Control samples were collected from personnel in our department and their families. The age distribution ranged from 25 to 50 years. Individuals with infectious diseases, or any other types of disorder, in particular allergic phenomena, were eliminated.

Thirty patients with disseminated malignancy, who had never yet been treated, were tested including: 4 melanomas, 5 adenocarcinomas of the breast, 4 squamous cell carcinomas of the lung, 4 adenocarcinomas of the lung, 1 pleural mesothelioma, 4 adenocarcinomas of the colon, 5 adenocarcinomas of the ovary, 1 ovarian dysembryoplastic tumor and 2 squamous cell carcinomas of the uterine cervix. Of these, 9 patients were examined before and after surgical excision of their tumor (these were thus localized early respectable tumors), 4 patients were tested before and 4 weeks after treatment with daily intravenous injections of Coryne-bacterium parvum (4 mg) (these patients were suffering from dis-seminated tumors), 11 patients were tested at the time of treatment by single or multiple plasmapheresis (35). These patients were tested before or immediately and 2 weeks after the end of their plasmapheresis therapy.

Parameters studied. The number of macrophages as well as the total number of migrating cells (polymorphonuclear and mononuclear cells), were examined because we felt that the test had a relative quantitative value inasmuch as it involved comparison between the various categories of subjects, or in time in the same patient, rather than the establishment of a very precise model of cell kinetics in an inflammatory reaction. In addition, great atten-tion was paid to avoid any variation in either the surface area of the abrasion (which was thus fixed by projection of the head of the drill onto the skin, without any movement) or the force of application of the glass plate. In order to eliminate the conse-quences of these approximations, only highly significant results were sought (Student's t test). Finally, the very narrow disper-sion of the results on either side of the mean would appear to be in favor of a statistically significant quantitative value.

RESULTS

Changes in cell response in supposedly normal controls. As has already been described by certain authors (14,20,51,38) the first slides examined showed marked mobilization of polymorpho-nuclear cells, essentially neutrophils, the number of which in-creased progressively being followed by a progressive decrease. Mononuclear cells, which consisted almost entirely of macrophages (38,71), were present from the third hr in very small quantities. Their number increased rapidly (Fig. 1) throughout the 48 hr of the test. After 12 hr, they were present in numbers equal to those of the polynuclears, then became far more numerous than the latter after 24 hr. These cells were large varying from 15 to 20 microns. Their basophilic cytoplasm contained azurophilic granules, and often several vacuoles. The nucleus was rounded, oval or elongated, but monomorphic. They were emigrated mono-cytes (38,71).

Comparison of the number of macrophages appearing in skin windows in normal controls and in patients with disseminated disease (Fig. 1, Table I). After 6 hr the number of macrophages migrating was less in the cancer patients than in the controls. This difference continued to increase at 12, 24 and 48 hr.

TABLE I

Means ± Standard Deviations of the Number of Macrophages Migrating to a Skin Window in Normal Controls and in Patients with Disseminated Malignant Disease. (Statistical Significance)

Time After Abrasion	Normal Controls	Patients Mean ± S. D.	Significance
3 hr	37.61 ± 14.02	29.52 ± 14.46	N.S.
6 hr	484.57 ± 120.22	205.14 ± 106.29	$p<0.01$
12 hr	2187.57 ± 673.85	685.72 ± 257.02	$p<0.01$
24 hr	3090.10 ± 935.22	827.00 ± 353.13	$p<0.001$
48 hr	4727.03 ± 896.23	1594.14 ± 576.37	$p<0.001$

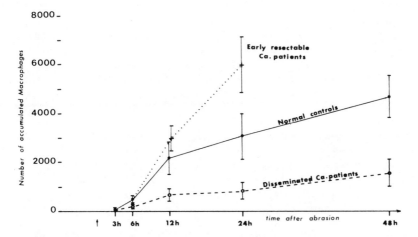

Fig. 1. Kinetics of macrophage migration to the skin window of 30 normal controls, 30 dissseminated cancer patients and 9 early resectable cancer patients. (Means ± S.D.)

By contrast, the number of polymorphonuclear cells did not notably differ between the normal and diseased subjects. Nevertheless, in the latter the migration of polymorphonuclear cells appeared to decrease less rapidly than in the normal subjects. This difference was, however, only slightly significant ($p < 0.5$ at 48 hr).

Subsequently, a study was made of the three intermediate time periods. At 3 hr, the exudate remained very poor and did not differ significantly. At 48 hr, cell migration took place much more in the form of agglomerates which made counting very difficult.

Study of cell migration in patients with localized tumors and effect of tumor removal (Fig. 1). This study involved 9 individuals with localized tumors including 5 patients with lung tumors (3 squamous cell carcinomas, 1 bronchial adenocarcinoma, and 1 oat cell carcinoma), 3 with adenocarcinomas of the breast and 1 with squamous cell carcinoma of the uterine cervix. Study of cell kinetics before surgery in these 9 patients revealed monocytic migration whch was importantly greater in comparison with the normal controls. Thus, at 24 hr the extremes of migration seen were 4,500 and 9,000. And at 24 hr, despite the small number of patients in this series, the difference was significant ($p < 0.01$) (Fig. 1).

Tumor excision which was considered oncologically satisfactory by the surgeon and histopathologist was associated in the majority of cases with a return to normal kinetics, i.e. identical with that of healthy individuals.

Changes induced by immunotherapy using C. parvum by intravenous administration (4 mg/day) for 4 weeks. Four patients with disseminated malignant disease, (2 melanomas, 1 disseminated carcinoma of the breast and 1 disseminated carcinoma of the colon) but who had previously received immunochemotherapeutic treatment, were tested. Changes in cell migration, as shown in Fig. 2a and 2b, were not perceptible before 24 hr. Up to 12 hr, there was no notable modification in the cellular exudate. By contrast, at 24 hr, in the 4 cases studied the number of macrophages had more than doubled. And in 3 cases out of 4 it exceeded the best figures from the normal control population. Nevertheless, the individuals studied had a previous inflammatory exudate which was relatively rich in 3 of them, possibly as a result of the nonspecific immunotherapy that they had received before in association with their chemotherapy.

Effects of plasmapheresis on the composition of the inflammatory exudate. The single plasmapheresis consisted of 1 session

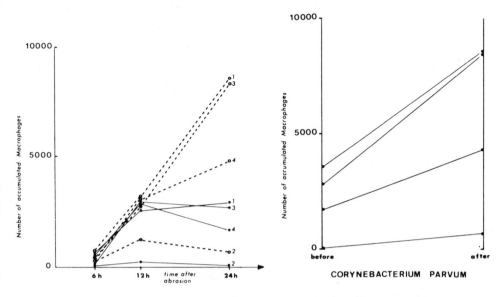

Fig. 2.   Kinetics of macrophage migration to the skin window of patients with neoplastic diseases having undergone daily intra-venous treatment for 4 weeks with <u>Corynebacterium parvum</u>.   The same patients have been tested before treatment (——) and after treat-ment (---).

Fig. 2B.   Changes in monocyte migration at the inflammatory site 24 hr after its creation in patients with neoplastic disease having undergone daily intravenous treatment for 4 weeks with <u>Corynebac-terium parvum</u>.

of plasma exchange of an average of 4.5 liters of plasma with fresh frozen plasma and reinjection of the leukocytes harvested after washing in saline. As shown by the Fig. 3, plasmapheresis increased considerably the level of monocyting migration in the patients herein tested. It was noted in one case that this im-provement in migration persisted, while in 3 cases the levels returned to those measured previously.

     The multiple plasmapheresis consisted of 6 sessions accord-ing to the procedure for single plasmapheresis. Results from 7 patients are shown in Fig. 4. In 2 cases there was a considerable increase in the number of monocytes migrating to the inflammatory site, but this returned to the previous level 15 days after the end of the series of plasmapheresis. One of these two patients showed evidence of spectacular regression of pulmonary metastases of a renal adenocarcinoma, demonstrated objectively by X-ray examination. In the 5 other patients, there was either a slight decrease in the number of macrophages migrating to the inflammatory site, or no change.

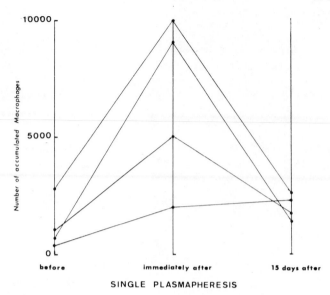

Fig. 3. Changes in monocyte migration at the inflammatory site
12 hr after its creation in patients with malignant disease having
undergone single plasmaparesis.

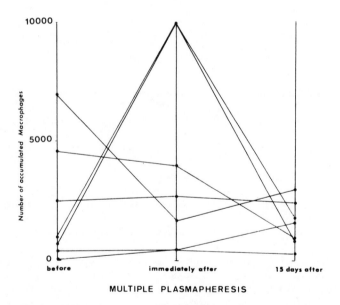

Fig. 4. Changes in monocyte migration at the inflammatory site
12 hr after its creation in patients with malignant disease
having undergone multiple plasmapheresis.

DISCUSSION

This study was made using Rebuck skin windows to evaluate the inflammatory reaction in vivo with special reference to the migration of monocytes to an inflammatory site created artificially and in a nonspecific manner. Quantitative information was collected in order to be able to assess any possible changes related to malignant disease, at different degrees of advancement, as well as those induced by ablation of the tumor or by immune therapy.

Numerous authors have carried out such a Rebuck test in various diseases (e.g., leukemia, agranulocytosis), and in various contexts (e.g., cancer patients receiving chemotherapy) most frequently using antigenic substances placed upon the abraded area, thereby provoking a delayed-type hypersensitivity reaction. Furthermore, up to the present time, two authors (14,20) have carried out such studies in patients with malignant disease using a nonspecific technique in order to study the inflammatory reaction of these patients, but these studies involved percentages of macrophages without any consideration of the cellularity, giving only a relative significance to the results obtained.

The results of the present study are in perfect agreement with those of animal experiments indicating an alteration in monocyte mobilization in an inflammatory area in tumor-bearing animals (4,50,58,60). Patients with widely disseminated tumors show evidence of marked alteration in monocytic migration. By contrast, in the 9 patients with localized tumors, we were surprised to find that monocytes arrived in greater number than that seen in the normal controls. The interesting results obtained in this special group of patients may represent a factor of favorable prognosis, indicative of their reticuloendothelial system being in a state of activation probably induced by the tumor. Nevertheless, these results should be viewed with caution inasmuch as the number of subjects tested was too small.

This may also indicate that impairments of this function occur only secondarily to extension of the disease. Similarly, this fact could be in favor of a block of anti-tumor reaction solely at a local-regional level when the tumor is at an early stage of its development, or possibly of selective block involving cytotoxic function (since the tumor is not rejected), but not their migratory function. Finally, with extension of the tumor, depression of this function is maximal. Increase in the level of certain glycoproteins, in parallel with tumor growth (35) would appear to be worthy of consideration in terms of the etiology of this block, since the in vitro chemotaxis of blood monocytes is depressed if they are incubated with high concentrations of orosomucoid comparable with the blood levels of this protein in patients with malignant disease (personal unpublished data).

Finally, immune therapy such as the one with C. parvum which
is known as a nonspecific stimulant of monocytic cells, may be
associated with a considerable improvement in monocyte response in
patients with disseminated malignant disease, this being quite in
agreement with data from the literature and largely justifying
the value of such stimulants in the treatment of malignancy.

It is of interest to note that treatment aimed at eliminating
factors blocking anti-tumor immune reaction may increase the level
of nonspecific inflammatory response which, on the one hand,
would appear to confirm hypotheses of a block of this anti-tumor
reaction by various factors and, secondly, justify continued research in this domain. But one cannot rule out, in the genesis
of this improvement, the possible additional effect of opsonins
as is the case with the administration of fresh plasma from normal donors.

Classical skin tests for the assessment of delayed-type
hypersensitivity to antigens such as tuberculin, candidin and
streptokinase were performed in all of these patients, whether
they were suffering from disseminated tumors, early resectable
tumors, or during various forms of treatment. The results obtained were widely variable, without any significant value in
terms of the different stages of extension of the disease. By
contrast, study of the cell reaction provoked by a cutaneous
abrasion was considered to be more closely correlated with the
clinical context. For these reasons it is felt that this test is
a valuable means of assessing the capability of the organism to
deal with neoplastic disease. In addition, it may represent a
useful tool in the monitoring of immune therapy.

SUMMARY

Leukocyte chemotaxis in response to a nonspecific stimulus
(skin abrasion) was studied in vivo using the Rebuck skin window
technique in 30 healthy volunteers and 30 untreated patients with
various metastatic malignancies as well as in 9 patients with
early resectable cancer. The absolute number of cells migrating
to the inflammatory site and the percentage of mononuclear cells
were recorded 3, 6, 12, 24 and 48 hr after initiation of the
stimulus. The influence of tumor removal, daily intravenous injections with C. parvum and single or multiple plasmapheresis
was studied in 9, 4, 4 and 7 patients, respectively. Major qualitative differences were observed between controls and advanced
cancer patients. Their was no difference in the absolute number
of cells between cancer patients and normal controls. In contrast, mononuclear cells appeared later in cancer patients than

in controls and were significantly decreased (p<0.001 at both 24 and 48 hr). In our 9 patients with early resectable cancer, there was an increase in the macrophage mobilization and tumor removal was associated with a return to normal values. The patients on i.v. C. parvum showed a striking increase in their number of mono-nuclear cells at 24 hr. Also, some patients on plasmapheresis showed an even more dramatic increase in the percentage of mono-nuclear cells at 6, 12 and 24 hr, over the baseline values. These quantitative differences observed in vivo are consistent with in vitro data suggesting that monocyte function is altered in patients with advanced cancer and indicate that immunological manipulation is capable of restoring monocyte function. The skin window technique offers a simple and convenient technique for monitoring monocyte function in cancer patients. When compared to the conventional skin tests the latter often give variable results.

ACKNOWLEDGEMENTS

We would like to thank Brinon Rémy, Mrs. Falconnet and Samak Martine for considerable help in this work, and Bereziat Francoise for typing the manuscript.

REFERENCES

1. Alexander, P. and Evans, R., Nature (Lond.) 232 (1971) 16.
2. Allison, A. C., Davies, P. and De Petris, S., Nature: New Biol. 232 (1971) 153.
3. Berken, A. and Benacerraf, B., J. Exp. Med. 123 (1966) 119.
4. Bernstein, I. D., Zbar, B. and Rapp, H. J., J.N.C.I., 49 (1972) 1641.
5. Bessis, M., Antibiol. and Chemother. 19 (1974) 361.
6. Bhisey, A. N. and Freed, J. J., Exp. Cell. Res. 64 (1971) 419.
7. Blumenstock, F., Saba, T. M., Weber, P. and Cho, E., Reticuloendothel. Soc. 19 (1976) 157.
8. Blumenstock, F.A., Saba, T. M. and Weber, P., J. Reticuloendothel. Soc. 23 (1978) 119.
9. Boetcher, D. A. and Leonard, E. J., J.N.C.I., 52 (1974) 1091.
10. Boyden, S., J. Exp. Med. 115 (1962) 453.
11. Currie, G. A. and Basham, C., J. Exp. Med. 142 (1975) 1600.
12. Currie, G. A. and Eccles, S. A., Br. J. Cancer, 33 (1976) 51.
13. Di Luzio, N. R., McNamee, R., Olcay, I., Kitahama, A. and Miller, R. M., Proc. Soc. Exp. Biol. Med., 145 (1974) 311.
14. Dizon, Q. S. and Southam, C. M., Cancer, 16 (1963) 1288.
15. Eccles, S. A. and Alexander, P., Nature, 250 (1974) 667.
16. Evans, R., Transplantation, 14 (1972) 468.
17. Evans, R. and Alexander, P., Nature, 236 (1972) 168.
18. Fauve, R. M., Hevin, B., Jacob, H., Gaillard, J. A. and

Jacob, F., Proc. Nat. Acad. Sci. (USA), 71 (1974) 4052.
19. Germain, R. N., Williams, R. M. and Benacerraf, B., J.N.C.I., 54 (1975) 709.
20. Goldsmith, H. S., Levin, A. G. and Southam, C. M., Surg. Forum., 16 (1965) 102.
21. Halpern, B. N., Biozzi, G., Stiffel, C., Mouton, D., Nature, 212 (1966) 853.
22. Harmel, R. P. and Zbar, B., J.N.C.I., 54 (1975) 989.
23. Hartwig, J. H. and Stossel, T. P., J. Biol. Chem., 250 (1975) 5696.
24. Haskill, J. S., Proctor, J. W. and Yamamura, Y., J.N.C.I., 54 (1975) 307.
25. Hausman, M. S., Brosman, S., Snyderman, R., Mickey, M. R. and Fahey, J., J.N.C.I., 55 (1975) 1047.
26. Hibbs, J. B., Science, 180 (1973) 868.
27. Hibbs, J. B., J.N.C.I., 53 (1974) 1487.
28. Hibbs, J. B., Transplantation, 19 (1975) 77.
29. Holtermann, O. A., Pascale, G. P. and Klein, E., J. Med., 3 (1972) 305.
30. Holtermann, O. A., Klein, E. and Casale, G., Cell Immunol., 9 (1973) 339.
31. Hortermann, O. A., Djerassi, L., Lisafeld, B. A., Elias, E. G., Papermaster, B. W. and Klein, E., Proc. Soc. Exp. Biol. Med., 147 (1974) 456.
32. Isa, A. M., and Sanders, B. R., Transplantation, 20 (1975) 296.
33. Israel, L., Depierre, A., Edelstein, R., Cros-Decam, J. and Maury, P., Panminerva Med., 17 (1975) 187.
34. Israel, L. and Edelstein, R., World. J. Surg. 1 (1977) 585.
35. Israel L., Edelstein, R., Mannoni, P., Radot, E., and Greenspan, E. M., Cancer, 40 (1977) 3146.
36. Israel, L. and Edelstein, R., Isr. J. Med. Sci., 14 (1978) 105.
37. Israel, L. and Edelstein, R., In: Treatment of cutaneous and subcutaneous metastatic tumors with intralesional glucan. Immune Modulation and control of neoplasia by adjuvant therapy. (Ed. M. A. Chirigos), Raven Press, N. Y., (1978) 249.
38. Jansa, P., Folia Haematol., Leipzig, 101 (1974) 213.
39. Jensen, J. A. and Esquenazi, V., Nature (Lond.) 256 (1975) 213.
40. Jones, J. T., McBride, W. H. and Weir, D. M., Cell Immunol. 18 (1975) 375.
41. Kay, A. B. and McVie, J. G., Br. J. Cancer, 36 (1977) 461.
42. Keller, R., J. Exp. Med. 138 (1973) 625.
43. Kindmark, C. O., Clin. Exp. Immunol. 8 (1971) 941.
44. Koppelmann, B. A., Moore, T. C., Lemmi, C. A. E. and Porter, D. D., Surgery, 78 (1975) 181.
45. Mackaness, G. B., J. Exp. Med. 120 (1964) 105.
46. McVie, J. G., Logan, E. C. and Kay, A. B., Europ. J. Cancer,

13 (1977) 351.
47. Mansell, P. W. A., Ichinose, M., Reed, R. J., Krementz, E. T.,
    McNamee, R. and Di Luzio, R. N., J.N.C.I., 54 (1975) 571.
48. Marti, J. H., Grosser, N. and Thomson, D. H. P., Int. J.
    Cancer. 18 (1976) 48.
49. Mosesson, M. W., Chen, A. G. and Huseby, R. M., Biochim. Bio-
    phys. Acta, 386 (1975) 509.
50. Normann, S. J. and Sorkin, E., J.N.C.I., 57 (1976) 135.
51. Paz, R. A. and Spector, W. G., J. Path. Bact., 84 (1962) 85.
52. Piessens, W. F., Churchill, W. H. and David, J. R., J.
    Immunol., 114 (1975) 293.
53. Pisano, J. C., Jackson, J. P., Di Luzio, N. R. and Ichinose,
    M., Cancer Res., 32 (1972) 11.
54. Rebuck, J. W. and Crowley, J. H., Ann. N. Y. Acad. Sci., 59
    (1955) 757.
55. Rocklin, R. E., J. Invest. Dermatol., 67 (1976) 372.
56. Saba, T. M., Aspecific opsonins. Proc. of 4th International
    Convocation on Immunology. In: Immune system and infectious
    diseases (Eds. F. Milgrom and E. Neter), S. Karger, Co. Basel,
    (1975) 489.
57. Saba, T. M. and Cho, E., J. Reticuloendothel. Soc., 22 (1977)
    583.
58. Synderman, R., Pike, M. C., Blaylock, B. L. and Weinstein, P.,
    J. Immunol. 116 (1976) 585.
59. Synderman, R., Meadows, L., Holder, W. and Wells, S., J.N.C.I.,
    60 (1978) 737.
60. Snyderman, R. and Pike, M. C., Science, 192 (1976) 370.
61. Synderman, R., Seigler, F. H. and Meadows, L., J.N.C.I., 58
    (1977) 37.
62. Stossel, T. R., N. Engl. J. Med., 290 (1974) 717.
63. Stossel, R. T., Field, R. J., Gotlin, J. D., Alper, C. A. and
    Rosen, F. S., J. Exp. Med., 141 (1975) 1329.
64. Van Loveren, H. and Den Otter, W., J.N.C.I., 53 (1974) 1057.
65. Van Oss, C. J., Gillman, C. F., Bronson, P. M. and Border,
    J. R., Immunol. Commun., 3 (1974) 329.
66. Ward, P. A., J. Exp. Med., 128 (1968) 1201.
67. Wellek, B., Hahn, M. and Opferkuch, W., Agents and Actions,
    6 (1976) 260.
68. Wilkinson, P. C., Nature (Lond.), 244 (1973) 512.
69. Wilkinson, P. C., Clin. Exp. Immunol., 25 (1976) 355.
70. Wood, G. and Morantz, R., J. Reticuloendothel. Soc., 22 (1977)
    58a.
71. Wulff, H. R. and Sparrevohn, S., Acta Path. et Microbiol.
    Scandinav., 68 (1966) 101.

PROTECTION FROM MALIGNANCY BY NONIMMUNE LYMPHOID CELLS

T. J. LINNA and K. M. LAM*

Department of Microbiology and Immunology, Temple
University School of Medicine, Philadelphia, PA. (USA)

The discovery of a lymphoid cell population, capable of killing
tumor target cells in vitro without previous immunization (2,4) has
generated much interest among scientists working on the influence
of the immune system on tumor development. The effector "natural
killer" (NK) cells in the in vitro assay lack the characteristics
of the major T cell, B cell, and macrophage populations (2,4).
These NK cells have receptors for the Fc portion of the IgG molecule
in man, and may also have Fc receptors in the mouse (2), although
this issue is still controversial (4). The NK cells, having the
"natural" ability to kill tumor target cells over a wide antigenic
range without previous immunization, have been proposed to have
an immunosurveillance function in malignancy (2,4). However,
virtually all work on NK cells has been performed in vitro, and
their in vivo relevance is therefore difficult to assess.

In Marek's disease, a naturally occurring, DNA virus-induced
malignancy of the fowl, the development of "natural" resistance to
the malignancy with age is well known. We have found that a
similar age-related resistance exists to a Marek's disease-relat-
ed tumor cell line, and that this resistance can be transferred
with lymphoid cells.

We will present data in this tumor model, showing that
animals are protected from a supralethal inoculation of malignant
cells by transferred lymphoid cells from donors isogeneic with the
recipients for the major histocompatibility (B) locus. The cells

---

*Present address: Department of Microbiology, School of Veterinary
 Medicine, Tuskegee Institute, Alabama (USA)

responsible for protection do not appear to belong to the major T
cell, B cell, and macrophage populations. We have previously
reported briefly on these findings (6), and we will now report on
further characterization of the cell population, including the
finding that these nonimmune effector cells are radiosensitive and
possess Fc receptors.

Thus, the cell capable of conferring protection from tumor
death in vivo in this tumor system appears very similar to the NK
cell described in rodents and in man.

MATERIALS AND METHODS

Animals. Hy-Line line SC chickens were used in these studies.
The SC chickens have B^2/B^2 as their major histocompatibility antigens. Fertile eggs were obtained from Hy-Line International, Des
Moines, Iowa, and incubated and hatched in a Jamesway 252B incubat-
or-hatcher. The animals were kept as a rule in conventional
quarters in thermostatically controlled brooders until 4 weeks
old, and thereafter in cages. One group of donors was housed in
a laminar flow room immediately after hatching until organ sampling,
with appropriate isolation precautions, for reasons stated below.

Tumor. The JMV tumor line, originally obtained by rapid
passage of the JM Marek's disease agent, was used in these studies.
This is a highly virulent lymphoid tumor cell line (12). It was
originally kindly given to us by Dr. M. Sevoian, University of
Massachusetts, Amherst, Mass. The line was passaged 3 times in
SC chickens and kept in liquid nitrogen until used.

General Experimental Protocol

Cell transfers. The experimental groups of chickens were
given 5×10^7 spleen cells intraperitoneally from 8-week-old donors,
isogeneic with the recipients for the major histocompatibility (B)
locus, on the day of hatching. The treatments of the spleen cell
populations are described below. The following day, the experimenta:
animals, untreated controls, and when applicable, controls receiving
non-treated spleen cells from non-treated donors, were given a
$10LD_{50}$ dose of JMV tumor cells intraperitoneally. The animals
were observed daily for mortality. Dead animals were autopsied
to confirm the JMV malignancy. The animals dying from causes
other than JMV malignancy were excluded from evaluation. In some
experiments, the timing between administration of spleen cells and
JMV cells was varied (see below).

Donor Lymphoid Cell Manipulations

Depletion of T cells. Normal spleen cells were treated with monospecific, differentially absorbed rabbit anti-chicken T cell serum, and guinea pig complement. The antiserum used killed 100% of thymocytes, but no bursa cells. The possibility that a minor T cell population has escaped destruction by the xeno-antiserum cannot be completely excluded.

Depletion of B cells. Normal spleen cells were treated with monospecific, differentially absorbed rabbit anti-chicken B cell serum and complement to destroy B cell population. The antiserum used killed 100% of bursa cells, but no thymocytes. Again, the possibility that some B cells may escape destruction by this anti-serum cannot be excluded. The additional method of depleting B cells by cyclophosphamide (CY) (9) was carried out by daily treat-ment of donors with 4 or 3 mg of CY i.p. for 3 or 4 days, respect-ively (Linna, Frommel, Good, 1972).

Depletion of phagocytic and adherent cells. Spleen cells were depleted of phagocytic cells by treatment with carbonyl iron and magnets, and of adherent cells by incubating cells at 37 C for 40 mins on plastic Petri dishes.

In vitro irradiation. The spleen cells were X-irradiated in vitro with a General Electric Maxitron 300 X-ray machine. The cells were given 650R or 1300R at a rate of 328R/min.

Enrichment and depletion of Fc receptor-bearing cells. Two methods were used for enrichment and depletion of Fc receptor-bear-ing cells. First, Fc receptor-bearing cells were rosetted with sheep erythrocytes (SRBC) sensitized with chicken anti-SRBC IgG (1). The Fc receptor-bearing, rosetting cell population was separated by centrifugation. The non-rosetting cell population was also sampled and used as the population depleted of Fc-receptor-bearing cells. Secondly, spleen cells were incubated on monolayers of SRBC sensizied with chicken anti-SRBC antibody on poly-L-lysine-treated plastic Petri dishes (3). Fc receptor-bearing cells attach-ed to the monolayer were harvested and used in cell transfers. The non-adherent cells were also used as cells lacking Fc receptors in cell transfer studies.

Evaluation of Data

The differences in tumor mortality between the different groups were evaluated using the Fisher-Yates exact test, with four-fold tables when applicable.

RESULTS AND DISCUSSION

The "natural," age-related resistance to field strains of
Marek's disease is well known. We have previously demonstrated
that a similar age-related resistance exists to a supralethal
challenge of the JMV leukemia. Seven-week-old animals were
resistant, while newly hatched animals were very sensitive to a
challenge with $10LD_{50}$ of JMV leukemia cells (6,7). We have found
that resistance to the JMV malignancy can be transferred with
spleen cells from normal, non-immunized, 8-week-old donors
isogeneic with the recipients for the major histocompatibility (B)
locus (6,7).

Although we have not had any cases of Marek's disease in our
colony, and are not using any vaccine against Marek's disease,
there is a remote possibility that the donor animals may have
been inadvertently exposed to the MD agent and consequently be
immune. Therefore, we compared the protective ability of cells
from donors raised in conventional quarters with cells from 8-week-
old donors, brought to a laminar flow isolation room immediately
after hatching, and reared in this room until used. Spleen cells
from laminar flow room-reared donors were as efficient in
conferring protection from tumor death as were spleen cells from
animals reared in conventional quarters (Table I). Thus, there
is no indication that the cells transferring protection from tumor
death would come from MD-exposed animals.

We have previously reported that surgical thymectomy of donors
on the day of hatching does not influence the ability of such spleen
cells to transfer protection at 8 weeks of age (6,7). In keeping
with this finding, thymus cells cannot confer resistance on a
statistically significant level (6,7). Since thymectomy at hatching, without adjunct treatment, does not accomplish complete depletion of the thymus-dependent cell population, the question of
participation of T cells was further studied by using donor cells,
depleted of T cells by treatment with anti-T cell serum (ATS) and
complement. Also this more profoundly T cell depleted population
was able to confer protection on a statistically significant level
(Table I). Thus, the cell population conferring protection does
not appear to be a major T cell population. However, the possibility that a T cell subset, not affected by newly hatched thymectomy or treatment with our anti-T cell serum and complement, cannot
be excluded. It is of interest to note in this context that the
level of protection conferred by the ATS-treated cells may be
somewhat, although not significantly, lower than protection conferred by untreated cells.

We have also previously reported that depletion of B cells by
surgical bursectomy of the donors at hatching did not influence

TABLE I

Effect of Treatment of Donor Chickens or Donor Spleen Cells on
the Protective Effect of Spleen Cells Against JMV-Induced Leukemia
in Newly Hatched Chickens

Treatment of donors or of spleen cells	No. cells given	No. deaths No. JMV inoculation	P[a]
Treatment of donor chickens:			
Raised in laminar flow room	5×10^7	1/20	< 0.002
Raised in conventional quarters	5×10^7	2/23	< 0.002
Controls	None	20/20	
Cyclophosphamide treated:			
4 mg/day for 3 days	5×10^7	3/20	< 0.002
3 mg/day for 4 days	5×10^7	6/19	< 0.002
Untreated	5×10^7	1/20	< 0.002
Controls	None	20/20	
Treatment of spleen cells:			
Anti-thymocyte serum and complement	5×10^7	12/25	0.05
Untreated	5×10^7	6/20	< 0.01
Controls	None	19/24	
Anti-bursa serum and complement	5×10^7	10/20	0.05
Anti-bursa serum and complement followed by anti-thymocyte serum and complement	5×10^7	10/20	0.005
Untreated	5×10^7	6/19	0.002
Controls	None	17/20	
Adherent cells depleted	5×10^7	7/10	< 0.01
Untreated	5×10^7	6/20	0.002
Controls	None	17/20	
Fc-receptor bearing cells (monolayer)	7×10^6	11/23	0.02
Fc-receptor depleted cells (monolayer)	5×10^7	18/19	Not significant
Whole spleen cells	5×10^7	10/20	< 0.05
Controls	None	16/18	
FC-receptor bearing cells (rosetting)	1×10^7	6/20	< 0.002
Fc-receptor depleted cells (rosetting)	5×10^7	14/20	Not significant
Whole spleen cells	5×10^7	1/20	< 0.002
Controls	None	16/18	

[a] P is determined by Fisher Yates Exact Probability Test with four-
fold tables, as compared with its respective controls.

the subsequent ability of their spleen cells to transfer protection (6,7). This incomplete but specific depletion of B cells was complemented by experiments in which a specific, profound defect of the bursa of Fabricius and of the B-cell system was accomplished by treatment with higher doses of cyclophosphamide in the newly hatched period (9). Also, spleen cells from such birds were able to confer protection (Table I). Spleen cells treated with mono-specific anti-B cell serum (ABS) and complement could also confer protection (Table I). Thus, a major B cell subset does not appear to be responsible for protection.

The participation of mature macrophages and adherent cells in protection was also evaluated. Neither exclusion of phagocytic cells by treatment of donor cells with carbonyl iron and magnets, nor exclusion of adherent cells by incubation on plastic (Table I), affected the ability of the donor cells to confer protection against leukemia. Thus, the cell population responsible for protection does not appear to be a mature macrophage-adherent cell. The participation of a promonocyte-promacrophage population, lacking the phagocytic and adherent properties of the mature cells, is difficult to exclude in this system, as in many others.

The cell transferring protection is radiosensitive, and/or needs to proliferate in the recipient, since donor cells irradiated with 650R in vitro can give only marginal protection, and cells irradiated with 1300R cannot protect to any significant extent.

Thus, the cell responsible for protection of recipient animals from tumor death does not appear to belong to the major T cell, B cell, or mature macrophage populations, but rather to the non-T, non-B, "third cell" population. In this probably heterogenous cell population, K cells (11,10,13) and "natural killer" cells (2,4,5) have been in the focus of special attention in recent years. K cells have IgG Fc receptors, necessary for their cytotoxic activity. NK cells have Fc receptors in man, and possibly also in rodents (2, 4). We studied whether the presence of Fc receptors for IgG on the donor cells has any influence on their capacity to transfer protection against tumor death. Using two methods for depleting and enriching the Fc receptors, we found that Fc receptor-carrying cells were capable of conferring protection to recipients on a statistically significant level, while cells lacking Fc receptors lacked protective capacity (Table I). The presence of complement receptors did not appear to have any bearing on the protective capacity of the cell population.

Thus, our data demonstrated that there is a nonimmune spleen cell population with the ability to protect from tumor death following challenge with a lethal dose of malignant MD-related lymphoid cells. The cell responsible for protection appeared to be a non-T, non-B, non-macrophage lymphoid cell with Fc receptors. This cell is apparently similar to the NK cell in man and rodents described by cytotoxic in vitro methodology. The exact identification of the protecting cell will have to await positive identification of the cell population, as is also the case with NK cells. For instance, the possibility is open that these cells could be a minor population belonging to the T cell lineage, as has been advocated for NK cells (2,4).

The cell type described by us also fits well with the characteristics of the K cells. The effector mechanism could therefore be as well of the K as of the NK type. It cannot be distinguished in vivo, whether the effector cell works directly on tumor cells, or with IgG antibody formed in response to tumor challenge. Actually, as K cells and NK cells are described to be similar in many respects (2,4), there is a possibility that the same cell population may use both effector mechanisms in vivo. Even in vitro, the question of contributions of antibody to the NK mechanism is not settled (2,4). Our results from in vitro work with this system are compatible with an NK-type affector mechanism (8).

ACKNOWLEDGEMENT

This work was supported by USPHS, NIH grant C A 13347 from the National Cancer Institute. We thank Dr. William McArthur, University of Pennsylvania, for helpful discussions on chicken lymphoid cell receptors, and demonstration of his technique for Fc and C receptors.

REFERENCES

1. Duncan, R. L., Jr. and McArthur, W. P. J. Immunol. 120 (1978) 1014.
2. Herberman, R. B. and Holden, H. T. In: Advances in Cancer Research (Eds. G. Klein and S. Weinhouse) Academic Press, New York, Vol. 27 (1978) 305.
3. Kedar, E., de Landazuri, M. O. and Bonavida, B. J. Immunol. 112 (1974) 1231.
4. Kiessling, R. and Haller, O. In: Contemporary Topics in Immunobiology (Eds. N. L. Warren and M. D. Cooper) Plenum Press, New York, Vol. 8 (1978) 171.
5. Koide, Y. and Takasugi, M. J. Nat. Cancer Inst. 59 (1977) 1099.
6. Lam, K. M. and Linna, T. J. Fed. Proc. (1977) 124.
7. Lam, K. M. and Linna, T. J. In: Advances in Comparative Leukemia Research 1977 (Eds. P. Bentvelzer, J. Hilgers and D. S. Yohn) Elsevier/North Holland Biomedical Press, Amsterdam (1978).

8. Lam, K. M. and Linna, T. J.   Submitted for publication.
9. Linna, T. J., Frommel, D. and Good, R. A.   Int. Arch.
    Allergy 42 (1972) 20.
10. MacLennan, I. C. M., Loewi, G. and Harding, B.   Immunol. 18
    (1970) 397.
11. Perlmann, P. and Permann, H.   J. Immunol. 108 (1972) 559.
12. Sevoian, M., Larose, R. N. and Chamberlain, D. M.   In:
    Proc. 101st Ann. Meet. A.V.M.A., Chicago (1964) 342.
13. Troye, M., Perlmann, P., Pape, G. R., Spiegelberg, H. L.,
    Naslund, I. and Gidlof, A.   J. Immunol. 119 (1977) 1061.

MODULATION OF THE TUMORICIDAL FUNCTION OF ACTIVATED MACROPHAGES BY BACTERIAL ENDOTOXIN AND MAMMALIAN MACROPHAGE ACTIVATION FACTOR(S)

J. B. HIBBS, J. B. WEINBERG, and H. A. CHAPMAN

Veterans Administration Hospital and University of

Utah Medical Center, Salt Lake City, Utah (USA)

Activated macrophage tumor cell killing can be modulated - enhanced or suppressed - by microenvironmental chemical signals. Our recent observations (21,6) as well as those of Russell et al. (34) suggest that tumor cell killing by activated macrophages is dependent on the local environment in which macrophages and tumor cells coexist. Activated macrophages are generally tumoricidal in vitro when cultured in medium supplemented with LPS-free fetal bovine serum (FBS) but these same macrophages do not kill tumor cells or do so inconsistently when cultured in medium supplemented with other types of serum. Macrophages representing four different functional states (within a continuum of macrophage differentiation) can be isolated from appropriate groups of mice and can also be generated in vitro by exposing the macrophages to appropriate stimuli (21,41) (see Fig. 1). (i) Normal resident macrophages are obtained from the peritoneal cavities of mice that have not received a sterile nonspecific inflammatory stimulant such as peptone or been infected with intracellular microorganisms such as Bacillus Calmette-Guérin (BCG) or toxoplasma. They do not respond effectively to chemical signals that induce the expression of tumor cell killing. (ii) Stimulated macrophages are obtained from mice injected intraperitoneally with 10% peptone, thioglycollate broth, or other sterile inflammatory stimulants. In vitro, normal macrophages acquire the stimulated state after culture for 48-72 hrs. When elicited in vivo stimulated macrophages are a mixed population of resident macrophages as well as macrophages recently derived from blood monocytes that migrated into the peritoneal cavity in response to an inflammatory stimulus. Stimulated macrophages do not kill tumor cells in culture medium containing FBS or other sera but become tumoricidal when exposed to large amounts of bacterial lipopolysaccharide (LPS) or lymphocyte super-

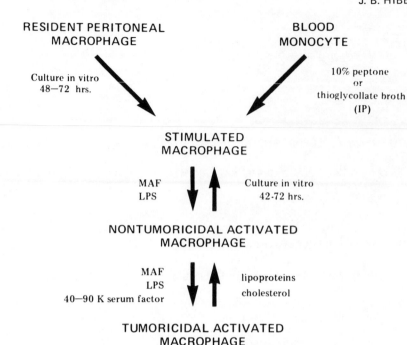

Fig. 1. Four functional states of macrophage differentiation.

natants with macrophage activating factor(s) (MAF) activity plus
small amounts of LPS. (iii) Nontumoricidal activated macrophages
are obtained from the peritoneal cavity of mice with chronic BCG
or toxoplasma infection, or are produced in vitro by exposure of
stimulated macrophages to MAF. Nontumoricidal activated macrophages have a markedly lowered threshold for induction of tumoricidal effect because picogram or nanogram quantities of LPS, low
concentrations of MAF, or the 40,000-90,000 dalton protein(s) of
serum fraction 3 induce tumor cell killing regardless of the kind
of serum in the medium. (iv) Tumoricidal activated macrophages
can also be obtained from the peritoneal cavity of mice with
chronic BCG or toxoplasma infection, but they kill tumor cells
regardless of the type of serum in the culture medium and without
added MAF or endotoxin. Such macrophages were only sporadically
obtained in our experiments. The probability of these highly
activated macrophages being obtained is increased by using toxo-
plasma-infected mice within 4-6 weeks after infection with the
microorganism or within 48-96 hrs after administering an intraperitoneal booster dose of toxoplasma (or a booster dose of BCG
in the case of BCG-infected mice). When observed in tissue culture, the tumoricidal activated state acquired by macrophage
exposure to in vivo or in vitro differention signals gradually

wanes with time (24-72 hrs). In addition, we have observed that
treatment with serum lipoproteins or enrichment of macrophage
membranes with cholesterol causes a reversible lowering of the
tumoricidal threshold from the tumoricidal activated to the nontumoricidal activated state (6). This differentiation sequence and
factors that influence it are summarized in Fig. 1 and suggest that
in vitro, and probably in vivo, a dynamic state exists among the
environmental chemical signals that can either increase or decrease
the probability for expression of macrophage-mediated tumor cell
killing.

   The concept of the macrophage activation response. These
findings that are schematically described in Fig. 1 gave us the
clue that the tumoricidal potential of activated macrophages is
not sharply delineated but instead controlled by a threshold that
is dependent on the net influences of antagonistic environmental
chemical signals. These observations have resulted in development
of the concept that the macrophage tumoricidal threshold and differentiation toward the tumoricidal state is regulated by an activation
response (21,6,41) (see Fig. 1). That a macrophage is undergoing
an activation response can be determined by an increased potential
for development and expression of nonspecific tumor cell killing
when compared to the relatively refractory resident peritoneal
macrophage.

   We define the activation response as an environmentally elicited
pleiotypic change in macrophage physiology that involves a lowering
of the tumoricidal threshold. The activation response occurs in
vivo during inflammatory or immunologic reactions and in vitro when
one or several inducing chemical signals are present in the local
environment. The tumoricidal threshold that regulates the macrophage cytotoxic effector system during the activation response has
several interesting characteristics: a) The tumoricidal threshold
is inversely related to the stage of macrophage differentiation
toward the tumoricidal state (21,41). b) The tumoricidal threshold
can be modulated, i.e., it can be increased as well as decreased
by environmental signals (21,6,41,7). c) There is evidence to
suggest that what we describe as a tumoricidal threshold is related, at least in part, to membrane organization, particularly macrophage membrane lipids (6,7).

   We plan to limit the remainder of the review to a discussion
of modulation of macrophage tumoricidal potential by LPS and MAF
elaborated by NaIO4-treated mouse peritoneal cells. We have
studied the effect of these two chemical signals in some detail
((21,41,42) and believe the results provide increased understanding
of how these two environmental factors interact to modulate the
macrophage activation response and tumoricidal threshold.

METHODS AND RESULTS

A detailed description of materials and methods for the
experiments reviewed here can be found elsewhere (41,42). Briefly,
LPS from Escherichia coli 0128:B12 extracted with phenol by the
Westphal method (43) was purchased from Sigma Chemical Co. (St.
Louis, MO). Lipid A was produced by acid hydrolysis of LPS
with 1% glacial acetic acid at 100 C for 2 hrs (14). The lipid A
was solubilized in 1% triethylamine at concentrations < 500 times
that to be used in the assays. Base hydrolysis of LPS was done
by using 1 N NaOH at 56 C for 90 mins followed by neutralization
with 1 N HCl and extensive dialysis against PBS. The Limulus
amebocyte lysate (LAL) assay used to detect the presence of LPS
was performed as described (10). Cell-free supernatants from
NaIO$_4$-treated peritoneal cells from BCG-infected mice were used
as a source of MAF. MAF was prepared by an adaptation of the
methods described by Bressler et al. (41,4). In vitro macrophage-
mediated tumor cell killing was quantitated by either visual cell
counting (41), or by measurement of ^{3}HTdR release from previously
labeled 3T12 tumor target cells (29). The cytotoxicity test
was performed as previously described (21,41). Pure macrophage
colonies were established from thioglycollate-induced peritoneal
exudate cells by methods previously described by Stewart et al.
(37). Gel chromatography was done in a sterile manner on a 2.5 x
60 cm G100 Sephadex column equilibrated in 0.15 M NaCl, 0.02%
sodium azide, 5 mM tris buffer at 4 C. Fractions of interest were
dialyzed against sterile LPS-free water, lyophilized, and reconstituted at desired concentrations in culture medium (DMM) for use
in the tumor cell killing assay. Macrophage migration inhibition
factor (MIF) activity was assayed by the method of Landolfo et al.
(26). ^{14}C-glucosamine incorporation into mouse peritoneal exudate
cells (PEC) was determined by a modification of the assay devised
by Hammond and Dvorak (17).

We previously defined activated but noncytotoxic macrophages
as nontumoricidal activated macrophages (21). In the experiments
reviewed here we obtained nontumoricidal activated macrophages
from the peritoneal cavity of mice with chronic BCG infection,
and we refer to them as BCG macrophages. Freshly explanted
resident peritoneal macrophages from normal mice are not made
tumoricidal by FBS, MAF, or LPS. However, macrophages from mice
that have received intraperitoneal (i.p.) 10% peptone or other
sterile inflammatory stimulants 72 hrs previously appear to have
entered an early phase of the activation response because they
are made tumoricidal by relatively large amounts of LPS or MAF
plus small amounts of LPS (21). We termed macrophages in this
early phase of the activation response stimulated macrophages
and identify them in this review as peptone-normal macrophages.

Endotoxin renders macrophages tumoricidal. LPS, in amounts as high as 10 ug/ml, did not make peritoneal macrophages from non-infected, normal mice tumoricidal (Fig. 2). However, macrophages from noninfected, normal mice that had received i.p. peptone were fully tumoricidal in the presence of relatively high concentrations of LPS. In general, 500 ng/ml LPS were required for this effect. However, there was some variability to this, and occasionally as little as 100 ng/ml or as much as 1000 ng/ml or greater of LPS were required to make these peptone-induced normal macrophages tumoricidal. The cause of this variability is unknown but is probably related to in vivo factors that affect the state of macrophage activation before their removal from the peritoneal cavity for in vitro cultivation and testing.

Peritoneal macrophages from BCG-infected mice were generally nontumoricidal in cytotoxicity assays supplemented with LPS-free adult serum. However, the presence of 1 ng/ml LPS (and occasional-ly 0.5 ng/ml LPS) throughout the assay made the macrophages fully tumoricidal. Pretreatment of the BCG macrophages with 50-150 ng/ml LPS for two hrs at 37 C also made them cytolytic for tumor cells. Macrophages from BCG-infected mice that had or had not received peptone intraperitoneally responded equally well to LPS.

LPS is capable of directly making macrophages tumoricidal in the absence of lymphocytes. The peritoneal cell monolayers consist of   90% macrophages as determined by phagocytosis of heat-killed Candida. The contaminating cells are lymphocytes, primarily B cells, which are more adherent than T cells (27,19). LPS is a B cell mitogen and can elicit MIF (or MAF) secretion from the B cells (45,44). It has been unclear whether LPS enhances the macrophage tumoricidal effect by a direct action on the macrophage, or by LPS-induced MAF secretion from the contaminating B cells. Peritoneal cell monolayers washed extensively were no less sensitive to the effects of LPS than were monolayers that were not washed. However, we could never be fully confident that this washing rinsed away all B cells.

The development by Stewart et al. (37) of a system for select-ively growing pure adherent macrophage colonies in liquid medium has made it possible to examine the effects of LPS on macrophages free of any contaminating lymphocytes. LPS was capable of making these cloned macrophages tumoricidal (Fig. 3). There was no spontaneous killing of tumor cells by these macrophages, but pretreatment of the colonies with $\geq$ 500 ng/ml LPS for 2 hrs, or the presence of $\geq$ 25-75 ng/ml LPS throughout the assay, resulted in a marked cytotoxic effect on the tumor cells in the areas of the macrophage colonies. Colony macrophages treated with 1% MAF for 2 hrs at 37 C in a preincubation were not tumoricidal. But the presence of as little as 1 ng/ml LPS subsequently added

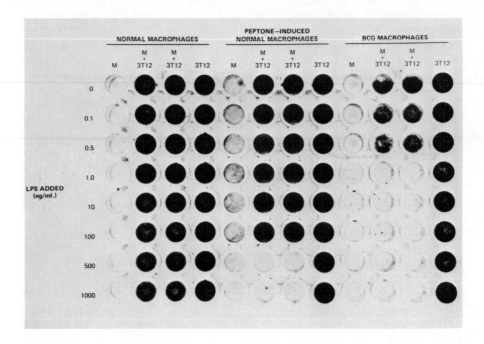

Fig. 2. Low power photograph of a Giemsa-stained microtiter
plate showing a tumor cell killing assay. Columns M, M + 3T12
and 3T12 represent chambers with macrophages, macrophages plus
3T12 cells, or 3T12 cells alone, respectively. The initial seed
of peritoneal cells for the M or M + 3T12 columns was 4 x 10^5 cells/
chamber, and the initial seed of tumor cells for the M + 3T12 or
3T12 columns was 6 x 10^3 cells/chamber. The 3T12 cell multilayers
are darkly stained and macrophages are not discernibly stained.
The normal macrophages do not become tumoricidal with 0-1000 ng/ml
LPS; the peptone-induced normal macrophages become tumoricidal
with $\geq$ 500 ng/ml LPS; and the BCG macrophages become tumoricidal
with $\geq$ 1 ng/ml LPS. Those chambers showing gross evidence of a
tumoricidal effect also show 4+ tumor cell killing (0-3 3T12 cells/
300X microscopic field as compared to an initial 3T12 seed of
33-37 3T12 cells/300X field) when quantitated by the cell-counting
assay.

(Reprinted from the Journal of Immunology, Ref. 41, with
permission of the publisher.)

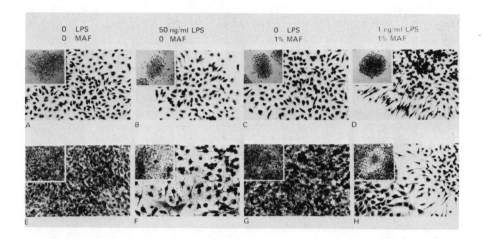

Fig. 3. Photomicrographs from Giemsa-stained chambers of a microtiter plate showing the effect of LPS and MAF on tumor cell killing
by cloned macrophages from C$_3$H/HeN mice. Cloned macrophage colonies
were used 20 days after initial seeding in this experiment. Chambers A through D contain macrophages alone, and E through H contain
macrophages and 3T12 tumor cells (6 x 10^3 cells/chamber initial
seed). The cultures were done in 10% adult bovine serum with or
without MAF and/or LPS present through the 60 hr assay. Macrophages with no additives (E), with 1% MAF (G), or with 1 ng/ml
LPS (not shown) are overgrown by the 3T12 cells, but macrophages
with 50 ng/ml LPS (F) or 1 ng/ml LPS and 1% MAF (H) are cytotoxic
to 3T12 cells in the area of the colonies. Magnifications are
92.8X with 14.5X for insets.

(Reprinted from the Journal of Immunology, Ref. 41, with permission
of the publisher.)

throughout the assay caused these MAF-treated macrophages completely to destroy the adjacent tumor cells.

These experiments show that pure colonies of cloned peritoneal
macrophages directly acquire nonspecific tumoricidal capability in
response to LPS, a chemical signal from a nonimmunological source.
This suggests that lymphocytes or their secretory products are not
obligate intermediates for the induction by LPS of macrophage
differentiation to the tumoricidal state.

The lipid moiety of LPS is responsible for the LPS effect on
macrophages. Lipid A, produced by mild acid hydrolysis of LPS,
was capable of making BCG macrophages tumoricidal. It was, in
general, slightly less potent than the parent, intact LPS, but

doses as low as 1 ng/ml of lipid A made the BCG macrophages
markedly tumoricidal (Table I). Alkaline treatment of LPS, which
cleaves and saponifies lipid A ester-linked fatty acids without
altering the antigenic polysaccharide (40), completely destroyed
the effect of LPS. Whereas 1 ng/ml of the native LPS made BCG
macrophages tumoricidal, doses as high as 1 µg/ml of base hydrolyz-
ed LPS did not make the BCG macrophages kill tumor cells. Polymyxin B sulfate, which forms a stable molecular complex with the
lipid A region of LPS (30) and blocks several effects of LPS in
vitro (23,5) and in vivo (32,11), markedly inhibited the effect
of LPS. When polymyxin B (0.1 to 25 ug/ml) was added to assay
cultures, LPS (1-100 ng/ml) was completely inhibited in its ability
to make BCG macrophages tumoricidal (Table II). BCG macrophages
from the lipid A-nonresponder strain (C3H/HeJ (39,36) were quite
resistant to the effect of LPS (Table III). Whereas macrophages
from BCG-infected C_3H/HeN mice were made tumoricidal by 1 ng/ml
LPS, 250-500 ng/ml LPS were required to render macrophages from
BCG-infected C_3H/HeN mice tumoricidal. Furthermore, pure, cloned
macrophages from C_3H/HeN and C_3H/HeJ mice responded unequally to
LPS. The presence of $\geq$ 50 ng/ml LPS in assays made C_3H/HeN colony
macrophages cytotoxic for 3T12 cells, but cloned macrophages from
C_3H/HeJ mice required $\geq$ 1000 ng/ml for this effect. If the
macrophages were first treated with 1% MAF, they were not tumoricidal, but the subsequent addition of $\geq$ 1 ng/ml LPS to C_3H/HeN
MAF-treated macrophages or $\geq$ 250 ng/ml LPS to C_3H/HeJ MAF-treated
macrophages resulted in marked tumor cell killing by these pure
macrophages. These results correlate with the findings of Chedid
et al. (8), who noted the inability to make C_3H/HeJ peritoneal
macrophages tumoristatic with LPS, and the resistance of C_3H/HeJ
peritoneal macrophages to the toxic effects of LPS noted by Glode
et al. (15). Peritoneal macrophages from BCG-infected mice of
other strains ($C_{57}Bl/6$, Balb/c, and National Institutes of Health
Swiss Webster) were made tumoricidal by LPS doses comparable to
those required to make macrophages from BCG-infected C_3H/HeN mice
kill tumor cells.

    Physiochemical and functional characteristics of MAF elaborat-
ed by $NaIO_4$-treated mouse peritoneal cells. As noted above, supernatants from $NaIO_4$-treated peritoneal cells contain MAF activity
as determined by the ability to induce macrophage differentiation
to the nontumoricidal activated state. By G100 Sephadex gel
chromatography, this MAF activity eluted in one fraction spanning
the molecular weight range 37,000-80,00 daltons (see Fig. 4).
This range roughly corresponds to that obtained for mouse MIF
by others (25). The MAF activity was stable to freezing at -20 C
and -70 C, and lyophilization. The activity was not affected by
heating at 56 C for 30 mins or 60 C for 60 mins, but it was totally abolished by heating at 80 C for 10 mins. The supernatants
were negative for LPS as assessed by the LAL assay. Polymyxin B,
an antibiotic that combines with the lipid portion of LPS and

TABLE I

Effect of Chemically Modified LPS on Tumor Cell Killing
by BCG Macrophages from C_3H/HeN Mice[a]

LPS added[c] (ng/ml)	Degree of tumor cell killing[b]		
	LPS type:		
	Native	Lipid A	Base hydrolyzed
0	0	0	0
1	4+	3+	0
10	4+	4+	0
100	4+	4+	0
1000	4+	4+	0

[a] 4×10^5 peritoneal cells per chamber.

[b] Tumor cell killing quantitated by visual cell counting. 4+ tumor cell killing signifies 0-3 tumor cells/300X microscopic field; 3+, 4-14 cells/field; 2+, 15-25 cells/field; 1+, 26-36 cells/field; and 0, a multilayer of tumor cells over the macrophages. For comparison, the initial tumor cell density (time 0) was 33-37 cells/300X field.

[c] LPS present throughout the 60 hr assay.

(Reprinted from the Journal of Immunology, Ref. 41, with permission of the publisher.)

TABLE II

Effect of Polymyxin B on LPS-Enhanced Tumor Cell Killing
by BCG Macrophages from C_3H/HeN Mice[a]

LPS added[b] (ng/ml)	Degree of Tumor Cell Killing (^{3}HTdR release[d])	
	Polymyxin B (ug/ml)[b,c]	
	0	25
0	4.5 ± 0.1%	0 ± 0.5%
50	57.9 ± 3.8%	0 ± 0.3%

[a] 4×10^5 peritoneal cells per chamber.

[b] Present throughout the 60 hr assay.

[c] PB has no effect on cell viability or growth rates at these concentrations.

[d] % release ± S.E.M. of quadruplicate samples.

(Adapted from the J. of Immunol., Ref. 41, with permission of the publisher.)

TABLE III

Comparison of the Effect of LPS on Tumor Cell Killing by
BCG Macrophages from C$_3$H/HeN and C$_3$H/HeJ Mice

LPS Added[b] (ng/ml)	Degree of Tumor Cell Killing[a]			
	Macrophage Source:			
	C$_3$H/HeN[c]		C$_3$H/HeJ[c]	
	2 x 10^5	4 x 10^5	2 x 10^5	4 x 10^5
0	0	0	0	0
1	1+	4+	0	0
10	3+	4+	0	0
50	4+	4+	0	0
100	4+	4+	0	1+
250	4+	4+	1+	3+
500	4+	4+	3+	4+

[a]Tumor cell killing assessed by visual cell counting (see legend
to Table I).
[b]LPS present throughout the 60 hr assay.
[c]Number of peritoneal cells per chamber.
(Reprinted from the Journal of Immunology, Ref. 41, with permission of the publisher.)

inhibits its activity, did not inhibit MAF (41). The ability to
abolish the activity by heating at 80 C for 10 mins, the negative
LAL assay, and the inability to alter the MAF activity with polymyxin B virtually exclude the possibility that the tumoricidal
enhancing qualities of this MAF preparation are due to contaminating LPA (41).

Although Haveman et al. (20) noted inhibition of the MIF activity in supernatants of specifically or nonspecifically stimulated
lymphocytes by diisopropyl fluorophosphate (DEP), David and Becker
(12) were unable to block MIF activity by DFP and other serine
esterase inhibitors. When our MAF preparation was treated overnight in 1 x 10^{-2} M DFP at room temperature, dialyzed against PBS
and then DMM, the MAF activity was unaltered as compared to untreated MAF similarly dialyzed.

The supernatants of NaIO$_4$-treated BCG PEC contained MIF activity when assayed using the agarose droplet technique of migration
quantitation. Table IV shows that the supernatants of NaIO$_4$-
treated BCG PEC when compared to supernatants of PBS-treated BCG
PEC were effective in inhibiting the migration of peritoneal cells

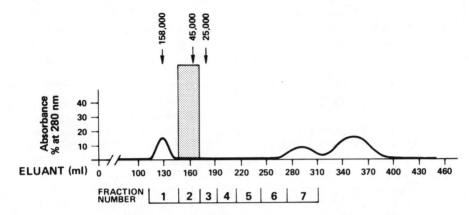

Fig. 4. Chromatography of supernatant from NaIO4-treated BCG
PEC on Sephadex G100 in 5 mM Tris, 0.15 $\underline{M}$ NaCl, 0.02% sodium azide
buffer, pH 7.4. The numbers 1-7 indicate the pooled fractions
tested for MAF activity. The curve shows the optical density
at 280 nm. The vertical arrows indicate elution points of aldo-
lase (158,000 daltons), ovalbumin (45,000 daltons), and chymotrypsinogen A (25,000 daltons). The shaded area denotes the fraction
that contained MAF activity (i.e., ability, in a 2-hr pretreatment,
to render peptone-normal macrophages tumoricidal when cultured
with 2 ng/ml LPS). (Weinberg and Hibbs, unpublished).

TABLE IV

MIF Activity of Supernatants from NaIO4-Treated BCG PEC

% supernatant[a]	Migration index[b]
0	1.00 ± 0.04
10	0.82 ± 0.10
20	0.50 ± 0.03
40	0.50 ± 0.02
80	0.51 ± 0.02

[a]Present throughout the 24-hr assay.
[b]Migration index $\pm$ S.E.M. for quadruplicate samples.

(From Weinberg and Hibbs, unpublished)

from mice that had received 1 ml sterile light mineral oil three
days previously. Also, peritoneal cells treated in suspension
at 4 C for 10 mins with 5×10^{-3} $\underline{M}$ NaIO$_4$/PBS had inhibited migration as compared to control, PBS-treated cells (migration index
of 0.56 ± 0.06).

Hammond $\underline{et}$ $\underline{al.}$ (17,18) have noted that MIF treatment of guinea
pig macrophages enhances their incorporation of glucosamine and
other sugars. Others have noted similar effects in murine systems
(2). Table V shows that the cell-free supernatants from NaIO$_4$-
treated BCG PEC slightly enhanced glucosamine incorporation, but
combination of supernatant with 10 ng/ml LPS increased the incorporation greater than the LPS or supernatant alone. These findings
indicate that soluble factors derived from NaIO4-treated BCG PEC
activate peritoneal macrophages as determined by enhancement of
glucosamine incorporation. The synergy between MAF and LPS in
promoting increased ^{14}C-glucosamine uptake by PEC is comparable
to the synergy noted in enhancing the tumoricidal capacity of
peritoneal macrophages or cloned macrophages. For example, a
2 hr pretreatment of peptone-normal macrophages with 1-25% (v/v)
of the cell-free supernatant from NaIO4-treated BCG PEC did not
make these cells tumoricidal. Likewise, the presence of 5 ng/ml
LPS in the cultures did not make the peptone-normal macrophages
kill the 3T12 cells. But if supernatant-treated peptone-normal
macrophages were cultured with 5 ng/ml LPS, they were tumoricidal
(see Table VI).

Many reagents are contaminated with LPS. Because of the
synergy between MAF and LPS, we believe it is important to demonstrate that the observed effect on the macrophage activation response attributable to preparations containing MAF is not partially
due to a second differentiation signal delivered by contaminating
LPS. Many commercially available reagents used commonly by
investigators contain enough LPS to affect significantly the
results of $\underline{in}$ $\underline{vitro}$ macrophage tumor killing assays (Table VII).
Useful tests that aid in determining if enhancing effects are due
to LPS are outlined in Table VIII.

                                DISCUSSION

These studies confirm the observations that LPS makes macrophages kill tumor cells, and demonstrate that differentiation
signals delivered by MAF and LPS are synergistic. The results
are also consistent with the notion that critical changes in the
composition and/or organization of membrane lipids accompany
macrophage differentiation to the tumoricidal state. Four
lines of experimental evidence suggest that the lipid region of
LPS is responsible for the LPS effect on macrophage tumor cell
killing. First, lipid A produced by acid hydrolysis of phenol-

TABLE V

Effect of Endotoxin or Supernatants from $NaIO_4$-Treated BCG PEC on ^{14}C-Glucosamine Incorporation into Peptone-Normal and BCG PEC

| | | ^{14}C-Glucosamine Incorporation (Stimulation index)[a] | | | |
| | | Peptone-Normal | | | BCG |
Pretreatment[b]	Present Through Assay	Expt 1	Expt 2	Expt 3	Expt 4
PBS	DMM	1.00 ± 0.08[d]	1.00 ± 0.04	1.00 ± 0.08	1.00 ± 0.07
PBS	LPS	1.80 ± 0.03[e]	1.47 ± 0.02[e]	1.98 ± 0.08[e]	1.56 ± 0.18[e]
PBS	MAF	1.15 ± 0.09	1.44 ± 0.02[e]	1.17 ± 0.11	1.46 ± 0.00[e]
PBS	LPS + MAF	4.38 ± 0.08[e]	3.51 ± 0.02[e]	2.35 ± 0.27[e]	2.74 ± 0.14[e]

[a] Stimulation index = experimental value ÷ control value (PBS – DMM).

[b] Pretreatment for 15 mins at 4 C in PBS or 5×10^{-3} $\underline{M}$ $NaIO_4$/PBS.

[c] 10 ng/ml LPS. 10% (v/v) supernatant of $NaIO_4$-treated BCG PEC (MAF).

[d] Stimulation index ± S.E.M. of six replicate samples.

[e] $p < 0.05$ by the paired t test as compared to controls (PBS – DMM).

(From Weinberg and Hibbs, unpublished.)

TABLE VI

Tumor Cell Killing by Peptone-Normal Macrophages Treated
with Endotoxin and/or Supernatants from NaIO$_4$-
Treated BCG PEC

% Supernatant (v/v)[a]	Degree of Tumor Cell Killing			
	0 LPS[b]		5 ng/ml LPS[b]	
	Cell Counting[c]	^{3}HTdR Release[d]	Cell Counting[c]	^{3}HTdR Release[d]
0	0	0.7 + 2.6%	0	1.2 + 1.5%
1.0	0	-0.5 + 1.5%	2+	16.7 + 1.8%
5.0	0	-2.2 + 0.6%	4+	39.9 + 3.8%
25.0	0	-2.1 + 1.0%	4+	49.8 + 4.4%

[a]Present only in 2-hr pretreatment with macrophages.
[b]Present through 60-hr assay after supernatant pretreatment.
[c]Tumor cell killing assessed by visual counting as described in
  footnote b of Table I.
[d]% ^{3}HTdR release + S.E.M. of quadruplicate samples.

(From Weinberg and Hibbs, unpublished)

extracted LPS has the same effect as the parent, intact LPS.
Second, base hydrolysis of LPS, which destroys its mitogenicity
and pyrogenicity (40) by cleavage and saponification of lipid A
ester-linked fatty acids, abolishes the ability of LPS to render
macrophages tumoricidal. Third, polymyxin B, which binds to the
lipid A part of LPS (30) and blocks several of its in vitro and
in vivo effects (23,11), inhibits the effect of LPS on macrophage tumor cell killing. And fourth, when compared with
macrophages from C$_3$H/HeN mice, macrophages from the lipid A-
nonresponder strain C$_3$H/HeJ mice (39,36) are relatively insensitive to the effect of LPS in this tumor cell killing
system. Alexander and Evans (1) were the first to demonstrate
that LPS and lipid A can make washed monolayers of peritoneal
macrophages cytotoxic for tumor cells in vitro.

There appears to be a synergistic effect between LPS and
MAF when they are added to macrophages derived from peritoneal exudates or to colonies of pure macrophages. For
example, if cloned macrophages are pretreated for 2 hrs with
1%-50% MAF, they are not cytotoxic to subsequently added tumor
cells. However, after a 2 hr preincubation with 1-5% MAF,
cloned macrophages become highly tumoricidal when 1-20 ng/ml
LPS are present in the culture medium throughout the cytotoxicity

TABLE VII

Results of Limulus Amebocyte Lysate Assay on Various Reagents[a]

Positive	Negative
Superoxide dismutase	L-histidine HCl
Horseradish peroxidase (Type II and VI)	Dimedone
Catalase (Sigma)	Catalase (Boehringer)
Xanthine oxidase (Grade IV)	Reduced glutathione (Grade IV)
Fetuin (Type I and II)	Sodium periodate
Alpha-1-antitrypsin	Imidazole (Grade III)
Bovine pancreatic inhibitor (Type III)	Dipalmitoylphosphatidylcholine
Ovomucoid (Type II-O)	Phorbol myristate acetate
Soybean trypsin inhibitor (Type I-S)	Tissue culture media powder (Gibco, Flow)
Bovine serum albumin	Dextran sulfate
Neuraminidase (Type VIII)	Fetal bovine serum (Sterile Systems)
Concanavalin A	Adult bovine serum (Sterile Systems)
Hemoglobin (Type IV)	
Porphobilinogen	
Fetal bovine serum (Gibco)	
Fetal bovine serum (Flow)	

[a]L-histidine HCl, dimedone, reduced glutathione, sodium periodate, and imidazole were tested at 5×10^{-3} M. Sera were tested after chloroform extraction. Tissue culture media powder was tested after formulation. All other agents were tested at 1 mg/ml (See Ref. 41 for sources of the reagents tested.)

(Reprinted from the Journal of Immunology, Reference 41, with permission of the publisher.)

TABLE VIII

Effect of Heat and Polymyxin B on MAF- and/or LPS-Induced
Tumor Cell Killing by BCG Macrophages from C_3H/HeN Mice[a]

Pretreatment Additive[c]	Degree of Tumor Cell Killing[b]	
	O PB	25 ug/ml PB[d]
DMM	0	0
MAF	3+	3+
Heated MAF	0	0
LPS	4+	0
Heated LPS	4+	0
MAF + LPS	4+	4+
Heated MAF + LPS	4+	0

[a]3×10^5 peritoneal cells per chamber.
[b]Tumor cell killing assessed by visual counting as described in
  footnote b of Table I.
[c]Macrophages treated at 37 C for 2 hrs with additives and then
  additives removed and macrophages challenged with tumor cells.
  MAF 5%, LPS 100 ng/ml. Heating at 80 C for 10 mins.
[d]Polymyxin B present in 2 hr pretreatment only.

(Reprinted from the Journal of Immunology, Ref. 41, with permission of the publisher.)

assay. When this combination is used, the cloned macrophages appear to become truly tumoricidal because no tumor target cells can
be found within the macrophage colonies. The synergistic effect
between MAF and LPS occurs when macrophages are pretreated with
MAF and then subsequently exposed to LPS or when MAF and LPS
are added concurrently to macrophages. If macrophages are
sequentially treated with LPS and then with MAF the marked synergistic effect is not noted. Time lapse cinematography has been
used to show that tumoricidal cloned macrophages lyse tumor target
cells (38). Others have also demonstrated tumor cell killing by
macrophage colonies (28), but this was specific killing by bone
marrow-derived macrophage colonies induced by a specific "macrophage cytotoxic factor," as opposed to the nonspecific killing
by peritoneal macrophage colonies induced by LPS or LPS and
MAF (41).

Freshly explanted normal resident peritoneal macrophages do
not reproducibly respond to LPS or MAF by differentiation to the
tumoricidal state (21,41). However, this relatively refractory

state is lost as macrophages begin to undergo an activation response. As macrophages differentiate toward the tumoricidal stage,
they exhibit a progressively lower threshold as determined by the
observation that less LPS is needed for eliciting a tumoricidal
response (41) (see Fig. 2). Indeed, it appears that differentiation
of macrophage monolayers toward the tumoricidal state parallels
their responsiveness to LPS in an inverse manner and that the
amount of LPS required to make them tumoricidal is a good index
of the level of activation existing prior to LPS exposure. In
our experience MAF-rich PEC supernatants generally induce in vitro
differentiation of stimulated macrophages or cloned macrophages
to the nontumoricidal activated rather than the tumoricidal
activated level (41). After MAF-rich lymphocyte supernatant
pretreatment of stimulated macrophage monolayers, the addition
of small amounts of LPS (1-10 ng/ml) makes these nontumoricidal
MAF-pretreated macrophages tumoricidal. This shows that MAF can
markedly lower the threshold for response to LPS without causing
macrophages to kill tumor cells in the absence of LPS. To
summarize at this point, qualitative changes in macrophage
physiology incurred in vitro during an inflammatory response --
acquisition of the stimulated differentiation state -- appears to
be a prerequisite for effective macrophage differentiation to the
tumoricidal state in response to LPS. Further changes in macrophage physiology are produced by exposure of stimulated macrophages or cloned macrophages -- which respond to differentiation
signals in a manner similar to stimulated macrophages -- to MAF
in vitro. MAF pretreatment markedly decreases the amount of
subsequently added LPS needed to induce macrophage differentiation to the tumoricidal stage (Fig. 3 and Table VI) which suggests
that membrane changes induced by MAF markedly increases the
sensitivity of macrophages to the second differentiation signal
delivered by LPS.

     During the past several years we have been attempting to
understand how environmental factors modulate the activation response at the level of macrophage membranes. It is our working
hypothesis that factors that regulate the macrophage activation
response ultimately influence the composition and/or organization
of membrane lipids (6,7,22). The association of certain classes
of phospholipids with membrane-bound enzymes, the ratio of un-
saturated to saturated fatty acids, and the cholesterol content and
distribution within membranes could be critical determinants of
macrophage membrane function. Similar dynamics underlying interactions between membrane lipids and proteins may be the basis for
the mechanism of lowering the macrophage tumoricidal threshold by
LPS. LPS has an affinity for membranes, and studies from several
laboratories suggest that stable LPS-cell membrane complexes are
formed via lipid-lipid hydrophobic interactions between lipid A
and membrane lipids (16,9,3,35,24). Furthermore, the recently
reported studied of Davies et al. (43) suggest that the binding of

the lipid A portion of LPS to the plasma membrane of peritoneal macrophages induces dynamic changes in plasma membrane organization. These cell surface changes appear to be triggered by a stable lipid A-membrane lipid association. Likewise, a lipid A-membrane lipid association producing biochemical-physiochemical changes in membrane organization could trigger a pleiotypic macrophage differentiation response that includes a lowering of the tumoricidal threshold.

In experiments described here we have shown that pure populations of cloned macrophages respond directly to a signal delivered by LPS by differentiating to the tumoricidal state. Ralph and his colleagues (31), also using a pure population of macrophages, demonstrated that LPS exposure of a macrophage cell line inhibited proliferation and induced secretion of colony stimulating activity. Taken together, these studies show that LPS can directly induce differentiation of macrophages. In our studies as well as those of Ralph et al. (31), lipid A produced responses identical to those of the intact LPS molecule. This suggests that the lipid A portion of LPS through hydrophobic interaction with macrophage membrane lipids could induce expression of differentiated functional responses. Our observations, described above, that less LPS or lipid A is required to induce macrophage differentiation to the tumoricidal state as macrophages progress along the differentiation continuum may suggest that sequential changes in macrophage membrane lipids are occurring as the differentiation process proceeds. Our speculation is that physiologic inducers of the macrophage activation response such as MAF cause an alteration in the composition and/or organization of membrane lipids that make macrophages more responsive to LPS or lipid A.

Clues to how LPS interacts with mammalian membranes may be found in experiments by Rothfield et al. (33). These workers studied the interaction of LPS and catalytic proteins from bacteria with phospholipid monolayers. Their results provide evidence that LPS and protein can each influence the activity of the other within a monolayer of phospholipid. For example, catalytically active proteins interact differently with a mixed LPS-phospholipid monolayer than with a monolayer composed solely of phospholipid. There is a marked difference in the surface potential when the protein interacts with the monolayer of pure phospholipid, while only a minor change occurs with the LPS-phospholipid monolayer. This suggests that protein interacts differently with phospholipid in the presence of LPS. In addition, the interaction of a small number of protein molecules with the pure phospholipid monolayer prevented subsequent penetration of LPS into the monolayer, while LPS continued to penetrate when a similar amount of protein was placed in a mixed LPS-phospholipid monolayer. These findings suggest that protein conformation may differ in the two situations and that LPS may have a dramatic influence on the interaction between phospholipids and a catalytically active protein. Mammalian membranes are a mosaic of many different lipids, and the lipid composition and physical state of various membrane regions may differ, i.e., domains of phase-separated and topographically organized lipids may exist within the membrane. It is possible that LPS interacting with the local lipid environment could influence phase separations within membranes as well as the conformational state and hence catalytic or receptor function of proteins within mammalian membranes.

Other studies from our laboratory provide evidence that expression of the activated macrophage nonspecific tumoricidal reaction may require acquisition of critical organization of macrophage membrane components including lipids. For example, the tumoricidal threshold of spontaneously tumoricidal activated macrophages is lowered to the nontumoricidal activated level by exposure to low density lipoprotein or cholesterol-rich liposomes (6). Likewise, when nontumoricidal activated macrophages are incubated for 2 hrs with low density lipoproteins or cholesterol-rich liposomes either before or while being incubated with either LPS (10-100 ng/ml), the 40,000-90,000 dalton serum factor, FBS, or MAF, the ability of these enhancing factors to induce differentiation to the tumoricidal activated stage is prevented. However, subsequent addition of LPS (5-10 ng/ml), the 40,000-90,000 dalton serum factor(s), or MAF during the 60 hr cytotoxicity assay fully restores the tumoricidal activity (6).(Chapman and Hibbs, unpublished observation). Thus, the enhancing effect of LPS, the 40,000-90,000 dalton serum factor(s), or MAF as well as the inhibitory effect of plasma lipoproteins and cholesterol-rich liposomes are reversible. Additional evidence for the possible importance of a critical composition and/or organization of membrane lipids in the response of macrophages to differentiation signals is demonstrated by our studies with the cholesterol binding polyene antibiotic Amphotericin B (7). Amphotericin B., like the 40,000-90,000 dalton serum factor, is capable of eliciting differentiation to the tumoricidal activated stage only if macrophage differentiation has previously progressed to the nontumoricidal activated stage either in vivo or by prior exposure to MAF in vitro. Since Amphotericin B binds to membrane cholesterol, we believe this is further evidence for the importance of membrane lipids in modulating macrophage differentiation in response to environmental signals. Taken together, these results demonstrate that the threshold for tumor cell killing, even at the highly differentiated nontumoricidal and tumoricidal activated stages, may be modulated by differentiation signals that are influenced by and in turn influence the organization -- including that of lipids -- of macrophage membranes. This suggests that the pleiotypic differentiation of macrophages induced by LPS or lipid A may have a similar genesis in hydrophobic interactions within membranes.

ACKNOWLEDGMENTS

This work was supported by the Veterans Administration (Washington, D. C.) and by the National Institutes of Health, (Bethesda, MD) Grants CA 14045 and CA 15811. We thank J. E. Brisbay, R. Christensen, M. W. Howlett, M. S. Knowlton, T. M. Sedlar, R. R. Taintor, Z. Vavrin, and C. Henderson for technical assistance during the course of studies reviewed here.

REFERENCES

1. Alexander, P. and Evans, R.   Nature New Biol. 232 (1971) 76.
2. Baughn, R. E. and Bonventre, P. F.   Inf. and Immun. 11 (1975) 313.
3. Benedetto, D. A., Shands, J. W. and Shah, D. O.   Biochim. et Biophys. Acta 298 (1973) 145.
4. Bressler, J., Krzych, U. and Thurman, G.   Fed. Proc. 35 (1976) 389.
5. Butler, T., Smith, E., Hammarstrom, L. and Moller, G.   Inf. and Immun. 16 (1977) 449.
6. Chapman, H. A., Jr. and Hibbs, J. B., Jr.   Science 197 (1977) 282.
7. Chapman, H. A., Jr. and Hibbs, J. B., Jr.   Proc. of Nat. Acad. of Scies. USA in press.
8. Chedid, L., Parant, M., Damais, C., Parant, R., Juy, D. and Galelli, A.   Inf. and Immun. 13 (1976) 722.
9. Ciznar, I. and Shands, J. W.   Infec. and Immun. 4 (1971) 362.
10. Cooper, J. F., Levin, J. and Wagner, H. N., Jr.   J. of Lab. and Clin. Med. 78 (1971) 138.
11. Corrigan, J. J., Jr. and Bell, B. M.   Infec. and Immun. 4 (1971) 563.
12. David, J. R. and Becker, E. L.   Europ. J. of Immunol. 4 (1974) 281.
13. Davies, M., Stewart-Tull, D. E. S. and Jackson, D. M.   Tiochim. et Biophys. Acta 508 (1978) 260.
14. Galanos, C., Luderitz, O. and Westphal, O.   Europ. J. of Biochem. 24 (1971) 116.
15. Glode, L. M., Jacques, A., Mergenhagen, S. E. and Rosenstreich, D. L.   J. of Immunol. 119 (1977) 162.
16. Hammerling, V. and Westphal, O.   Europ. J. of Biochem. 1 (1967) 46.
17. Hammond, M. E. and Dvorak, H. F.   J. of Exp. Med. 136 (1972) 1518.
18. Hammond, M. E., Selvaggio, S. S. and Dvorak, H. F.   J. of Immunol. 115 (1975) 914.
19. Handwerger, B. S. and Schwartz, R. H.   Transpl. 18 (1974) 544.
20. Hammerling, V. and Westphal, O., Europ. J. of Biochem. 1 (1967) 46.

21. Hibbs, J. B., Jr., Taintor, R. R., Chapman, H. A., Jr. and Weinberg, J. B. Science 197 (1977) 279.
22. Hibbs, J. B., Jr., Chapman, H. A., Jr. and Weinberg, J. B. J. of the Reticuloendothel. Soc. in press.
23. Jacobs, D. M. and Morrison, D. C. J. of Immunol. 118 (1977) 21.
24. Kabir, S. and Rosenstreich, D. L. Infec. and Immun. 15 (1977) 156.
25. Kuhner, A. L. and David, J. R. J. Immunol. 116 (1976) 140.
26. Landolfo, S., Herberman, R. B. and Holden, H. T., J. Immunol. 118 (1977) 1244.
27. Loughman, B. E., Farrar, J. J. and Nordin, A. A. J. Immunol. 112 (1974) 430.
28. Meerpohl, H. G., Lohmann-Matthes, M. L. and Fischer, H. Europ. J. Immunol. 6 (1976) 213.
29. Meltzer, M. S., Tucker, R. W., Sanford, K. K. and Leonard, E. J. J. Nat. Canc. Inst. 54 (1975) 1177.
30. Morrison, D. C. and Jacobs, D. M. Immunochem. 13 (1976) 813.
31. Ralph, P., Broxmeyer, H. E. and Nakoing, I. J. Exp. Med. 146 (1977) 611.
32. Rifkind, D. and Palmer, J. D. J. Bacteriol. 92 (1966) 815.
33. Rothfield, L., Romeo, D. and Hinckley, A. Fed. Proc. 31 (1972) 12.
34. Russell, S. W., Doe, W. F. and McIntosh, A. T. J. Exp. Med. 146 (1977) 1511
35. Shands, J. W., Jr. J. Infec. Dis. 128 Supplement 1 (1973) 189.
36. Skidmore, B. J., Chiller, J. M. and Weigle, W. O. J. Immunol. 118 (1977) 274.
37. Stewart, C. C., Lin, H. and Adles, C. J. Exper. Med. 141 (1975) 1114.
38. Stewart, C. C., Adles, C. and Hibbs, J. B., Jr. J. Reticuloendothel. Soc. 24 (1978) 106.
39. Sultzer, B. M. Nature 219 (1968) 1253.
40. Tripodi, D. and Nowotny, A. Ann. N. Y. Acad. Scies. USA 133 (1966) 604.
41. Weinberg, J. B., Chapman, H. A., Jr. and Hibbs, J. B., Jr. J. Immunol. 121 (1978) 72.
42. Weinberg, J. B. and Hibbs, J. B., Jr. submitted for publication.
43. Westphal, O., Luderitz, O. and Bister, F. Zeitschrift fur Naturforsch. 7b (1952) 148.
44. Wilson, J. M., Rosenstreich, D. L. and Oppenheim, J. J. J. Immunol. 114 (1975) 388.
45. Yoshida, T., Sonozaki, H. and Cohen, S. J. Exper. Med. 138 (1973) 784.

STUDIES ON THE ENDOTOXIN INDUCED TUMOR RESISTANCE

A. NOWOTNY and R. C. BUTLER

University of Pennsylvania and
Albert Einstein Medical Center
Philadelphia, Pennsylvania   (USA)

Bacterial endotoxin have been demonstrated to produce a variety of antitumor effects including the enhancement of non-specific resistance to tumors (2,10,16,23) and the hemorrhage and necrosis of solid subcutaneous tumors (15,18). Our laboratories originally reported in 1972 that the pretreatment of mice with endotoxin enhanced the level of nonspecific resistance to challenge with the TA3-Ha murine ascites tumor (10). More recently, we demonstrated that the antitumor effects of LPS in the enhancement of tumor resistance and in tumor hemorrhage could be mediated by soluble factors released into the serum following endotoxin treatment (3,3). The study we are reporting here was designed to further explore the immunologic mechanisms involved in the enhancement of resistance to this tumor. This includes an evaluation of the roles of different immunologic cell types and of some of the immunomodulatory factors produced in response to endotoxin.

MATERIALS AND METHODS

Mice. Young adult female mice were used exclusively. Strain A/J and C3H/HeJ mice were obtained from R. B. Jackson Memorial Laboratories, (Bar Harbor, ME). ICR and C57B1/6J mice were purchased from the Skin and Cancer Hospital, Temple Univ. (Philadelphia, PA). Balb/c nu/nu mice were provided for these studies by generous donation of Dr. Chungming Chang, National Cancer Institute, (Bethesda, MD). Mice were housed in groups of 10 and fed ad libitum with Purina mouse chow.

Tumors. The nonspecific TA3-Ha ascites tumor was originally isolated as a spontaneous mammary adenocarcinoma and was provided

455

by Dr. S. Friberg, Karolinska Institute, (Stockholm, Sweden). The tumor was subsequently maintained by serial passage through female A/J mice. The transplantable Sarcoma 37 tumor was originally isolated as a spontaneous lymphosarcoma in C3H mice by Gardner. It was maintained as an ascites tumor in female ICR mice.

Endotoxins. Lipopolysaccharides (LPS) were obtained from Serratia marcescens 08 by trichloroacetic acid extraction and from Salmonella minnesota S1114 and Salmonella minnesota R5 by the phenol/water procedure. Endotoxic glycolipids were isolated from rough mutants of Salmonella minnesota R595, Salmonella typhimurium 1102, Escherichia coli D31m4, and E. coli D21f2 by chloroform/ methanol extraction, as described previously (7). Polysaccharide-rich preparations (PS) were obtained from Serratia marcescens 08 endotoxin by hydrolysis with 1 M HCl at 100 C for 30 min, as described elsewhere (14).

Tumor protection assay. The tumor protection assay was designed to be an approximate measure of the degree of resistance of a mouse to a given tumor challenge dose as evidenced by the ability to survive tumor-associated mortality. The general format for enhancing tumor resistance (TUR) was to inject an agent such as LPS i.p. one day prior to i.p. challenge with viable TA3-Ha cells. The number of viable tumor cells in the challenge dose is indicated for each experiment (23).

Tumor hemorrhage assay. Sarcoma 37 tumor was harvested from the ascites form and washed with sterile saline. Female ICR mice were injected subcutaneously with 0.1 ml of a 1:1 dilution of packed Sarcoma 37 cells. Seven days later when the tumors were approximately 0.7 to 1.0 cm in diameter the mice were treated with an i.v. injection of LPS or post-endotoxin serum. Twenty-four hours after treatment the tumors were observed for hemorrhage extending over at least 25-50% of the tumor surface. This visual evaluation was confirmed by autopsy, after 48 hr.

Preparation of spleen cells. Mice were pretreated with 25 µg S. marcescens LPS i.v. 24 hr prior to the harvesting of spleens. Single cell suspensions of normal or LPS pretreated splenocytes were prepared in Eagle's MEM (GIBCO) supplemented with 10% fetal calf serum and antibiotics. Nonadherent spleen cell suspensions were prepared by incubation of whole spleen cell suspensions at 37 C for 1 hr in a Falcon plastic tissue culture flask. After 1 hr the non-adherent cells were gently resuspended and decanted into another flask for a second 1 hr incubation period. This process was repeated for a total of 3 one hr periods.

Treatment with carrageenan. Carrageenan Seakem 9 from Marine Colloids, Inc., (Rockland, ME.) was suspended in 0.9% sterile saline and sonicated at high power with a Branson Sonifier

to make a fine dispersion. Mice received i.p. injections of 3 mg
carrageenan on days -4, -1 and +1 with respect to the day of tumor
challenge.

Infection with BCG. Bacillus Calmette-Guerin (BCG) vaccine
was obtained from the University of Illinois Medical Center. For
injection the lyophylized BCG was reconstituted with 1 ml sterile
water and injected i.p. into mice at a dose of approximately 2 x
10^6 viable BCG.

Preparation of post-endotoxin serum. Post-endotoxin serum
was prepared by collecting blood 2 hr after i.p. injection of 20
µg of either LPS or PS. Some post-endotoxin sera were obtained
from mice which had been preinfected with BCG 18 days before
stimulation with either LPS or PS.

Determination of CSF levels. The CSF content of the post-
endotoxin sera was determined by the bone marrow colony formation
assay in semisolid agar by the method described by Bradley and
Metcalf (1).

Measurement of endotoxin levels. The level of residual endo-
toxin-treated splenocytes was estimated by the Limulus lysate
assay as described by Levin et al. (12). The endotoxin content
of different endotoxic preparations was measured by the chick
embryo lethality assay. Intravenous injection of endotoxin into
11-day-old chick embryos was carried out by the method of Smith
and Thomas (19).

RESULTS

Enhancement of tumor resistance by LPS. Pretreatment of mice
with Serratia marcescens LPS i.p. one day before challenge with
approximately 3 TD_{50} of TA3-Ha cells i.p. significantly enhanced
the rate of survival from tumor related mortality. As shown in
Table I, LPS enhanced tumor resistance (TUR) over a dose range of
1 to 50 µg.

Table II demonstrates that prophylactic pretreatment with
either single or repeated doses of LPS was much more effective
than treatment which began one day after implantation of the
tumor i.p. However, repeated post-treatment with LPS did produce
a moderate therapeutic effect in enhancing rejection of the tumor.

The route of injection of the LPS was important. As Table
III shows, systemic pretreatment with LPS administered i.v. was
much less effective than the local i.p. injection if the tumor
was given in the same anatomical location (23).

TABLE I

Endotoxin Dose-Response Curve

Pretreatment	% Survival[a]	P	CSF Titer (cfu/10^5 cells)
None	0		75
0.1 µg S. marcescens LPS	20		90
1 µg LPS	90	<.001	168
10 µg LPS	80	<.001	197
25 µg LPS	70	<.005	244
50 µg LPS	80	<.001	
100 µg LPS	40		

[a]Mice were challenged with 200 viable TA3-Ha cells i.p. on day 0.

TABLE II

Effect of Repeated Administration of LPS

µg LPS/Dose	Days of Administration	% Survival[a]	P
None		10	
20 µg	-1	75	<.001
20 µg	-5,-4,-3,-2,-1	85	<.001
20 µg	+1,+3,+5,+7,+9	45	<.005

[a]Mice were challenged with 2000 TA3-Ha cells i.p. on day 0.

TABLE III

Systemic Versus Local Stimulation
of Tumor Protection by LPS

Pretreatment (day - 1)	Route	% Survival[a]	P
None		0	
10 µg S. marcescens LPS	i.v.	20	<.05
10 µg S. marcescens LPS	i.p.	55	<.005

[a]Mice were challenged with 2000 TA3-Ha cells on day 0.

To determine whether the enhanced tumor resistance by endotoxic bacterial preparations was really due to the LPS molecule
as opposed to contaminants such as bacterial nucleic acid or protein, preparations from sequential steps in the purification of
LPS were assayed for both endotoxicity and antitumor activity.
As shown in Table IV, preparations with the highest endotoxicity
were consistently the most active in TUR, whereas the preparations
with low endotoxicity had little effect on survival.

TABLE IV

Comparison of Phenol.Water and TCA Extracts of
S. marcescens LPS -- Stages of Purification

Endotoxin Fraction[a]	Chick Embryo LD$_{50}$	CSF Titer	% Sur- vival[b]
Saline		31	0
TCA Extract (Crude)	0.25 µg	146	40
TCA, MeOH ppt.	0.40 µg	111	30
TCA, MeOH supn.	1 µg	51	0
TCA, MeOH ppt., UC ppt.	0.01 µg	105	50
TCA, MeOH ppt., UC supn.	0.33 µg	89	20
Phenol/Water Extract (Crude)	0.15 µg		40
P/W, MeOH ppt.	0.017 µg		50
P/W, MeOH supn.	0.60 µg		30
P/W, MeOH ppt., UC ppt.	0.032 µg		40
P/W, MeOH ppt., UC supn.	0.58 µg		0

[a]Endotoxins were prepared and purified as described by Nowotny (7).
[b]Mice were challenged with 120 TA3-Ha cells i.p. on day 0.

Supporting the role of the LPS molecule in the antitumor
effects of endotoxic preparations was the observation that endotoxin treatment did not affect the rate of survival of LPS-non-
responder C3H/HeJ mice as shown in Table V.

A variety of different smooth endotoxins and rough endotoxic
glycolipids were tested for the ability to stimulate enhanced
TUR and CSF production, as shown in Table VI. While complete LPS
from several smooth strains of S. minnesota and E. coli were consistently active in producing both of these effects, the glycolipids of rough Re strains were divided. Some glycolipids, such
as E. coli D31m4, D21f2 and F515, were more active than whole E.
coli LPS. In contrast, the S. minnesota R5, R7, and R595 glyco-

lipids displayed decreasing activity with decreasing polysaccharide chain length. S. typhimurium 1102 GL was endotoxic but was
completely inactive in TUR and CSF stimulation.

TABLE V

Endotoxin Does Not Protect C3H/HeJ Mice from Tumor

Pretreatment (Day - 1)	Challenge Dose	% Survival
None	500 TA3-Ha	70
25 μg S. marcescens LPS	500 TA3-Ha	70
None	1000 TA3-Ha	27
25 μg S. marcescens LPS	1000 TA3-Ha	32

TABLE VI

Tumor Protection by Smooth and Rough Endotoxins

Pretreatment (25 g on day -1)	% Survival[a]	P	CSF Stimulation Index
None	5		1.0
S. minnesota S1114	67	< .001	4.5
S. minnesota R5	60	< .005	3.6
S. minnesota R7	40	< .025	1.3
S. minnesota R595	27		1.0
None	12		1.0
E. coli 08 LPS	36	< .025	
E. coli 0111 LPS	40	< .025	
E. coli K12 LPS	30		2.4
E. coli D21fs GL	56	< .001	3.1
E. coli D31m4 GL	66	< .001	2.7
E. coli F515	64	< .001	
S. typhimurium 1102 GL	8		1.0

[a]Mice were challenged with 2000 TA3-Ha cells i.p. on day 0.

The nontoxic PS fraction produced by acid hydrolysis of LPS produced only a slight enhancement of TUR when given to normal mice, as shown in Table VII. However, BCG preinfected mice were much more responsive to the effects of PS and this combined treatment with both BCG and PS produced an enhancement of TUR above the level of either agent alone.

TABLE VII

Effect of BCG Infection Followed by Treatment
with LPS or PS on Resistance to Tumor

Treatment (days -4, -3, -2, -1, 0)	% Survival[a]	p vs. saline	p vs. BCG
None	12		
25 µg _S. marcescens_ LPS	65	< .001	
25 µg _S. marcescens_ PS	10		
25 µg _E. coli_ PS	35	< .05	
25 µg _S. typhimurium_ PS	20		
BCG preinfected (-18 days)	50	< .005	
BCG + 25 g LPS	91	< .001	< .025
BCG + 25 g _S. marcescens_ PS	70	< .001	
BCG + 25 g _E. coli_ PS	90	< .001	< .01

[a]Mice were challenged with 3000 TA3-Ha cells i.p. on day 0.

Cell types involved in TUR. The endotoxin induced enhancement of resistance was transferrable by splenocytes from pretreated donors. Table VIII shows that the adoptive transfer of 1×10^7 splenocytes from LPS pretreated donors to syngeneic recipient mice transferred a significant degree of tumor resistance. The transfer of untreated normal splenocytes produced no antitumor effect. Furthermore, when the adherent cell population was removed from the LPS-primed splenocytes prior to adoptive transfer, the resultant lymphocyte-rich nonadherent cell population was still capable of producing enhanced resistance.

Table IX demonstrates that LPS could enhance TUR in the complete absence of T-cell activity. Athymic BALB/c nu/nu nude mice which were pretreated with LPS showed an elevated level of tumor rejection.

TABLE VIII

Adoptive Transfer of Tumor Protection
by LPS-Treated Splenocytes

Species	Treatment of Transferred Cells	No. of Cells	% Survival	P
C57B1/6J		None	10^b	
"	Normal Spleen Cells	10^7	0	
"	LPS-Treated Spleen Cells[a]	10^7	45	< .025
"	Normal Nonadhering Spleen Cells	10^7	10	
"	LPS-Treated Nonadhering Cells	10^7	35	< .05
ICR		None	0^c	
"	Normal Nonadhering Spleen Cells	10^7	10	
"	LPS-Treated Nonadhering Cells	10^7	50	< .05

[a]Donor mice were injected i.v. with 25 µg S. marcescens LPS one
day before spleen cell transfer (.001 µg residual LPS/10 cells).
[b]Mice were challenged with 7×10^4 TA3-Ha cells i.p.
[c]Mice were challenged with 2000 TA3-Ha cells i.p.

TABLE IX

Endotoxin Induces Tumor Protection
in Athymic BALB/c nu/nu Mice

Pretreatment (-1 hr)	Challenge Dose	% Survival	P
None	500 TA3-Ha	10	
10 µg S. marcescens LPS	500 TA3-Ha	70	< .005

In the experiment shown in Table X, mice were pretreated
with carrageenan i.p. to produce a depletion of phagocytic cells
in the peritoneal cavity. This treatment abolished the ability
of LPS to stimulate tumor resistance above normal control levels.

Soluble factors involved in antitumor effects of endotoxin.
The role of soluble serum factors in the antitumor effects of
LPS were studied by the transfer of 2 hr post-endotoxin serum

from LPS treated donor mice. These sera contained virtually no
residual endotoxicity (.001 µg/ml by the Limulus lysate assay).

TABLE X

Effect of Carrageenan on Endotoxin Protection from Tumor

Treatment	% Survival[a]	p vs. Saline
Saline	30	
25 µg E. coli D31m4 GL (Day -1)	63	< .01
3 mg Carrageenan (Days -4, -1, +1)	13	
Carrageenan + E. coli D31m4	33	

[a]Mice were challenged with 2000 TA3-Ha cells i.p. on day 0.

Treatment with post-endotoxin serum induced a moderate enhancement of resistance to tumor as shown in Table XI. Post-PS sera
were similarly capable of stimulating enhanced resistance. The
preinfection of serum donors with viable BCG enhanced the subsequent ability of mice to release resistance-stimulating factors
in response to LPS or PS. Myeloid colony stimulating factor (CSF)
was detectable in both post-LPS and post-PS sera. The quantities
of CSF in the various sera were roughly proportional to the resistance enhancing capacity of each serum preparation.

These same post-LPS and post-PS sera also contained factors
responsible for mediating a second antitumor effect of LPS - the
hemorrhage and necrosis of solid subcutaneous Sarcoma 37 tumors
following i.v. injection of the sera. As shown in Table XII, the
preinfection of serum donors with BCG also enhanced the producor
PS.

DISCUSSION

In agreement with numerous reports in the literature we have
observed that endotoxin produces antitumor activity in two different systems -- the enhancement of nonspecific resistance to the
Ta3-Ha ascites tumor (2,10,16,23) and the hemorrhage and necrosis
of solid subcutaneous Sarcoma 37 tumors (15,18). In studying the
optimal conditions for the enhancement of tumor resistance (TUR)
by endotoxin, we found that S. marcescens LPS was effective over
a dose range of 1 to 50 µg when administered one day before tumor
challenge. Repeated pretreatment with LPS slightly enhanced the

TABLE XI

Post-Endotoxin Serum Enhances Resistance to Tumor

Treatment (0.5 ml i.v.)	% Survival	P	CSF Stimulation Index
Saline	33		1.0
Normal Serum	40		1.6
Post-LPS Serum[a]	75	< .01	8.7
Post-PS Serum	66	< .01	7.7
BCG Serum, Post-LPS[b]	100	< .001	15.6
BCG Serum, Post-PS	95	< .001	14.4
BCG Serum[c]	50		3.0

[a]Post-LPS and post-PS sera were collected 2 hr after i.p. injection of either LPS or PS from Serratia marcescens.
[b]Post-LPS and post-PS sera were collected from mice that had been infected with 2 x 10[7] BCG i.p. 18 days before treatment with LPS of PS.
[c]BCG serum was collected from mice 18 days after infection with 2 x 10[7] BCG.

TABLE XII

Sarcoma 37 Tumor Hemorrhage by Post-Endotoxin Sera

Treatment (0.5 ml i.v.)	% Tumors Hemorrhaged	P
Saline	9	
Normal Serum	12	
Post-LPS Serum	36	< .01
Post-PS Serum	45	< .005
BCG Serum, Post-LPS	67	< .005
BCG Serum, Post-PS	76	< .001
BCG Serum	28	
20 μg LPS	70	< .005

protective effect. However, even a single prophylactic treatment with LPS was much more effective than repeated therapeutic LPS treatments beginning one day after tumor implantation.

In agreement with the observations of Parr et al. (16) using a different tumor model, the local stimulation of the immune system by injection of LPS i.p. in the same site as the subsequent tumor challenge was significantly more active in enhancing TUR than systemic i.v. treatment which did, however, provide a slight degree of protection.

Crude endotoxin preparations are heterogeneous in that they contain not only LPS but also measurable amounts of nucleic acid and protein. By examining sequential steps in the process of purification of crude TCA or phenol/water extracted endotoxin preparations, we found that both the ability to induce the release of CSF and the ability to enhance TUR were linked most strongly to the endotoxic fractions. In contrast, preparations such as the methanol soluble supernatants which contain a large proportion of the contaminants had little activity in either of these effects.

Additional support for the activity of the LPS molecule as opposed to contaminants was the observation that endotoxin treatment did not stimulate TUR in C3H/HeJ mice. Many previous reports demonstrated that this strain of mouse is specifically deficient in its capacity to respond immunologically to the LPS molecule (8,21).

One of the common misconceptions in endotoxin literature is that the lipid moiety (Lipid A) is the same for all endotoxins. We have previously reported that a variety of heptoseless rough mutant (RE) endotoxic glycolipids could be differentiated both on the basis of chemical structure and also in the biological effectiveness of the lipid moiety (13). In the present report these Re glycolipids were evaluated for the ability to enhance TUR and to stimulate CSF release. Three different E. coli Re glycolipids were each highly active in stimulating both of these biological effects. In contrast, the Re glycolipids from S. minnesota R595 and S. typhimurium 1102 were inactive in both assays. In view of these results one cannot assume that all lipid moieties represent a single molecular species.

In the comparison of different S. Minnesota endotoxin structural mutants ranging from whole LPS through the R5 (Rc) and R7 (Rd) mutants to the heptoseless R595 GL, it was observed that the effectiveness in enhancing TUR and CSF decreased with decreasing polysaccharide chain length. This suggested that one or more of the active sites for the induction of these biological effects may reside in the polysaccharide portion of the LPS molecule in

this species of endotoxin. Consistent with this hypothesis, lipid-
free nontoxid PS preparations derived from certain strains of LPS
could provide a marginal but significant resistance to the TA3-Ha
tumor. These PS preparations were also active in CSF induction.
It was very interesting to note that the preinfection of mice
with BCG induced a strong response to subsequent stimulation with
either LPS or PS.

In initial steps towards determining the immunologic mechanism
involved in the enhancement of TUR by LPS we attempted to passively
transfer this nonspecific resistance from endotoxin treated donor
mice. The i.p. administration of 10^7 endotoxin pretreated spleen
cells to tumor recipients transferred a significant degree of
antitumor activity (23). Furthermore, if the transferred endotoxin
treated spleen cell suspensions were depleted of adhering cells
such as macrophages, the resultant nonadhering cell population
could still transfer some resistance. The adherence procedure
utilized has been demonstrated to remove more than 99% of the
phagocytic cells from a cell suspension (9). Therefore, it is
apparent that the transfer of TUR is not solely due to the transfer
of activated macrophages, but rather, that an activated lymphocyte
population may be responsible for transferring the resistance.

There is evidence that macrophages also play a role in TUR.
Treatment of mice with carrageenan prior to treatment with endotoxin prevented an increase in resistance over the level of saline
treated controls. A variety of studies have indicated that carrageenan is specifically cytotoxic to macrophages (11,17). Since
carrageenan can specifically deplete the macrophage population in
vivo, it would appear that macrophages play an essential role in
this mechanism of tumor resistance.

Since it was observed that macrophage depleted cell suspensions could transfer nonspecific resistance, lymphocytes are probably involved in the resistance mechanism. However, in these
studies T cells played no essential role in the endotoxin-induced
enhancement of TUR as demonstrated by the protection of athymic
BALB/c nu/nu nude mice from tumor by endotoxin. In contrast, there
is some circumstantial evidence indicating a role for the B cell
based upon the lack of response of C3H/HeJ mice. Coutinho (8)
demonstrated that the lack of responsiveness of C3H/HeJ mice to
endotoxin was due to a specific defect in the B cell rather than
to any defect in the response capacity of either macrophages or T
cells.

There is some indirect support for an immunologic model involving interaction between B cells and macrophages in the response
to endotoxin. Wilton et al. (22) found that cultured macrophages
could only be activated by LPS if B cells were added to the cultures.
The addition of T cells had no effect. In addition, cell-free

supernatants from endotoxin-stimulated B cells, but not from T
cells, could stimulate the macrophages. Therefore, endotoxin
could only stimulate B cells to release macrophage activating factors (MAF), which is very similar if not identical with macrophage
migration inhibitory factor (20).

One cannot exclude another possibility, namely that the endotoxin activated macrophages release B cell activating components.
If this macrophage activation occurs in in vivo, as it is the case
if we take endotoxin pretreated donor spleen cells, all the B cells
we obtained are already activated. Therefore, they may not require
the simultaneous transfer of macrophages for adoptive TUR. If
carrageenan treatment depletes macrophages in vivo, subsequent
endotoxin injection will not produce active B cells. Therefore,
adoptive transfer of TUR by spleen cells will not be possible. The
results reported here support this latter possibility.

We have, in fact, demonstrated that endotoxin-induced soluble factors are capable of mediating the antitumor effects of endotoxin. This role of soluble factors in TUR has been recently discussed in detail by Butler et al. (3,5). Briefly, we found that
post-endotoxin serum, containing negligible residual LPS, could
transfer nonspecific resistance. Post-PS serum also contained
factors capable of mediating this effect. The preinfection of
serum donors with BCG primed the donor mice to produce more highly
active serum in response to LPS or its nontoxic PS component. One
lymphokine which is released into the serum in response to both LPS
and PS is CSF which can stimulate the proliferation of monocyte
and granulocyte precursors in vivo (20). There was a consistent
relationship between the induction of high CSF levels and the induction of strong resistance to tumor which suggests a possible
role for CSF or CSF-like components in endotoxin-induced TUR (3).

In addition, these post-endotoxin sera also contained tumor
necrotizing factor (TNF) which was originally described by Carswell
et al. (6). As with TUR, post-endotoxin serum from BCG infected
mice was more potent in producing tumor hemorrhage than the serum
from uninfected donors. Perhaps the most significant new finding
of this particular study was that the nontoxic PS was as effective
as whole LPS in stimulating the release of TNF.

From these studies it appears that post-endotoxin serum may
contain a wide variety of factors responsible for a variety of
effects of LPS. We have recently reported that these sera also
contain factors capable of enhancing the in vitro antibody
response to SRBC by mouse splenocytes (4). These factors in the
post-endotoxin sera may play the most important role in the endotoxin-induced immune enhancement.

SUMMARY

In summary, this report has discussed the immunologic mechanisms involved in the enhancement of nonspecific resistance to tumor by endotoxin. The optimal conditions for tumor protection involved pretreatment with approximately 25 µg LPS administered at the site of subsequent tumor challenge. In an attempt to relate endotoxin structural components to the ability to enhance TUR, a variety of whole LPS's, endotoxic glycolipids and PS preparations were compared. While all of the intact LPS's and several of the glycolipids were effective in enhancing TUR, some endotoxic glycolipids were totally inactive although they were equally toxic. Some lipid-free PS preparations were also active although less than whole LPS. Evidence was presented to suggest that mechanism for enhancement of TUR involves B cells and macrophages but not T cells. The mechanism also involves the production of soluble factors which are released into the serum of mice in response to LPS or PS. These factors can transfer and mediate the antitumor effects of LPS. The preinfection of mice with BCG enhanced the activity of LPS and PS in the production of antitumor activity.

ACKNOWLEDGEMENTS

The authors gratefully acknowledge the generous help of Dr. C. Chang who made the BALB/c nude mice available for these experiments.   This work has been supported by PHS grant CA-16934-14.

REFERENCES

1. Bradley, T. R., Metcalf, D. Aust. J. Biol. Med. 44 (1966) 287.
2. Braun, W. J. Infect. Dis. 128 (1973) S118.
3. Butler, R. C., Abdelnoor, A. M. and Nowotny, A.   Proc. Natl. Acad. Sci. 75 (1978) 2892.
4. Butler, R. C., Friedman, H. and Nowotny, A.   J. Res. 23 (1978) 331.
5. Butler, R. C. and Nowotny, A. IRCS Med. Sci. 4 (1976) 206.
6. Carswell, E. A., Old, L. J., Kassel, R. L., Green, S., Fiore, N. and Williamson, B. Proc. Natl. Acad. Sci. 72 (1975) 3666.
7. Chen, C. H., Johnson, A. G., Kasai, N., Key, B., Levin, J. and Nowotny, A.   J. Infect. Dis. 128 (1973) S43.
8. Coutinho, A. Scand. J. Immunol. 5 (1976) 129.
9. Cowing, C., Lukic, M. and Leskowitz, S. J. Immunol. 123 (1975) 61.
10. Grohsman, J and Nowotny, A. J. Immunol. 109 (1972) 1090.
11. Herberman, R. B., Nunn, M. E., Holden, H. T. and Larvin, D. H. Int. J. Cancer 16 (L975) 230.
12. Levin, J., Poore, T. E., Zauber, N. P., Oser, R. S. New Engl. J. Med. 283 (1970) 1313.

13. Ng, A-K, Butler, R. C., Chen, C. H. and Nowotny, A. J. Bact. 126 (1976) 511.
14. Nowotny, A., Behling, U. H. and Chang, H. L. J. Immunol. 115 (1975) 199.
15. Nowotny, A., Golub, S. and Key, B. Proc. Soc. Exp. Biol. Med., 136 (1971) 66.
16. Parr, I., Wheeler, E. and Alexander, P. Br. J. Cancer 27 (1973) 370.
17. Rios, A and Simons, R. L. Transplantation, 13 (1972) 343.
18. Shear, M. J. J. Natl. Cancer Inst. 4 (1944) 461.
19. Smith, R. I., Thomas, L. J. Exp. Med. 104 (1975) 217.
20. Stanley, E. R., Hansen, G., Woodcock, J. and Metcalf, D. Fed. Proc. Am. Soc. Exp. Biol. 34 (1975) 2272.
21. Watson, J., Riblet, R. J. Exp. Med. 140 (1975) 1147.
22. Wilson, J. M., Rosenstreich, D. L. and Oppenheim, J. J., J. Immunol. 114 (1975) 388.
23. Yang, C., Nowotny, A., Infect. Immun. 9 (1974) 95.

A MACROPHAGE CHEMOTAXIS INHIBITOR PRODUCED BY NEOPLASMS:

CHARACTERIZATION OF ITS BIOLOGICAL ACTIVITY

R. SYNDERMAN and M. C. PIKE

Laboratory of Immune Effector Function of the Howard
Hughes Medical Institute in the Division of Rheumatic
and Genetic Diseases, Departments of Medicine and
Microbiology and Immunology, Duke University Medical
Center, Durham, North Carolina (USA)

There is considerable evidence to suggest that the immune
system provides some resistance to the development and spread
of neoplasms (12,22). The ability of neoplastic cells to ab-
rogate certain of the host's immunological defense mechanisms
may be pivotal in determing whether or not a neoplasm is successful in overcoming host resistance. The role of macrophages
as potential effectors of tumor cell destruction in vitro and
in vivo is well documented (1,2,3,5,11), and factors derived
from neoplasms which depress the function of these cells could
be expected to alter tumor-host relationships in favor of tumor growth (4,7,8,10,14). We have previously shown that most
humans with cancer have abnormalities of monocyte function (14,
20) and that murine neoplastic cells contain and release an extremely potent factor(s) which is capable of depressing the
mobilization of macrophages to inflammatory sites in vivo (10,14,
19). This factor also diminishes the chemotactic responsiveness
of macrophages in vitro (10,14). The present report further
characterizes the biological activity of the macrophage chemotaxis inhibitor (MCI) and describes its effects on several other
important functions of macrophages.

MATERIAL AND METHODS

Mice. Male C3Heb/Fej mice, 7-9 weeks old, were purchased
from Jackson Laboratories, Bar Harbor, Maine.

Inflammatory agents. Phytohemagglutinin (PHA, Burroughs-
Welcome Co., Research Triangle Park, North Carolina) was stored
at - 70 C as a 2 mg/ml solution in isotonic saline until used.
Where indicated, mice were injected intraperitoneally (i.p.) with
2.0 ml of sterile nonpyrogenic saline containing 35 μ PHA (19).
Proteose peptone (Difco Laboratories, Detroit, Mich.) was dissolved in deionized water to make a 9% solution (w/v), autoclaved
and, where indicated, mice were injected i.p. with 2.0 ml (18).
Concanavalin A (Con A, Pharmacia Fine Chemicals, Piscataway, New
Jersey) was stored frozen at - 70 C at a concentration of 2 mg/ml
in isotonic saline. Immediately prior to use, Con A was diluted
to 25 μg/ml in sterile saline and, where indicated, mice were injected i.p. with 2.0 ml.

Preparation of MCI and normal tissues filtrates. MCI was prepared as follows (10,14). Hepatoma 129 tumor cells ($H-2^k$) were
suspended to a concentration of 5×10^7 cells/ml in medium RPMI
1640 (Grand Island Biological Co., Grand Island, N. Y.) and disrupted by sonication using a Sonic Dismembranator, for 3-6 min
until no intact cells could be detected by light microscopy. The
suspension was then centrifuged for 10 min at 12000 g, the supernatant collected and subjected to ultrafiltration through Amicon
Centriflo 25 cones. The <25,000 M.W. filtrate was collected, ali-
quoted and stored at -70 C until used. Normal tissue filtrates
were prepared by standardizing C3H liver or spleen to contain the
same packed volume of tissue per ml of RPMI 1640 as did the tumor
cells. The tissues were then homogenized, sonicated and subjected
to the same centrifugation and ultrafiltration as that described
for the tumor cells. The effect of MCI and the normal tissue filtrates on the various macrophage functions was tested as follows.
MCI and normal tissue filtrates were diluted to contain the equivalent amount of protein as that contained in the filtrate derived
from 10^6 Hepatoma 129 cells/ml. Two-tenths ml of these solutions
or dilutions thereof were injected subcutaneously in the thighs of
groups of four C3H mice.

Quantification of macrophage accumulation in vivo. Macrophage
accumulation in response to an i.p. injection of an inflammatory
agent was quantified as described previously (19). Briefly, 24
hr after subcutaneous injection of tumor filtrates or control materials, groups of 4 mice were given i.p. injections of PHA, Con A
or proteose peptone 2 or 3 days before being sacrificed by CO_2 as-
phyxiation. The skin was then retracted to expose the abdominal
wall, 9.0 ml of RPMI 1640 containing 10% heat-inactivated (56 C
for 30 min) fetal calf serum (RPMI-FCS) vigorously injected into
the peritoneal cavity and approximately 8 ml of medium containing
cells was immediately withdrawn. Following quantification of the
total and differential white cell counts for the individual peritoneal cavities, portions of the cells within groups were pooled,
centrifuged for 10 min at 350 g, 4 C and resuspended in the appropriate medium for the different functional assays. Differential

counts were determined using a modified Wright-Geimsa stain (Diff-Quik, Harleco, Gibbstown, N. J.) and a nonspecific esterase stain (Technicon Inst. Corp., Tarrytown, N. Y.).

Quantification of macrophage chemotaxis in vitro. Macrophage chemotaxis was quantified by a modification of methods described previously (18). Pooled peritoneal macrophages from normal mice receiving the various inflammatory agents or no stimulant, or mice receiving s.c. injections of MCI or the tissue filtrates followed by i.p. injection, of the inflammatory agents or no stimulant were suspended in Gey's balanced salt solution containing 2% bovalbumin (Flow Labs, Rockville, Md.) and 0.01M HEPES buffer (Calbiochem, La Jolla, California), pH 7.0 (GBSS) to a concentration of 2.0×10^6 macrophages/ml. Four-tenths ml of cells suspension was placed in the upper compartment of a modified Boyden chamber (13) and separated from the chemotactic stimulus, 3% activated mouse serum (AMS) (18) in the lower compartment by a 5.0 μ polycarbonate (Nuclepore) filter (Wallabs, San Rafael, California). All assays were performed in triplicate and chambers containing cells and stimulants were incubated for 4 hr in 37 C humidified air. Following incubation, the chambers were emptied, filters removed, fixed in ethanol and stained with hematoxylin. Chemotaxis was scored as the number of macrophages which migrated completely through the filter in 20 oil immersion microscopic fields (1540X) ± S.E.M.

Radiolabelled antibody coated sheep erythrocytes (^{51}CrShEA). Sheep erythrocytes were collected in sterile Alsever's solution (1:1), washed three times in gelatin Veronal buffer containing optimal amounts of Ca^{+2} and Mg^{+2} (GVB^{++}) (6) and resuspended to 10^9 cells/ml in GVB^{++}. One ml of cell suspension was incubated with 50 μCi of Na^{51}CrO$_4$ (200-500 Ci/g chromium, New England Nuclear Corp., Boston, Mass.) and 0.01 ml of IgG sheep cell hemolysin (kindly provided by Dr. Wendall Rosse, Duke University Medical Center, Durham, N. C.) for 1 hr at 37 C. Following incubation, the cells were washed 3 times with GVB^{++} and resuspended to 5×10^7 cells/ml in RPMI-FCS for use in the phagocytosis assay.

Phagocytosis assay. The pooled peritoneal cell suspensions from untreated mice or from mice treated with various inflammatory stimulants were standardized to contain 8×10^5 macrophages/ml in RPMI-FCS, and 0.5 ml of each cell preparation dispensed into a well of 16 mm diameter tissue culture plate (Linbro Scientific Co., Hamden, Ct.) All Assays were performed in triplicate. Following incubation for 3 hr at 37 C in 5% CO_2, 95% humidified air, the monolayers were washed twice with RPMI-FCS to remove nonadherent cells. ^{51}CrShEA (0.5 ml) were then added to each well and incubated an additional 60 min at 37 C, after which time the supernatant fluid was aspirated, the monolayers washed once with RPMI-FCS and the bound extracellular ^{51}CrShEA lysed using ammonium chloride potassium buffered (ACK) lysing medium (0.15M NH$_4$Cl, 0.01 M KHCO$_3$, 0.0001M EDTA). Following two additional washes, the mac-

rophage monolayers were dissolved in 0.6 ml of 0.5% sodium dodecyl
sulfate. Five tenths ml of the dissolved cells from each well
were counted for radioactivity using a Biogamma Counter (Beckman
Instruments, Fullerton, California). Results are expressed as
counts per min (cpm) minus background cpm ± S.E.M.

Macrophage adherence assay. The cell preparations were suspended to contain 8 x 10^5 macrophages/ml in RPMI and incubated
with 10 μc/ml $Na^{51}CrO_4$ for 1 hr at room temperature. Following 3
washes with medium, the cells were resuspended to 8 x 10^5 macro-
phages/ml in RPMI-FCS and 0.5 ml aliquots dispensed into each well
of 16 mm diameter Linbro tissue culture plates. Following incubation for 3 hr at 37 C, 5% CO_2, CO_2, 95% humidified air, the cells
were washed twice to remove nonadherent cells. The adherent cells
were then dissolved in 0.6 ml SDS, 0.5 ml aliquots removed, placed
in vials and the radioactivity counted. Adherence index (A.I.) is
expressed as:

$$A.I. = \left(\frac{\text{cpm in adherent fraction}}{\text{total available cpm}}\right) \times 100 \pm S,E,M.$$

RESULTS

Effect of MCI on macrophage accumulation induced by various
inflammatory stimulants. We previously showed that the subcutaneous injection of MCI in the thighs of mice depressed macrophage
accumulation into the peritoneal cavity in response to an injection of PHA (10,14). To determine whether MCI produced the same
effect when other inflammatory agents were used, groups of mice
were given s.c. injections of various dilutions of MCI, normal
tissue filtrates or nothing, followed 24 hr later by an i.p. injection of PHA, Con A, proteose peptone or no stimulant. Forty-
eight hr after having received PHA or Con A, or 72 hr after having
received peptone or no stimulant, the mice were sacrificed, and
the total number of macrophages recovered from the individual
peritoneal cavities quantified. Table I illustrates that a dose
of MCI corresponding to that obtained from 2 x 10^5 hepatoma cells
produced inhibition of macrophage accumulation varying from 44 to
75% when compared to animals given no s.c. injection. Decreasing
doses of MCI produced correspondingly reduced amounts of inhibition of macrophage accumulation induced by all the inflammatory
agents tested. Subcutaneous injection of MCI caused no significant
decrease in the number of resident macrophages found in the peritoneal cavities of mice receiving no inflammatory stimulant i.p.

In order to eliminate the possibility that MCI inhibited macrophage accumulation in vivo by sequestering macrophages at its

TABLE I

Inhibition by MCI of Macrophage Accumulation Induced
by Various Inflammatory Agents

Mice Injected s.c. with:[1]	Number of Macrophages ($\times 10^6$) Recovered from the Peritoneal Cavities of Mice Injected i.p. with:[2]			
	Con A	Peptone	PHA	No Stimulant
MCI[3]	3.6±0.2	2.0±0.2	4.0±0.2	1.9±0.3
MCI (1:10)	3.9±0.4	3.2±0.5	4.9±0.2	1.7±0.2
MCI (1:1000)	6.7±0.5	5.8±0.8	5.7±0.6	2.0±0.2
Liver filtrate[4]	8.1±0.6	7.5±0.9	7.4±0.5	2.5±0.3
Spleen filtrate[4]	7.4±1.0	7.9±0.8	7.4±0.7	2.1±0.2
No injection	8.0±1.0	7.9±0.5	7.1±0.8	1.9±0.3

1) Groups of mice were injected s.c. with 0.2 ml of the indi-
    cated concentrations of MCI or the tissue filtrates 24 hr
    before receiving i.p. injections of inflammatory stimulants.

2) Mice were injected i.p. with the indicated inflammatory sti-
    mulant or no stimulant 48 hr (PHA, Con A and no stimulant)
    or 72 hr (peptone) before being killed. The peritoneal cavi-
    ties were then exposed, lavaged with Gey's BSS and the total
    and differential white cell counts determined for the indi-
    vidual peritoneal cavities. The numbers indicate the average
    number of macrophages recovered from the peritoneal cavities
    of mice within groups ± S.E.M.

3) MCI stock solutions contained the equivalent of 2×10^5 Hepa-
    toma 129 cells/0.2 ml RPMI 1640.

4) Liver and spleen filtrates were diluted to contain an amount
    of normal tissue equivalent to 2×10^5 Hepatoma 129 cells/0.2
    ml RPMI 1640.

s.c. injection site, the inflammatory nature of MCI itself was investigated. Groups of mice were given i.p. injections of 2.0 ml
sterile saline containing ten times the maximum amount of MCI
tested s.c. for inhibition of macrophage accumulation. A corresponding concentration of the liver filtrate was used as a control.
Mice were sacrificed 2 days later and the total number of macrophages present in the individual peritoneal cavities of these
mice receiving no injections were determined. The number of
macrophages recovered from the peritoneal cavities of mice injected i.p. with the normal liver filtrate was approximately 50%
greater than the number obtained from untreated mice. Injection of
MCI i.p. caused a slight decrease in the number of macrophages recovered from the peritoneal cavities when compared to untreated
mice (MCI treated = $2.5 \pm 0.1 \times 10^6$; liver filtrate treated - 4.9
$\pm 1.5 \times 10^6$, untreated = $3.1 \pm 0.4 \times 10^6$) indicating that MCI has
no inflammatory activity in vivo.

Effect of administration of MCI in vivo on the chemotactic
responsiveness of peritoneal macrophages in vitro. The presence
of a growing neoplasm in the thighs of mice was previously shown
to depress the in vitro chemotactic responsiveness of the resident
peritoneal macrophages and also of those induced by i.p. PHA administration (16,21). We therefore sought to determine if MCI caused
a similar effect on macrophage chemotactic responsiveness. Groups
of C3H mice were given s.c. injections of various dilutions of MCI,
the normal tissue filtrates or no injection, followed 24 hr later
by i.p. injection of the three different inflammatory stimulants
or no stimulant. Forty-eight or 72 hr later, the mice were sacrificed, and the recovered macrophages tested for their chemotactic
responsiveness to AMS in vitro. Table II illustrates that the injection of doses of MCI equivalent to that derived from 2×10^2 to
2×10^5 hepatoma cells caused a dose dependent inhibition of chemotactic responsiveness in vitro regardless of the inflammatory
agent used to elicit the peritoneal macrophages. In addition, the
injection of MCI in vivo caused a dramatic depression of the in
vitro chemotaxis of the resident peritoneal macrophages (27 to 83%).
The injection of normal liver and spleen filtrates caused no depression of the in vitro chemotactic responsiveness of any of the
cell preparations tested.

Effect of MCI on the phagocytic and adherence abilities of
peritoneal macrophages. To determine the effect of MCI on another
macrophage function, the phagocytic ability of resident macrophages
or macrophages elicited by various inflammatory agents was tested
using mice treated s.c. with MCI, normal tissue filtrates or no
filtrate. In contrast to the depression of macrophage migratory
function noted in animals treated with MCI, the ability to phagocytize ^{51}CrShEA by macrophages from the same animals was markedly
enhanced (Table III). An enhancement of peritoneal macrophage
phagocytosis of up to 159% was noted in animals treated with MCI

TABLE II

Effect of In Vivo Administration of MCI on the
In Vitro Chemotactic Responsiveness
of Macrophages

Mice Injected s.c. with:[1]	Chemotactic Responsiveness of Macrophages Induced by i.p. Injection of:[2]			
	PHA	Con A	Peptone	No Stimulant
MCI[3]	106±12	184±2	178±20	14±11
MCI (L:10)	168±34	218±6	234±16	41±4
MCI (1:1000)	196±12	300±22	348±32	61±3
Liver filtrate[4]	242±12	342±18	384±8	81±28
Spleen filtrate[4]	254±26	328±12	392±10	81±16
Nothing	224±6	342±6	374±12	84±2

1)   Groups of 4 mice were injected s.c. with 0.2 ml of the indi-
     cated dilutions of MCI or tissue filtrates 24 hr before re-
     ceiving i.p. injections of inflammatory stimuli.

2)   Mice were injected i.p. with the indicated inflammatory sti-
     mulant or no stimulant 48 hr (PHA, Con A and no stimulant)
     or 72 hr (peptone) before being killed. The peritoneal
     cavities were then lavaged, portions of the individual
     exudates pooled within groups and the cells standardized
     to contain 2×10^6 macrophages/ml in Gey's BSS for quantifi-
     cation of chemotaxis (see Methods). Chemotactic responsive-
     ness is expressed as macrophages per 20 oil immersion (1540X)
     fields ± S.E.M. migrating completely through the filter.

3)   MIC stock solutions contained the equivalent of 2×10^5 Hepa-
     toma 129 cells/0.2 ml RPMI 1640.

4)   Liver and spleen filtrates were diluted to contain an amount
     of normal tissue equivalent to 2×10^5 Hepatoma 129 cells/
     0.2 ml RPMI 1640.

followed 24 hr later by any of the three inflammatory agents. The most dramatic effect on phagocytosis, however, was noted in resident peritoneal macrophages from mice treated with MCI (Table III), where enhancement of phagocytosis ranged from 184 to 231%. The injection of normal tissue filtrates produced no significant effect on the phagocytic response of macrophages.

Since the phagocytosis assay used in these studies depends on the ability of the cells to adhere to plastic tissue culture plates (17), it was necessary to determine whether the enhancement of phagocytosis seen in macrophages from animals treated with MCI was due to increased adherence of the peritoneal macrophages. To test this possibility, macrophages from animals receiving s.c. injections of MCI, normal tissue filtrates or no injection, followed 24 hr later by i.p. Con A were labeled with ^{51}Cr, washed extensively and allowed to adhere to tissue culture plates for an incubation time indentical to that employed in the phagocytosis assay. Table IV illustrates that there were no substantial differences in the A.I. of macrophages obtained from treated or untreated mice. Similarly, no differences were observed in the A.I. of cells from MCI treated or untreated mice when PHA, proteose peptone or no stimulant were used to elicit the macrophages (Data not shown). These results indicate that macrophages from MCI-treated mice have an enhanced ability to phagocytize ^{51}CrShEA, which contrasts markedly with their impaired directed migratory responses both in vivo and in vitro. Enhancement of phagocytosis by peritoneal macrophages from mice bearing growing tumors has previously been noted (15).

DISCUSSION

The relative biological importance of immune function in providing resistance against tumor development and spread is not yet clearly understood; however, there is substantial evidence that macrophages may be instrumental in this resistance (1,2,3,5,11). The finding that substances produced by tumors are capable of hindering the migration of macrophages to inflammatory sites in vivo suggests that anti-inflammatory properties of altered cells may be selected for in the genesis of clinically apparent neoplasms (4,7,8,10,14). The present report further characterizes the biological consequences of a tumor derived anti-inflammatory factor, MCI (10,14), on several functions of macrophages. MCI was found to inhibit the migration of macrophages into the peritoneal cavities of mice injected with PHA, Con A or proteose peptone. Mitogens such as PHA are not of themselves chemotactic in vitro and probably exert their inflammatory effects in vivo by stimulating lymphocytes to produce lymphokines. The nonspecific inflammatory stimulant proteose peptone does, however, possess intrinsic chemo-

TABLE III

Effect of In Vivo Administration of MCI on the
Phagocytic Response of Macrophages

Mice Injected with:[1]	Phagocytosis (cpm) of ^{51}CrShEA by Macrophages Induced by i.p. Injection of:[2]			
	Con A	Peptone	PHA	No Stimulant
MCI[3]	12,646±200	3,670±64	4,898±95	674±28
MCI (1:10)	11,890±159	4,591±58	5,392±187	764±26
MCI (1:1000)	9,165±189	3,402±91	2,501±37	657±36
Liver filtrate[4]	8,647±206	2,179±46	2,086±158	212±13
Spleen filtrate[4]	8,282±167	1,802±131	2,726±171	238±19
No injection	8,681±195	1,949±56	2,081±24	231±18

1) Groups of 4 mice were injected s.c. with 0.2 ml of the indicated concentrations of MCI, tissue filtrates or normal saline before receiving i.p. injections of inflammatory stimuli.

2) Mice were injected i.p. with the indicated inflammatory stimulant or no stimulant 48 hr (PHA, Con A or no stimulant) or 72 hr (peptone) before being killed. The peritoneal cavities were then lavaged, portions of the individual exudates pooled within groups and the cells standardized to 8 x 10^5 macrophages/ml for quantification of phagocytosis (see Methods). Results are expressed as ingested counts per min (cpm) ± S.E.M.

3) MCI stock solutions contained the equivalent of 2 x 10^5 Hepatoma 129 cells/0.2 ml RPMI 1640.

4) Liver and spleen filtrates were diluted to contain an amount of normal tissue equivalent to 2 x 10^5 Hepatoma 129 cells/0.2 ml RPMI 1640.

TABLE IV

Effect of In Vivo Administration of MCI
on Macrophage Adherence

Mice Injected s.c. with:[1]	Adherence Index (A.I.)
MCI[3]	55.0±1.2
MCI (1:10)	51.8±1.4
MCI (1:1000)	61.4±2.3
Liver filtrate[4]	51.0±0.7
Spleen filtrate[4]	54.2±4.4
No injection	50.9±1.2

1) Groups of 4 mice were injected s.c. with 0.2 ml of the indicated concentrations of MCI or the tissue filtrates 24 hr before receiving i.p. injections of Con A.

2) Mice were injected i.p. with Con A 48 hr before being killed. The peritoneal cavities were then exposed, lavaged with Gey's BSS, portions of the individual exudates pooled within groups and the cells standardized to 8×10^5 macrophages/ml for quantification of adherence (see Methods). Results are expressed as Adherence Index (A.I.):

$$= \frac{\text{counts per min (cpm) } ^{51}\text{Cr labeled macrophages adhered to tissue culture dish}}{\text{total available cpm}} \times 100$$

3) MCI stock solutions contained the equivalent of 2×10^5 Hepatoma cells/0.2 ml RPMI 1640.

4) Liver and spleen filtrates were diluted to contain an amount of normal tissue equivalent to 2×10^5 Hepatoma 129 cells/ 0.2 ml RPMI 1640.

tactic activity for macrophages and PMNs in vitro (unpublished).
It therefore seems unlikely that MCI depresses macrophage accumulation in vivo solely through an inhibition of lymphokine production, since MCI was equally effective in inhibiting macrophage
migration in vivo and chemotaxis in vitro when PHA, Con A or proteose peptone were used as inflammatory stimulants. Indeed, in
the absence of an inflammatory stimulus, MCI caused severe depression of the in vitro chemotactic responsiveness of resident peritoneal macrophages. These data suggest that MCI exerts its effects
on macrophage migration by directly affecting the macrophage.

    In contrast to chemotaxis, MCI or whole tumor cells (15) pro-
duced an opposite effect on the phagocytic ability of macrophages.
Doses of MCI which caused depression of macrophage accumulation
in vivo and chemotaxis in vitro produced no effect on adherence
but enhanced the phagocytic response of macrophages from the same
animals. The effects of MCI or tumor cell implants (15) on phagocytosis were observed with all inflammatory stimuli tested, but
the most dramatic effects were found in the resident peritoneal
macrophages. The cells most responsive to the effects produced
by MCI on phagocytosis appear to be the resident peritoneal macrophages, since enhancement levels in macrophages elicited by inflammatory stimuli were considerably less, probably reflecting the dilution of resident peritoneal cells by newly arrived macrophages
from the blood.

    The significance of MCI's reciprocal effects on macrophage
migration and phagocytosis is not clear at this time. MCI may
have differing effects on as yet undefined subpopulations of macrophages or may arrest monocytes and macrophages at a stage in
their development during which they are most phagocytically active
but less chemotactically responsive. It should be noted, however,
that inflammatory agents such as PHT, Con A and proteose peptone
which enhance the phagocytic activity of peritoneal macrophages
also enhance the chemotactic responsiveness of these cells.
Another possible explanation for the divergent effects of MCI on
macrophage function is that MCI affects a specific metabolic pathway
in such a way as to produce enhancement of phagocytosis and depression of chemotaxis. Such an effect is indeed seen in human monocytes when adenosine metabolism and S-adenosyl L-methionine-mediated
methylation is blocked by factors which cause accumulation of adenosine and S-adenosyl hemocysteine. The relationship of the effects
of MCI to adenosine metabolism and methylation is now under investigation.

    Whatever the mechanism by which MCI acts, it is certain that
tumors produce a factor(s) which profoundly alters the ability of
macrophages to function normally both in vivo and in vitro. This
alteration of macrophage function produced by a factor from neoplastic cells could affect the ability of such cells to survive

the surveillance of the immune system and permit them to develop
into lethal neoplasms.

SUMMARY

Murine neoplastic cells have been shown to contain and release
a potent factor which depresses macrophage accumulation in vivo
and chemotactic responsiveness in vitro. Since this factor may
be important in allowing neoplasms to escape macrophage-mediated
surveillance, its biological activity in vivo was further characterized. Mice were injected with various doses of the macrophage
chemotaxis inhibitor (MCI) subcutaneously and tested for their
responsiveness in vivo to several different inflammatory agents
given intraperitoneally. Macrophage accumulation caused by phyto-
hemaglutinin, Concanavalin A and proteose peptone were all depressed by MCI derived from as few as 200 tumor cells. The in vitro
chemotactic responsiveness of the recovered macrophage was also
depressed as was the chemotactic responsiveness and resident peritoneal macrophages from mice treated with MCI but not given an inflammatory stimulus. In contrast to its effects on chemotaxis,
the administration of MCI to mice produced an enhancement of macrophage phagocytosis, most dramatically seen in the resident peritoneal macrophages. The paradoxical effects of MCI on macrophage
chemotaxis and phagocytosis are identical to the effects of growing neoplasms in mice. The ability of macrophages from mice
treated with MCI to adhere to plastic was not altered. These
findings demonstrate that murine neoplasms contain a factor capable
of markedly altering the host's macrophage function in vivo and in
vitro. The data also suggest that the factor acts directly on
the macrophage and that its effect on chemotaxis and phagocytosis
are different.

REFERENCES

1.   Cleveland, R. P., Meltzer, M. S., and Zbar, B., J. Natl. Can.
      Inst., 52 (1974) 1887.
2.   Evans, R., and Alexander, P., Nature, 236 (1972) 168.
3.   Evans, R., Transplantation, 14 (1972) 568.
4.   Fauve, R. M., Hevin, B., Jacob, H., Gaillard, J. A., and
      Jacob, F., Proc. Nat. Acad. Sci., U. S. A., 71 (1974) 4052.
5.   Hibbs, J. B., Jr., Lambert, L. H., Jr., and Remington, J. S.,
      Nature (New Biology), 235 (1972) 48.
6.   Mayer, M. M., In: "Experimental Immunochemistry", (Ed. E. A.
      Kabat and M. M. Mayer), Charles C. Thomas, Springfield,
      Illinois, 2nd ed. (1961) 133.
7.   Normann, S. J., and Sorkin, E., Cancer Res., 37 (1977) 705.
8.   North, R. J., Kirstein, P. P., and Tuttle, R. L., J. Exp.

Med. 143 (1976) 559.

9. Pike, M. C., Kredich, N. K., and Synderman, R., Clin Res., 26 (1978) 25A.
10. Pike, M. C., and Synderman, R., J. Immunol., 117 (1976) 1243.
11. Shin, H. S., Hayden, M., Langley, S., Kaliss, N., and Smith, M. R., J. Immunol., 114 (1975) 1255.
12. Smith, R. T., and Landy, M., "Immune Surveillance", Academic Press, New York, (1970).
13. Synderman, R., and Pike, M. C., In: "In Vitro Methods in Cell-Mediated and Tumor Immunity", (Eds. B. R. Bloom and J. R. David) Academic Press, New York, New York, (1976) 651.
14. Synderman, R., and Pike, M. C., Science, 192 (1976) 370.
15. Synderman, R., and Pike, M. C., Am. J. Path. 88 (1977) 727.
16. Synderman, R., Pike, M. C., Blaylock, B. L., and Weinstein, P., J. Immunol., 116 (1976) 585.
17. Synderman, R., Pike, M. C., Fischer, D., and Koren, H., J. Immunol., 119 (1977) 2060.
18. Synderman, R., Pike, M. C., McCarley, D., and Lang, L., Infec. Immun., 11 (1975) 488.
19. Synderman, R., Seigler, H. F., and Meadows, L., J. Natl. Can. Inst., 58 (1977) 37.
20. Synderman, R., and Stahl, C., In: "The Phagocytic Cell in Host Resistance", (Eds. J. A. Bellanti and D. H. Dayton), Raven Press, New York, (1975) 267.
21. Stevenson, M. M., and Meltzer, M. S., J. Natl. Can. Inst., 57 (1976) 847.
22. Waldmann, T. A., Strober, W., and Blaese, R. M., Ann. Int. Med., 77 (1972) 606.

ENHANCEMENT OF TUMOR GROWTH BY PERITONEAL MACROPHAGES OF NORMAL AND TUMOR-BEARING MICE

A. GABIZON and N. TRAININ

Department of Cell Biology, The Weizmann Institute

of Science, Rehovot (ISRAEL)

Macrophages appear to play an important role on host-tumor inter-actions. In in vivo models, large numbers of macrophages have been shown to present in a variety of solid tumors (1,8,6). The reason for their presence and their action on tumor growth are, however, not clear. Data suggestive of a stimulatory effect on tumor growth have been reported (2). In vitro, activated macro-phages exert a cytotoxic effect on many tumor cell lines (3,5).

The specific aim of these studies was to investigate the effect of non-activated macrophages on the growth of tumor cells in in vivo transfer tests. Our results indicate that macrophages stimulate the initiation of tumor development.

MATERIALS AND METHODS

Animals and tumors. Two-6 month-old inbred C_3H/eB, $(C_3H/eB$ x $C_{57}Bl/6)F_1$ and Balb/c mice were used in these experiments. Tumor cells were derived from a chemically-induced fibrosarcoma of C_3H/eB mice and a radiation-induced lymphoma of Balb/c mice, both of them serially transplanted in syngeneic mice. After subcutaneous injection to syngeneic or F_1 hosts both tumors gave rise to palpable nodules which grew progressively and metastasized until death of the host.

Cell preparation. Tumors were removed, minced and trypsinized (0.25% trypsin) for 30 min at 37 C and the cells washed and counted by the trypan blue exclusion test. Peritoneal exudate cells (PEC) were harvested by repeated peritoneal washings with cold phosphate buffered saline (PBS). In most of the experiments, PEC were obtain-

485

ed from mice injected i.p. with 3 ml of Thioglycollate (29.8 gr/l,
Difco) 5 days previously. Thyoglycollate-induced PEC contained
more than 80% of macrophages by morphological criteria. In some
experiments, PEC and spleen cells were obtained from fibrosarcoma-
bearing C₃H/eB mice. A macrophage-enriched cell suspension was
prepared in the following way: PEC were cultured for 2 hr in
plastic Petri dishes in the presence of Eagle's medium + 10% fetal
calf serum. Non-adherent cells and cells detached by a 10 min
treatment with trypsin (0.25%) were discarded. The remaining
adherent cells were recovered by careful scrubbing with a rubber
policeman, washed twice in E.M. and then checked in the Winn test.

Winn assay. In vivo testing was done following the Winn
assay (7). The final suspension of PEC or spleen cells in E.M. was
mixed with tumor cells at the indicated ratios and immediately
injected subcutaneously into the interscapular space of syngeneic
recipient mice. A control group of mice was injected with tumor
cells only. Animals were regularly palpated and the day of tumor
appearance as well as the final tumor incidence were recorded.

Statistical analysis. P values were calculated by the Student's
t test.

RESULTS

Enhancing effect of PEC from normal mice on tumor growth. When
PEC from normal mice were added to an inoculum of tumor cells, a
significant and reproducible enhancement of tumor growth was
observed. The tumor enhancing effect was expressed by a shorter
latency period (i.e., time from tumor injection to tumor appearance) in mice injected with PEC + tumor cells, as compared to control
mice injected with tumor cells only. Table I presents 3 of such
experiments with the fibrosarcoma of C₃H/eB mice. Table II indicates that the enhancing effect of PEC was also observed with a second
syngeneic tumor model, a lymphoma of Balb/c mice. Moreover, PEC
from athymic nude mice possessed the same tumor enhancing activity
as their heterozygous littermates, (Table II) indicating that the
phenomenon of tumor enhancement was not dependent on T cells in
this particular model.

Unstimulated macrophages mediate the tumor-enhancing effect.
The above experiments were carried out with thyoglycollate-
induced PEC. We then investigated whether normal resident peritoneal cells manifest tumor-enhancing activity. Fig. 1 shows that
PEC from normal mice or thyoglycollate-injected mice enhanced
tumor growth almost to the same degree. Therefore, thyoglycollate
stimulation does not seem to be related to the tumor-enhancing
properties of PEC. Macrophages purified by adherence to Petri

TABLE I

Enhancement of Tumor Growth by Peritoneal Exudate Cells[a] (PEC)

		Mean Day of Tumor Appearance (Final Tumor Incidence)
Expt. 1 (	Tumor cells[b] only	24 ± 1 (8/9)
	Tumor cells + PEC[c]	19 ± 1 (9/9)
Expt. 2 (	Tumor cells only	30 ± 4 (5/5)
	Tumor cells + PEC[c]	21 ± 1 (10/10
Expt. 3 (	Tumor cells only	24 ± 1 (8/8)
	Tumor cells + PEC[c]	16 ± 2 (8/9)

Expt. 1: $p < 0.05$
Expt. 2: $p < 0.025$
Expt. 3: $p < 0.025$

[a]Thioglycollate-induced PEC from normal C_3H/eB mice.
[b]5×10^4 cells from a chemically-induced fibrosarcoma were injected s.c. into syngeneic C_3H/eB mice with or without PEC.
[c]Tumor cell: PEC ratio was 1:40

dishes were tested in the same experiment and found to cause tumor
enhancement (Fig. 1). Their effect was quite comparable to that
of unfractionated PEC.

Enhancing effect of PEC from tumor-bearing mice on tumor growth.
We have shown previously that after s.c. implantation of 5×10^4
fibrosarcoma cells into C_3H/eB mice, the in vivo antitumor response of spleen cells follows a characteristic biphasic pattern
(4). Indeed we found that spleen cells from animals at an early
stage of tumor growth transferred together with tumor cells into
syngeneic recipients protected against the tumor (Protective period).
Subsequently the protective activity declined leading to a 2nd
phase in which spleen cells caused tumor enhancement (Enhancing
period). We were now interested in comparing the activity of PEC
and spleen cells from the same tumor-bearing mice. As seen in
Fig. 2, tumor growth was enhanced to a similar extent by PEC from
normal mice and PEC from tumor-bearing mice in the Protective period.
In contrast, to PEC, spleen cells from the same tumor-bearing mice
caused the expected tumor-inhibitory effect. The possibility that
changes in the activity of PEC with regard to tumor growth could
be expressed in a later stage was investigated by comparing the
activity of PEC obtained from tumor-bearing mice $3\frac{1}{2}$ weeks and $6\frac{1}{2}$

TABLE II

Enhancement of the Growth of a Lymphoma by Peritoneal Exudate
Cells[a] (PEC)

		Mean Day of Tumor Appearance ± S.E. (Final Tumor Incidence)
Expt. 1	Lymphoma cells[b] only	25 ± 1 (9/9)
		(p < .0005)
	Lymphoma cells + PEC[c] (Balb/c)	18 ± 1 (9/9)
Expt. 2	Lymphoma cells only	22 ± 1 (9/9)
	Lymphoma cells + PEC[c] (Balb/c nu/+)	16 ± 0 (9/9) (p < .0125)
	Lymphoma cells + PEC[c] (Balb/c nu/nu)	16 ± 1 (9/9) (p < .05)

[a]Thyoglycollate-induced PEC from normal Balb/c mice.
[b]10^5 cells of a radiation-induced lymphoma were injected s.c.
 into syngeneic Balb/c mice with or without PEC.
[c]Lymphoma cell: PEC ratio was 1:25.

weeks after tumor inoculation. As shown in Fig. 3, PEC from tumor-
bearing mice stimulated tumor growth to the same degree independently of the stage of tumor growth.

DISCUSSION

    The present experiments indicate that macrophages are capable
of enhancing tumor growth in in vivo transfer tests. These results
raise the possibility that tumor-infiltrating macrophages exert a
similar stimulatory effect on in situ tumor growth. In the same
tumor model in which we have shown that lymph node (unpublished
data) and spleen T lymphocytes (4) possess an in vivo inhibitory
effect on tumor growth, macrophages from tumor-bearing mice caused
tumor enhancement. The interplay of these opposed activities of
the lymphoreticular system may be important in the understanding
of host-tumor interactions during the course of tumor growth.

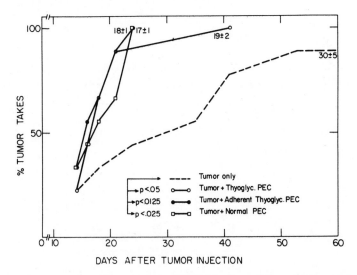

Fig. 1. Effect of thyoglycollate-induced PEC (Thyoglyc. PEC), unstimulated PEC (Normal PEC) and macrophage-enriched PEC (Adherent Thyoglyc. PEC) on tumor growth. 5 x 10^4 tumor cells were injected either alone or together with PEC in a 1:40 cell ratio. Recipients were normal (C$_3$H/eB x C$_{57}$Bl/6 F$_1$ mice).

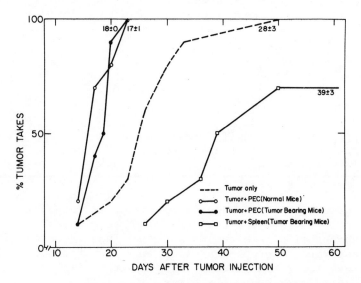

Fig. 2. Effect of PEC and spleen cells from tumor-bearing mice in the Protective period (3-4 weeks after tumor inoculation) on tumor growth. 5 x 10^4 tumor cells were injected either alone or together with PEC or spleen cells in a 1:50 cell ratio. Recipients were normal C$_3$H/eB mice.

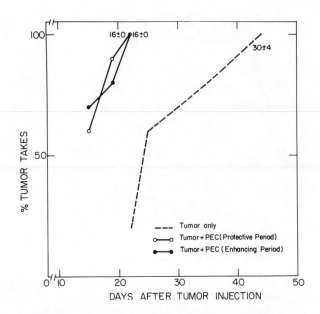

Fig. 3.   Effect of PEC from tumor-bearing mice 3½ weeks after tumor
inoculation (Protective period of spleen cells) and 6½ weeks after
tumor incoulation (Enhancing period of spleen cells) on tumor growth.
5 x 10⁴ tumor cells were injected either alone or together with PEC
in a 1:40 cell ratio.   Recipients were C_3H/eB mice.

SUMMARY

    The effect of peritoneal macrophages on tumor growth was
investigated in an in vivo transfer assay (Winn test).   A significant acceleration of tumor appearance was observed in animals injected with tumor cells together with peritoneal exudate cells (PEC)
from normal mice, as compared to animals injected with tumor cells
alone.   Macrophages were shown to be the cells responsible for tumor
enhancement.   PEC from tumor-bearing mice also caused a strong
tumor-enhancing effect in the Winn test.   These results indicate
that non-activated macrophages can enhance tumor growth in in vivo
transfers and raise the question of whether a similar effect takes
place in the primary host of a tumor.

REFERENCES

1. Evans, R. Transpl. 14 (1972) 468.
2. Evans, R. Brit. J. Canc. 35 (1977) 557.
3. Evans, R. and Alexander, P. Nature 228 (1970) 620.
4. Gabizon, A., Small, M. and Trainin, N. Int. J. Canc. 18 (1976) 813.
5. Hibbs, J. B., Jr., Lambert, J. H., Jr. and Remington, J. S. Nature New Biol. 235 (1972) 48.
6. Szymaniec, S. and James, K. Brit. J. Canc. 33 (1976) 36.
7. Winn, H. J. J. Immunol. 86 (1961) 228.
8. Wood, G. W., Gillespie, G. Y. and Barth, R. F. J. Immunol. 114 (1975) 950.

MACROPHAGE INVOLVEMENT IN LEUKEMIA VIRUS-INDUCED TUMORIGENESIS

M. BENDINELLI, D. MATTEUCCI, A. TONIOLO, and H. FRIEDMAN

Institute of Microbiology, University of Pisa (Italy),
and Department of Microbiology and Immunology, Albert
Einstein Medical Center, Philadelphia (USA)

Macrophages (MØ) play a pivotal role in viral infections. The
interaction of virus with these cells may lead to different results
in terms of both virus destiny and MØ function and survival, and may
ultimately determine the outcome of the encounter between the virus
and the entire host. Indeed, an inverse relationship has been observed in several experimental models between the ability of mononuclear phagocytes to restrain the virus and viral pathogenicity and
persistence (3).

As discussed by others in this book and elsewhere (39,1,2), MØ
exert crucial functions also in host defenses against neoplasia,
and their antitumor functions can be markedly influenced by tumor-
induced changes. As a matter of fact, a number of similarities
appears to exist between the antiviral and antitumor functions of
MØ. This is not surprising because in either case MØ have to deal
with cells presenting modifications of the external membrane. New
surface antigens are a common finding in tumor cells and in virus-
infected cells they occur even more frequently than hitherto believed
(43). It has also been speculated that the antitumor activities of
MØ might be philogenetically linked to the antimicrobial defense
mechanism of lower animals which is mainly in the "pseudopodia" of
MØ (2).

From this informational background it is reasonable to infer
that MØ should be profoundly involved in the pathogenesis of virus-
induced leukemias (VIL). On theoretical ground, MØ should influence,
and be influenced by, both viral infection and tumor growth and their
overall antileukemia activity should be the result of the interplay
of both nonspecific and immunological mechanisms. After all, the
key function of immune surveillance in defense against virus-induced

neoplasms has never been questioned. Moreover, in the case of
VIL the interaction of the host with the leukemia virus (LV)
should facilitate the antitumor functions of MØ since leukemic cells
share surface antigens with the inducing virus (4) and MØ can be
rendered tumoricidal even by unrelated viral infections or by
immune responses to unrelated antigens (1,25). Nevertheless, evidence for the involvement of MØ in VIL is scanty. Very little is
known about the intervention of MØ in spontaneous VIL and the
results obtained in experimental models concern mainly short-
incubation VIL that are thought not to occur in nature.

MØ AS TARGETS FOR LV REPLICATION AND LV-INDUCED TRANSFORMATION

That LV may replicate in MØ has been clearly demonstrated in
recent studies with the avian tumor system (28,30). Cultures of
both embryonic and adult chicken MØ could easily be infected with
leukosis, leukemia and sarcoma viruses. Myeloblastosis, myelo-
cytomatosis, and sarcoma virus-infected MØ, though exhibiting
normal immune and nonimmune phagocytosis, also presented signs of
transformation, while erythroblastosis and lymphoid leukosis virus-
infected cells did not. The relevance of these observations to the
in vivo situation, in regard to the infecting cycles of avian LV
as well as to host defenses against these viruses, is not known.

Murine LV replication in MØ has been investigated less systematically. Type C particles budding from the membrane of MØ were
observed in mice infected with Gross, Moloney and Rauscher LV and
taken to indicate that MØ actually support LV replication (69,27),
but the subsequent finding that mouse MØ can be activated to
produce endogenous retrovirus (33) coupled with the great variety
of stimuli which can lead to retrovirus derepression has weakened
this deduction considerably. However, peritoneal MØ obtained
from Friend leukemia complex (FLC)-infected mice have been shown
to release virus in culture (40,44) even for prolonged periods (50)
and in the latter study normal peritoneal MØ could be infected in
vitro. In addition, we have unpublished evidence that spleen MØ
are among the first cells to replicate FLC in the mouse.

MØ AS EFFECTOR CELLS IN NATURAL RESISTANCE TO LV

Two lines of evidence can be considered under this heading.
The first is the observation that treatments which impair MØ
activity reduce resistance to murine LV. Anti-MØ serum and RES
blocking substances, such as colloidal gold or carbon, have given
somewhat equivocal results (19,12,5,36) (not surprisingly, because
the first poses specificity problems and blockade is never
complete), but a clear indication emerges from the use of MØ
toxins endowed with high selectivity such as silica and carrageenan.

Silica has been shown to enhance FLC-induced leukemia (38) and carrageenan Rauscher leukemia complex (RLC)-induced leukemia (36).

The second line of evidence is the repeatedly observed inhibition of VIL by MØ-activating biologic and synthetic immunostimulants. These include Bordetella pertussis (59), Toxoplasma gondii, Besnoitia jellisoni (31), Corynebacteria (37, BCG (60), Freund's complete adjuvant (32), phytohemagglutinin (42), natural (statolon) or synthetic double stranded RNA (45), pyran copolymer (57), thioglycolate (62). Friend, Rauscher and spontaneous AKR leukemias in the mouse and Kirsten leukemia in the rat have been inhibited. For most of the above listed agents the relationship between VIL-inhibiting and MØ-activating properties is only correlative, but in the case of statolon and pyran copolymer the finding that silica treatment of the recipients abolished the protective action (57,67,68) provides direct evidence that MØ are indeed involved in resistance. In the pyran investigation (57), mice could also be protected by infusion of adherent peritoneal exudate cells (PEC) obtained from donors treated with the drug. In contrast, glycogen-elicited or resident peritoneal cells were ineffective, suggesting that the degree of MØ activation may be critical. The mechanism by which pyran-activated PEC protected was not investigated but the involvement of soluble factors was considered feasible. The possibility that MØ-active agents exert their beneficial effect by counteracting the MØ impairment which may occur in VIL (see below) should also be considered.

MØ INVOLVEMENT IN IMMUNE RESISTANCE TO LV

Another possible mechanism whereby MØ-active agents might protect against VIL is by potentiating or restoring MØ functions needed in the afferent and efferent limbs of immune response.

That MØ may be important in the efferent limb of immune response to VIL is suggested by the finding that the anti-Friend leukemia effect of transfused immune spleen cells is markedly reduced by treating the recipients with silica and is reintegrated by statolon (68). MØ have been shown to acquire antitumor activity from specifically immune lymphocytes in vitro (26) and in vivo (70). Spontaneous regression of Friend leukemia in mice is highly dependent on normally functioning immune mechanisms (21). Thus the observation that treatment of leukemic mice with MØ-toxic agents prevents both spontaneous (44) and statolon-induced regression (41) and that infusion of low numbers of normal peritoneal MØ induces regression of an otherwise progressing Friend leukemia (44) constitutes further strong evidence for key effector functions of MØ in immune resistance to VIL.

A role for MØ in the afferent limb of immune response against
LV antigens is indicated by recent in vitro attempts to sensitize
lymphocytes against radiation LV-associated antigens. While direct
antigen application was ineffective, sensitization could be
achieved by incubating lymphocytes with antigen-fed MØ (63).

MØ IMPAIRMENT IN VIL

That MØ functions may be damaged during VIL has been shown in
mice infected with FLC or RLC. The rate of carbon clearance was
either unchanged or enhanced in these animals but the amount of
carbon cleared per unit of spleen and liver weight was reduced
(51,24,58). Splenic uptake of xenogeneic red cells was also
depressed in FLC-infected mice (66). However, spleen and liver
uptake of particulate materials is not an adequate index of MØ
function in Friend and Rauscher leukemias because these organs
are the primary target in these diseases and any change of RES
function may be either secondary, or obscured by, organ architecture alterations caused by leukemic infiltration.

MØ impairment has, however, been confirmed by studying phagocytic cells resident in the peritoneal cavity (40,44,18). In FLC-
infected mice these MØ presented virus antigen on the surface and
exhibited a depression of certain functions (immune phagocytosis,
ability to spread on glass, motility), while others were unchanged (nonimmune phagocytosis, formation of EA rosettes). In
RLC-infected mice nonimmune and immune phagocytosis was normal
but intracellular killing of bacteria was reduced.

Two caveats should be kept in mind in this context. The first
is that viral preparations maintained by serial passage in mice
are often contaminated with LDH virus, unless purposely freed of
it, and that this passenger replicates in MØ and impaires MØ
functionality (56). However most of peritoneal MØ alterations
mentioned above were either confirmed with LDH virus-free LV
(40) or intimately correlated with productive LV infection of the
MØ (44). The second caveat is that MØ present at different
anatomical sites may be functionally heterogeneous (65) and in VIL
might also behave differently. For instance, we have found that
splenic MØ taken from mice infected with FLC or with its lymphatic
leukemia component (Rowson-Parr isolate, RP-LLV) have enhanced
ability to phagocytize opsonized sheep red cells (SRC).

MØ IN LV-INDUCED IMMUNODEPRESSION

In general, MØ may contribute to the pathogenesis of an immunodepressed status in two different ways: they can be deficient
in their ability to cooperate with lymphoid cells in the generation

of immune responses (54), or they can act as suppressor cells
limiting the responsiveness of lymphocytes (49). There is evidence
that in the immunodepression that often, if not always, accompanies
VIL (20) MØ can be involved in either way.

MØ as suppressor cells. In retrospect, the first indication
this type of MØ involvement was probably obtained studying the
development of SRC-lytic antibody-forming cells (PFC) by peritoneal
cells in vitro, a phenomenon which appears to be due to antigen-
independent differentiation of precommitted lymphocytes (13).
Peritoneal cells obtained from mice with advanced Friend leukemia
produced numbers of PFC reduced to a higher extent than expected
on the basis of the concomitant fall in the proportion of lymphocytes (6). Moreover, MØ depleted lymphocytes from normal and
leukemic mice were equally active (7), suggesting that in the
latter animals MØ were in fact inhibiting the reactivity of lymphocytes.

Subsequent studies have clearly established that MØ act as suppressor cells in various physiological and pathological conditions
(49) and also in the course of oncornavirus-induced tumorigenesis.
The clearest example of the latter situation comes from mice bearing
primary tumors induced by Moloney sarcoma virus. These animals
were immunodepressed and contained in the spleen suppressor cells
which nonspecifically inhibited lymphocyte reactivity to various
antigens and mitogens as well as the generation of a specific anti-
tumor response in vitro. The responsible cells were characterized
as MØ, because they were radioresistant, phagocytic, adherent and
susceptible to carrageenan (35,29). Although maximal suppressive
activity paralleled the peak size of the tumor, it is not known
whether the suppression-inducing stimulus was the tumor itself,
the sarcoma virus or its helper LV. Suppressor cells are, in
fact, induced by the latter virus but their nature has not been
fully characterized (17). Also not characterized are the suppressor cells described in various organs of leukemic AKR mice (55).
Unequivocal evidence for a suppressor function of MØ in VIL has
been recently obtained in studies with a LV originally isolated
from a chemically induced thymic lymphoma. Animals injected with
this virus exhibited depressed B cell functions and concomitantly
presented in the spleen MØ (identified on the basis of radio-
resistance, adherence and phagocytic activity) which suppressed
the antibody response of normal lymphoid cells in vitro (53).

Cells endowed with suppressive activity are also implicated
in FLC-induced leukemia (34,8). We have characterized the spleen
cells from mice in the early stages of infection with FLC or RP-
LLV which depress the in vitro antibody response of normal lymphoid
cells (Table I). They were identified as B lymphocytes acting
through the mediation of virus, though in FLC-infected mice
suppressor cells with non-B, non-T and non-MØ properties were also

TABLE I

Characterization of Suppressor Cells in the Spleen of
FLC- or RP-LLV-Infected Mice

Treatment of infected cells		RP-LLV Day -7	FLC Day -7	FLC Day -5
None		+	+	+
Freezing-thawing		−	−	
Sonication		−	−	
U.V. irradiation	120 ergs/mm^2	+	+	
	600 ergs/mm^2	±	±	
No depletion	adherence to plastic surface	+	+	
	adherence to glass wool	+	+	+
	incubation with silica	+	+	
	incubation with carrageenan	+	+	
T-cell depletion	adherence to nyloon wool	+	+	+
	anti-theta serum + C	+	+	
B-cell depletion	adherence to nylon wool	−	±	−
	anti-Ig serum + C	−	+	−
Incubation with antiviral antibody		−	−	
Supernatant of infected cell cultures		−	−	

Spleen cells from normal Balb/c mice were SRC-stimulated in vitro
in the presence of graded numbers of syngeneic infected spleen
cells treated as indicated. PFC were assayed on the 4th day.
Suppressive activity: + maintained, ± reduced, − abolished.
Further details in (9).

present and tentatively identified as leukemic cells. A major
contribution of MØ could be excluded (9). This conclusion is in
keeping with the results in Fig. 1; shows that the addition of
splenic adherent cells from uninfected or RP-LLV-infected mice
exerted no significantly different effects on the antibody response of normal spleen cells.

Defect in the auxiliary functions of MØ. The possibility that
a deficit of the collaborative functions of MØ contributes to LV-
induced immunodepression was investigated by two different approaches studying the in vitro PFC response of spleen cells from mice
infected with viruses of the FLC.

In the first approach, adherent and non-adherent spleen cells

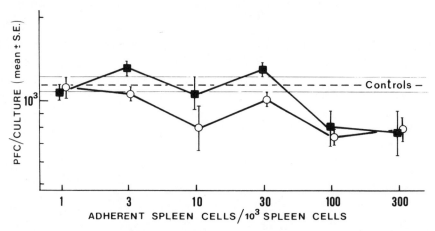

Fig. 1. Effect of normal (■) or RP-LLV-infected (O) MØ-enriched
spleen cells on in vitro antibody response by normal lymphoid cells
Spleen cells from normal Balb/c mice were SRC-stimulated alone or
in the presence of adherent syngeneic spleen cells (48) added at
the initiation of cultivation. PFC assayed on the 5th day.

from normal or 7-day FLC-infected mice were cross-recombined. As
shown by Table II, infected MØ-depleted non-adherent cells responded normally or near-normally when SRC-stimulated in mixed cultures
with uninfected MØ-rich adherent cells, and the response of normal
nonadherent cells mixed with infected adherent cells was also in
the normal range. These results are somewhat different from those
of other workers who, by using the same strains of mice and virus,
found that the non-adherent fraction of FLC-infected spleens was
hyporesponsive even if mixed with normal adherent cells (22). The
discrepancy can be explained by differences in the timing of infection or more probably in the efficiency of the separation procedures.
However, recently the same authors have ascertained that T-helper
and B-precursor lymphocytes are not affected by FLC, and came to
the conclusion that the impairment must be located in some collaborative step (23).

    In the second approach PEC from normal mice were added to
cultures of infected spleen cells (8,61,10). Unless otherwise
stated, PEC were elicited from syngeneic mice 3-5 days before
collection with 2 ml of 2% proteose peptone. Fig. 2 shows that
PEC induced a dose-dependent potentiation of the PFC response
developed by FLC- or RP-LLV-infected spleen cells, while the response of uninfected spleen cells was either not significantly
affected or diminished depending on the PEC dosage. It is important to notice, however, that the reversal of immunodepression was
complete only very occasionally. Even in the presence of the most
favorable proportion of PEC (60/10^3 spleen cells), the response
of FLC-or RP-LLV-infected cells in the experiments summarized in

TABLE II

In Vitro Antibody Response of Recombined Adherent and Non-
Adherent Spleen Cells from Normal or FLC–Infected Mice

Cells Cultured	PFC/Culture (mean ± S.E.)
Normal non-adherent	‹10
Normal adherent	‹10
Normal adherent + normal non-non-adherent	492 ± 39
FLC non-adherent	20
FLC adherent	‹10
FLC adherent + FLC non-adherent	178 ± 9
Normal adherent + FLC non-adherent	438 ± 25
FLC–adherent + normal non-adherent	482 ± 62

Spleen cells from normal or 7-day infected Balb/c mice were
separated into adherent and non-adherent fractions (48). The separated populations were then recombined as indicated and SRC-
stimulated. PFC assayed on the 5th day.

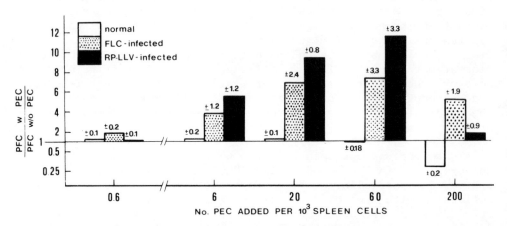

Fig. 2. Effect of PEC on in vitro antibody response by spleen cells
from uninfected, FLC- or RP-LLV-infected mice. Spleen cells from
Balb/c mice infected 5 days earlier or uninfected were SRC-stimulated alone or in the presence of PEC. PFC assayed on the 5th day.
Each bar represents the mean ± S.E. of 5-6 experiments. Further
details in (8).

Fig. 2 averaged, respectively, 60 ± 17 and 80 ± 5% of the uninfected controls. Properties and distribution of the cells which
exhibited restorative activity leave little doubt that the
effector cells were MØ (Table III).

TABLE III

Restorative Activity of Various Uninfected Cell Additions
on the In Vitro Antibody Response of RP-LLV-Infected Spleen Cells

Cell Type Added	Restored
PEC	++
Plastics-adherent PEC	++
T cell-depleted PEC (anti-θ + C)	++
Heated PEC (30 min at 56 C)	−
Resident peritoneal cells	+
Spleen cells	−
Adherent spleen cells (48)	+
Thymus cells	−
SRC-educated T cells (8)	−
Bone marrow cells	−

Spleen cells from Balb/c mice RP-LLV-infected 5-7 days earlier were
SRC-stimulated in the presence of graded numbers of the cell types
indicated. PFC assayed on the 5th day. Numbers in parenthesis
refer to papers in which technical details can be found.

    Thus either approaches clearly evidenced a deficit of MØ
collaborative functions in mice infected with FLC viruses. Though
the auxiliary function of MØ in the induction of the immune responses is generally agreed upon, the mechanisms involved are still
controversial (54,49,52). As studied in antibody responses in vitro,
these may include a) promoting of lymphoid cell viability, b) antigen handling and/or processing, c) antigen presentation, d) mediation of T-B cell cooperation, and e) amplification of B cell responses via soluble factors. In a series of experiments we have
attempted to identify the MØ function(s) impaired by infection.
The restorative activity of PEC was markedly reduced by a few hr
delay in the time of addition to infected cells (Fig. 3a) and
abolished by heating at 56 C per 30 min (Table III), but exhibited
a remarkable resistance to U.V. radiation (Fig. 3b). In certain
cases U.V. radiation actually potentiated the restorative activity
This occurred when PEC were precultured for 1 day before addition
to the infected spleen cells (Table IV). Since in vitro cultivation
increases MØ activation, U.V. treatment before culture may have
prevented excess activation. That the level of activation is

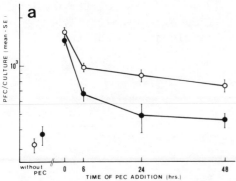 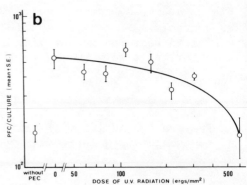

Fig. 3a. Effect of PEC added at various times on in vitro antibody response by spleen cells from FLC– (●) or RP–LLV–infected (0) mice. Spleen cells from Balb/c mice infected 7 days earlier were SRC–stimulated and supplemented with PEC (60/10³ spleen cells) at various times from the initiation of cultivation. PFC assayed on the 5th day.

Fig. 3b. Effect of U.V. irradiated PEC on in vitro antibody response by RP–LLV–infected spleen cells. Spleen cells from Balb/c mice infected 7 days earlier were SRC–stimulated alone or in the presence of PEC (60/10³ spleen cells) irradiated (12 ergs/mm²/sec) immediately before cultivation. PFC assayed on the 5th day.

TABLE IV

Enhancing Effect of U.V. Radiation on the Ability of Precultured PEC to Reintegrate the In Vitro Antibody Response of RP–LLV–Infected Spleen Cells

Cells Added	PFC Culture (mean ± S.E.)
None	148 ± 8
PEC precultured	493 ± 18
PEC 300 ergs/mm², then precultured	1473 ± 7
PEC 600 ergs/mm², then precultured	873 ± 52

Spleen cells from Balb/c mice RP–LLV–infected 7 days earlier were SRC–stimulated alone or in the presence of PEC (6 x 10⁴ spleen cells) which had been precultured for 1 day. PEC were U.V. irradiated (12 ergs/mm²/sec) before precultivation. PFC assayed on the 5th day.

critical is suggested by the results in Fig. 4: a certain degree
of activation was clearly needed for optimal restorative activity
but PEC elicited by strong irritative stimuli were ineffective
or even inhibitory at doses which were still restorative with
moderately activated PEC.

Table V lists agents which were tested for their ability to
substitute for the addition of MØ in restoring the immune responsiveness of infected spleen cells. Agents known for their ability
to mimick the viability-and activation-promoting function of MØ,
such as 2-mercaptoethanol and PEC culture supernatants, or to substitute for T-cell help, such as Con A-conditioned medium, were not
effective. Restorative activity was associated only with agents
known to curtail the need for the accessory function of MØ in in
vitro antibody response to SRC, such as LPS or allogenetic-
conditioned medium. A substantial reversal of suppression could
also be obtained by stimulating the infected cells with a very
large dose of antigen.

Taken together these results indicate that the MØ deficit
which contributes to the depressed in vitro responsiveness does
not reside in the lymphocyte-viability-and activation-promoting
functions but in the events needed for an efficient antigen presentation. This interpretation also accounts for the above
finding that uninfected nonadherent spleen cells reponded normally
when mixed with infected adherent spleen cells (Table II). In
this cell mixture most probably the infected MØ provided the
viability-promoting function, while the antigen-presentation
function, which requires few cells (52), was probably due to
those residual MØ in the non-adherent uninfected population which
inevitably remain after any MØ-depletion procedure.

Attempts were also made to evaluate the relevance of these
in vitro findings to events occurring in the intact host (10,16,11).
Fig. 5 shows that the inoculation of PEC simultaneously with
the antigen markedly potentiated the antibody response of RP-LLV-
infected mice, though exerting little or no effect on the response
of normal mice. In keeping with what observed in vitro, the response did not exhibit a complete recovery since in the animals
treated with 2×10^6 PEC it averaged $37 \pm 6\%$ of the uninfected
controls in three different experiments, and the active cells
were identified as MØ on the basis of their adherence properties.
However, in contrast to the in vitro results, in our hands the
inoculation of PEC at doses ranging from 2×10^5 - 2×10^7 had no
effect on the antibody response of FLC-infected mice. Moreover,
spleen cells from RP-LLV-infected mice gave greatly reduced responses, as compared to uninfected cells, when transferred into
γ-irradiated syngeneic recipients which might have themselves
provided MØ functions, and their responsiveness was not modified
by the simultaneous inoculation of PEC (Table VI). It would,

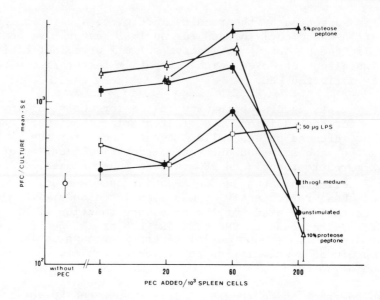

Fig. 4. Effect of PEC elicited by various treatments on in vitro antibody response by RP-LLV-infected spleen cells. Spleen cells from Balb/c mice infected 7 days earlier were SRC-stimulated alone or in the presence of peritoneal cells which had been elicited by i.p. inoculating the indicated substances 5 days earlier. PEC assayed on the 5th day.

TABLE V

Restorative Activity of Various Additions on the In Vitro
Antibody Response of RP-LLV-Infected Spleen Cells

Addition	Conditions	Restoration
Extra dose of SRC (8)	100x	+
Sonicated SRC (14)	1 x ⟶ 10x	−
2-Mercaptoethanol (8)	$1 \times 10^{-4} \longrightarrow 2 \times 10^{-5}M$	−
E. coli LPS (8)	5 ug or 10 ug	++
Con A conditioned medium (64)	50%	−
Allogeneic conditioned medium (47)	50%	+
Syngeneic conditioned medium (47)	50%	−
PEC supernatant (15)	3% ⟶ 50%	−
Dialyzed PEC supernatant (15)	3% ⟶ 50%	−

Spleen cells from Balb/c mice RP-LLV-infected 5-7 days earlier
were SRC-stimulated in the presence of teh indicated substances,
PFC assayed on the 5th day. Numbers in parenthesis represent
references in which technical details can be found.

TABLE VI

Effect of PEC on In Vivo Antibody Response of Irradiated Mice
Reconstituted with Spleen Cells from RP-LLV-Infected Donors

Mice Reconstituted With	PFC/Spleen (mean ± S.E.)
No cells	69 ± 12
Normal spleen cells	4730 ± 595
RP-LLV-spleen cells	608 ± 176
RP-LLV-spleen cells + 1 x 10^5 PEC	750 ± 275
RP-LLV-spleen cells + 3 x 10^5 PEC	560 ± 148
RP-LLV-spleen cells + 1 x 10^6 PEC	743 ± 153
1 x 10^6 PEC	75 ± 21

Balb/c mice (6 per group) received 650 R γ-irradiation and after
20 hr were i.v. inoculated with 3 x 10^7 syngeneic spleen cells
mixed with 1 x 10^8 SRC and with the indicated number of PEC. PFC
assayed 8 days later. Spleen cell donors infected 5 days before
sacrifice.

therefore, appear that a MØ deficit play some role in the immunodepression observed in the intact animal, as also suggested by
data showing that the antibody response to antigens which show
little or no MØ-dependence is relatively resistant to suppression
(23,11), but in order to establish how important this role is,
further studies are needed.

CONCLUSIONS

In recent years it has become evident that MØ intervenes in
immunological and nonimmunological phenomena in many previously
unperceived fashions. It is as a consequence of this progressing
knowledge that we are now beginning to realize that these cells
are involved in virus-induced leukemogenesis in a variety of ways,
and that the basic property of phagocytosis and virus inactivation
per se might not be the most important.

It is an easy forecast that in the next few years much more
information about the nature and the significance of MØ activity
in the pathogenesis of virus-induced leukemias will become available.
The many functions that are being attributed to MØ in nontumor
virus infections and in neoplasia "continually open new fields to
our vision" (Pasteur). At the present time it would be premature
to draw conclusions on even to offer some speculations. At this
stage, it is only apparent that there is a need for much further

work. Hopefully, future research will not only allow a more
coherent and integrated view of MØ contribution to this important
area of tumorigenesis but also provide hints to the comprehension
of the mechanisms which regulate the coexistence of endogenous
viruses and their hosts.

ACKNOWLEDGEMENTS

The expert technical assistance of Mrs. Luciana Montagnani is
gratefully acknowledged. This work was supported in part by
a grant from the Italian National Research Council (Progetto
finalizzato virus, CT 77,00248.84).

REFERENCES

1. Alexander, P. Ann. Rev. Med. 27 (1978) 207.
2. Alexander, P. Brit. J. Canc. 33 (1976) 344.
3. Allison, A. C. Transplant. Rev. 19 (1974) 3.
4. Bauer, H. Adv. Canc. Res. 20 (1974) 275.
5. Bendinelli, M. and Batt, G. Virol. Immunol. 66 (1973) 1.
6. Bendinelli, M. Immunol. 14 (1968) 836.
7. Bendinelli, M. In: Immunity and Tolerance in Oncogenesis
    (Ed. L. Severi) Division of Cancer Research, Perugia (1970)
    623.
8. Bendinelli, M., Kaplan, G. S. and Friedman, H. J. Natl. Canc.
    Inst. 55 (1975) 1425.
9. Bendinelli, M., Matteucci, D. and Toniolo, A. Submitted for
    publication.
10. Bendineeli, M., Toniolo, A. and Friedman, H. Ann. N. Y.
    Acad. Sci. 276 (1976) 431.
11. Bendinelli, M., Campa, M., Toniolo, A. and Garzelli, C. J.
    Gen. Virol. 39 (1978) 243.
12. Buchman, V. M., Radzichovskaya, R. M., Svet-Moldavsky, G. J.,
    Kozlova, M. D., Mikaelian, S. E. and Levin, V. J. Biomed. 19
    (1973) 335.
13. Bussard, A. E. and Pagès, J. M. Ann. Immunol. 127C (1976)
    583.
14. Byrd, W., Feldman, M. and Palmer, J. Immunol. 27 (1974) 331.
15. Calderon, J., Kiely, J-M., Lefko, J. L. and Unanue, E. R.
    J. Exp. Med. 142 (1975) 151.
16. Ceglowski, W. S. and Friedman, H. Proc. Soc. Exp. Biol. Med.
    148 (1975) 808.
17. Cerny, J., Grinwich, K. D. and Stiller, R. A. J. Immunol.
    119 (1977) 1097.
18. Cox, K. O. and Keast, D. J. Natl. Canc. Inst. 50 (1973)
    941.
19. Dallenbach, F. D., Stichs, H. P., Muller, B. and Gerber, H.
    Verh. Dtsch. Ges. Path. 55 (1971) 294.

20. Dent, P. B. Progr. Med. Virol. 14 (1972) 1.
21. Dietz, M., Furmanski, P., Clymer, R. and Rich, M. A. J.
    Natl. Canc. Inst. 57 (1976) 91.
22. Dracott, B. N., Wedderburn, N. and Salaman, M. H. J. Gen.
    Virol. 14 (1972) 77.
23. Dracott, B. N., Wedderburn, N. and Doenhoff, M. J. Immunol.
    34 (1978) 679.
24. Elliott, S. C. and Schloss, G. T. Infected. Immun. 3 (1971)
    217.
25. Evans, R. and Alexander, P. In: Immunobiology of the Macro-
    phage (Ed. D. S. Nelson) Academic Press, (1976) 535.
26. Evans, R. and Alexander, P. Nature 228 (1970) 620.
27. Feldman, D. G., Dreyfuss, Y. and Gross, L. Cancer Res. 27
    (1967) 1792.
28. Gazzolo, L., Moscovici, M. G., Moscovivi, C. and Vogt, P. K.
    Virology 67 (1975) 553.
29. Glaser, M., Kirchner, H., Holden, H. T. and Herberman, R. B.
    J. Natl. Canc. Inst. 56 (1976) 865.
30. Graf, T., Royer-Pokora, B., Meyer-Glauner, W., Claviez, M.,
    Gotz, E. and Beug, H. Virol. 83 (1977) 98.
31. Hibbs, J. B., Lambert, L. H. and Remington, J. S. J. Infect.
    Dis. 124 (1971) 587.
32. Hibbs, J. B., Lambert, L. H. and Remington, J. S. Proc. Soc.
    Exp. Biol. Med. 139 (1972) 1053.
33. Huebner, K. and Croce, C. M. J. Virol. 18 (1976) 1143.
34. Kateley, J. R., Kamo, I., Kaplan, G. S. and Friedman, H. J.
    Natl. Canc. Inst. 53 (1974) 1371.
35. Kirchner, H., Chused, T. M., Herberman, R. B., Holden, H. T.
    and Laurin, D. H. J. Exp. Med. 139 (1974) 1473.
36. Knyszynski, A. and Danon, D. J. Reticuloendothel. Soc. 22
    (1977) 341.
37. Kouznetzova, B., Bizzini, B., Chermann, J. C., Degrand, F.,
    Prevot, A. R. and Raynand, M. Recent Results Cancer Res.
    47 (1974) 275.
38. Larson, C. L., Ushijima, R. N., Baker, R. E., Baker, M. B.
    and Gillespie, C. A. J. Natl. Canc. Inst. 48 (1972) 1403.
39. Levy, M. H. and Wheelock, E. F. Adv. Canc. Res. 20 (1974)
    131.
40. Levy, M. H. and Wheelock, E. F. J. Immunol. 114 (1975) 962.
41. Levy, M. H. and Wheelock, E. F. J. Reticuloendothel. Soc.
    20 (1976) 243.
42. Lozzio, B. B., Brown, A. and Hewins, J. P. Exp. Hemat. 2
    (1974) 16.
43. Macfarlan, R. T., Burns, W. H. and White, D. D. J. Immunol.
    119 (1977) 1569.
44. Marcelletti, J. and Furmanski, P. J. Immunol. 120 (1978) 1.
45. Marx, P. A. and Wheelock E. F. Ann. N. Y. Acad. Sci. 276
    (1976) 502.
46. Metzler, C. M., Kostyk, T. G. and Gershon, R. K. J. Immunol.

117 (1976) 1295.

47. Mishell, R. I., Lucas, A. and Mishell, B. B.   J. Immunol. 119 (1977) 118.
48. Mosier, D. E.   Science 158 (1967) 1573.
49. Nelson, D. S.   In: Immunobiology of the Macrophage (Ed. D. S. Nelson) Academic Press, New York (1976) 235.
50. Odaka, T. and Kühler, K.   Naturforschg. 20 (1965) 473.
51. Old, L. J., Benacerraf, B., Clarke, D. A., Carswell, E. A. and Stockert, E.   Cancer Res. 21 (1961) 1281.
52. Pierce, C. W. and Kapp, J. A.   In: Immunobiology of the Macrophage (Ed. D. S. Nelson) Academic Press, New York (1976) 1.
53. Roder, J. C., Tyler, L., Ball, J. K. and Singhal, S. K.   Cell. Immunol. 36 (1978) 128.
54. Roelants, G. E.   In: B and T Cells in Immune Recognition (Eds. F. Floor and G. E. Roelants) John Wiley, London (1977) 103.
55. Roman, J. M. and Golub, E. S.   J. Exp. Med. 143 (1976) 482.
56. Rowson, K. E. K. and Mahy, B. W. J.   Virol. Monogr. 13, Springer-Verlag, Wien, (1975)
57. Schuller, G. B. and Morahan, P. S.   Cancer Res. 37 (1977) 4064.
58. Seidel, H. J. and Nothdurft, W.   J. Reticuloendothel. Soc. 19 (1976) 173.
59. Sinkovics, J. G., Ahearn, M. J., Shirato, E. and Shullenberger, C. C.   J. Reticuloendothel. Soc. 8 (1970) 474.
60. Siegel, B. V. and Morton, J. I.   Blood 29 (1967) 585.
61. Specter, S., Patel, N. and Friedman, H.   Proc. Soc. Exp. Biol. Med. 151 (1976) 163.
62. Strauss, R. R., Friedman, H., Mills, L. and Zayon, G.   Nature 255 (1975) 343.
63. Treves, A. J., Feldman, M. and Kaplan, H. S.   J. Natl. Canc. Inst. 58 (1977) 1527.
64. Waldman, H., Poulton, P. and Desaymard, C.   Immunol. 30 (1977) 723.
65. Walker, W. S. In: Immunobiology of the Macrophage (Ed. D. S. Nelson, Ed.) Academic Press, New York (1976) 91.
66. Wedderburn, N. and Salaman, M. H.   Immunol. 15 (1968) 439.
67. Wheelock, E. F., Toy, S. T., Weislow, O. S. and Levy, M. H. Prog. Exp. Tumor Res. 19 (1974) 396.
68. Wirth, J. J., Levy, M. H. and Wheelock, E. F.   J. Immunol. 117 (1976) 2124.
69. Yumoto, T., Recher, L., Sykes, J. A. and Dmochowski, L. Natl. Canc. Inst. Mon. 22 (1966) 107.
70. Zarling, J. M. and Tevethia, S. S.   J. Natl. Canc. Inst. 50 (1973) 149.

FUNCTIONAL HETEROGENEITY AND T CELL-DEPENDENT ACTIVATION OF MACROPHAGES FROM MURINE SARCOMA VIRUS (MSV)-INDUCED TUMORS

H. T. HOLDEN, L. VARESIO, T. TANIYAMA and P. PUCCETTI

Laboratory of Immunidagnosis, National Cancer Institute,

Bethesda, Maryland (USA)

Tumor growth may induce a wide variety of cellular immune responses in the host (see Ref. 5 for review). Furthermore, the generation and effector phases of each type of response may involve participation and interaction between different subpopulations of lymphoid cells.

In an attempt to learn more about these complex interactions, we have been examining host immune functions in animals bearing MSV-induced tumors. Although our initial studies have employed peripheral lymphoid cells (13,9,2,12), recently we have been examining the functional activity of host cells isolated from the tumor since this may be more relevant to the regression or progression of the tumor. T cells with high levels of cytolytic antitumor activity (6,3) and macrophages with both cytostatic (6,16) and cytolytic activity against tumor cells (16,18) have been recovered from MSV-induced tumors. Macrophages from these tumors, however, are capable of opposing effects on neoplastic growth, since they can also suppress the generation of cellular immune responses (6).

In this report we will summarize our recent findings on the functional activity of macrophages isolated from the tumor and on the interactions of macrophages with T cells. Macrophages from the tumor will be shown to suppress the function of T lymphocytes, inhibiting proliferation-independent production of MIF and MAF. Reciprocally, in mice bearing MSV-induced tumors, T cells (or factors from these cells) appeared to be required for macrophages to become cytolytic. We have also obtained evidence for functional heterogeneity of cytolytic macrophages within MSV-induced tumors.

509

MATERIALS AND METHODS

Animals. $C_{57}Bl/6$ conventional and NIH Swiss nude mice were obtained from the Division of Research Services, National Institutes of Health, and from the Mammalian Genetics and Animal Production Section, Division of Cancer Treatment, National Cancer Institute (Bethesda, Maryland).

Tumors. Eight- to 12-week-old mice were injected intramuscularly in the leg with either the regressor (MSV) or progressor (MSV-H) stock of the Moloney strain of murine sarcoma virus (virus preparation and characterization were outlined in Ref. 13). Tumors appeared at 6-8 days after inoculation. In conventional mice injected with MSV, tumors reached maximum size at 14 days and subsequently regressed by 21-25 days. Tumors induced in conventional mice by MSV-H or in nude mice by MSV usually grew progressively and caused death of the animal in 21-75 days.

Allogeneic immunization. $C_{57}Bl/6$ mice were injected i.p. with 10^7 RL♂1 ascites tumor cells, a Balb/c radiation-induced lymphoma, and immune spleen cells for MIF and MAF production were harvested 10-17 days later.

Tissue culture. RBL-5, a $C_{57}Bl/6$ Rauscher virus-induced lymphoma, was adapted to tissue culture and maintained in stationary suspension culture in RPMI 1640 medium supplemented with 10% fetal calf serum as previously described (7).

Preparation of peritoneal exudate cells (PEC) and cells from the tumor (CfT). PEC were obtained from normal or MSV injected mice by washing the peritoneal cavity with 10 ml of cold Hanks' balanced salt solution (BSS) containing 5-10% fetal calf serum (and sometimes 100 U/ml of heparin) 3-4 days after injection of 2.5 ml of light mineral oil (MIF assays) or 1 ml of 10% thioglycollate (macrophage mediated cytotoxicity), or 1 day after injection or 1 ml of fetal calf serum (MAF assay). CfT were prepared from minced MSV-induced tumors by successive 15-20 min treatments with 0.125% collagenase at 37 C.

Treatment of effector populations. T cells were depleted by treatment with anti-Thy 1,2 antibody plus rabbit complement as previously described (8). Adherent cells were obtained by plating PEC or CfT in plastic Petri dishes for 2-3 hrs. Nonadherent cells were removed by vigorous washing and the adherent cells harvested using a rubber policeman. Rayon wool column and iron/magnet treatments (9), and 1 g velocity sedimentation of cells (6), were performed as reported earlier.

^{51}Cr release assay. Macrophage-mediated cytolysis was measured in an 18 hr ^{51}Cr release assay with RBL-5 target cells (16).

Baseline release was determined by using an equal number of syngeneic thymus cells in place of effector cells.

Growth inhibition assay. Macrophage-mediated cytostasis was
determined in a 48 hr growth inhibition assay (10) by measuring
^{3}H-thymidine uptake by RBL-5 target cells.

Production of MIF. MIF production was measured by the indirect
agarose droplet assay (12). Spleen cells taken from animals 14
days after inoculation with MSV were depleted of macrophages and
stimulated with puromycin-treated RBL-5 cells. Supernatants were
harvested from cultures of spleen cells, incubated alone or in the
presence of different cell preparations from the tumor, and
assayed for MIF on normal, light mineral oil-induced PEC. Supernatants from C_{57}B1/6 alloimmune spleen cells were tested in a similar manner. Migration inhibition greater than 15% was considered
positive (12).

Production of MAF. Supernatants prepared as described above
for MIF were tested for MAF as described by Ruco and Meltzer (17)
except that we employed at 18 hr ^{51}Cr release assay with RL♂1
target cells.

RESULTS AND DISCUSSION

Previously we had found that T lymphocytes obtained from the
spleen of mice 14 days after inoculation with MSV were cytolytic
for tumor cells (13) and produced MIF when stimulated by intact
tumor cells (12). Since we also knew that cytolytic T lymphocytes
are present within the tumor of these animals (6), it was of interest to determine whether CfT also could produce MIF. Therefore,
CfT and spleen cells from the same MSV-tumor-bearing mice were
tested for their ability to produce MIF (Table I). Spleen cells,
as expected, were positive whereas the CfT did not produce
detectable levels of MIF. Because a large percentage of the CfT
were macrophages and because macrophages have been reported to be
suppressive for several immune functions, these cells were depleted
by the iron/magnet technique or by passage over rayon wool columns
as well as by the iron/magnet technique. No activity was detected
in the macrophage depleted Cft while the level of MIF produced by
the spleen cells remained essentially the same.

Although the CfT still did not produce MIF after macrophage
depletion, it was still possible that suppressor cells at the tumor
site were responsible for inhibiting the immune function. To test
this hypothesis, we measured lymphokine production by spleen cells
from MSV-immune mice, cultured with RBL-5 tumor cells in the
presence or absence of CfT. Supernatants from cultures to which
10% CfT had been added were not positive for MIF activity (Table II).

TABLE I

Comparison Between MIF Production from Spleen Cells and
from Cells from the Tumor

Responders[a]	Percent Migration Inhibition		
	No Treatment	Iron/Magnet	Iron/Magnet + Rayon Column
ISC	38	49	32
CfT	10	6	4
NSC	3	-10	3

[a]Immune spleen cells (ISC) and cells from the tumor (CfT were
removed 14 days after injection of MSV. Normal spleen cells
(NSC) were tested as a control.

TABLE II

Suppression of MIF Production by Cells from MSV Tumors
and Characteristics of the Suppressor Cells

	Suppressor[a] Cells	Treatment	% Migration Inhibition
Exp. No. 1	None	--	43
	10% CfT	--	10
	10% CfT	Rayon wool column + iron/magnet	40
Exp. No. 2	None	--	34
	10% aCfT	Media	-2
	10% aCfT	Complement	5
	10% aCfT	Anti-Thy 1.2 + C	-1

[a]Cells added to cultures of immune spleen cells plus RBL-5
cells.

Suppressor activity of the CfT was removed by sequential treatment
with the iron/magnet and rayon wool column techniques while the
activity of adherent CfT was not affected by treatment with anti-
Thy 1.2 plus complement. These data indicate that the cells
suppressing MIF production were adherent, phagocytic, and were
probably macrophages and not T cells. Adherent cells from the tumor
(aCfT) often had quite high suppressor activity with complete suppression of MIF production noted at concentrations of cells as low
as 1.5% while adherent PEC (aPEC) from normal mice had no activity.

   To further evaluate the interaction between suppressor cells
and responding T cells, the kinetics of MIF production was compared
with the ability of macrophages to suppress when added at different
times after the initiation of culture. Multiple cultures of MSV
immune spleen cells with RBL-5 were set up. Some of these cultures
were harvested at different times, while in others, 10% aCfT were
added at various times and the cultures were then harvested at 24 hrs.
MIF activity was first detectable after 6-8 hrs (Fig. 1), and the

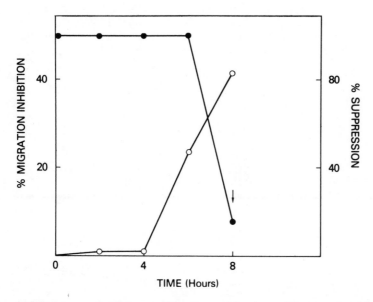

Fig. 1. Kinetics of MIF production and the effect of addition
of macrophages at different times. The times shown represent the
hr after initiation of culture at which supernatants were harvested
from culture of immune spleen cells plus RBL-5 tumor cells (O) or
at which aCfT were added to the stimulated cultures (●). In the
cultures with aCfT, supernatants were harvested for MIF at 24 hrs.

ability of the aCfT to suppress MIF production was markedly diminished if they were added after 6-8 hrs of culture. These results
indicate that macrophages can suppress the initiation of MIF production but cannot turn it off after it has begun.

   Macrophage-mediated suppression has generally been associated
with immune responses that are proliferation dependent (14).
However, Bloom et al. (1) demonstrated that MIF production was not
dependent on proliferation of the responding cells. To confirm
this and to extend our observations, MSV immune spleen cells (ISC)
were depleted of macrophages (dISC), treated with mitomycin C to
block proliferation, and then stimulated with RBL-5 tumor cells
(Table III). When supernatants of mitomycin C-treated cultures were
compared to controls, similar levels of MIF activity were detected.
Furthermore, the MIF production in both cultures was equally susceptible to the suppressive activity of the aCfT. Therefore, MIF production was not proliferation dependent and, consequently, the
macrophages must be exerting their suppressive effect through
another mechanism.

   Hence, macrophages from the tumor are capable of suppressing
both proliferation-dependent and proliferation-independent immune
responses. In light of this finding, it was not too surprising
that we were unable to show MIF production in the lymphocytes
isolated from the tumor. However, the possibility still exists
that even though cytotoxic T cells are found within the MSV-induced
tumors, the T lymphocytes that produce lymphokines do not migrate
to that site.

TABLE III

Suppressive Effect of Adherent Cells from MSV-Induced Tumors
(aCfT) on MIF Production by Mitomycin C-Treated Immune
Spleen Cells

| Responder Cells | Treatment | Percent Migration Inhibition | |
		Control	aCfT Added
dISC[a]	None	35	2
dISC	Mitomycin C	30	-3

[a]Macrophage depleted MSV-immune spleen cells.

Two other questions were addressed regarding the suppression of MIF production by macrophages from the tumor: a) Was the suppressive activity antigen specific and b) was the production of other lymphokines similarly affected by the suppressor cells? Data concerning both these issues are presented in Table IV. Spleen cells from $C_{57}Bl/6$ mice immunized with MSV or with allogeneic tumor cells (RLo1) were cultured with cells bearing the appropriate antigen, with or without the addition of 10% aCfT. The supernatants from each culture were tested for both MIF and MAF. Production of both lymphokines was suppressed by a CfT regardless of whether the cells were responding to tumor-associated antigens or alloantigens.

Macrophages isolated from MSV-induced tumors also can display potent cytostatic or cytolytic effects on tumor cells. Previously we have shown that the macrophages from the tumor that mediate cytoastasis were heterogeneous in size, as determined by 1 g velocity sedimentation (6). We have now examined the distribution profile of cytolytic activity found in regressing and progressing tumors of conventional mice and in progressing tumors of nude mice. Single cell suspensions were prepared from 14 day regressor tumors or from 60 day progressor tumors of conventional mice and treated with anti-Thy 1.2 plus complement before they were subjected to 1 g velocity sedimentation. Progressively growing tumors from nude mice were handled in the same manner but without the anti-Thy 1.2 plus complement treatment. Each fraction was tested for cytolytic activity and the data were normalized to percent activity per fraction (6). The profile of the cytolytic activity in the 14 day regressor (Fig. 2) was very similar to that described earlier for the cytostatic activity. Major peaks occurred at 4 mm/hr and at 5-6 mm/hr.

TABLE IV

Suppression of MIF and MAF Production by Adherent Cells
from the Tumor (aCfT)

Immune Spleen Cells	Stimulator Cells	Suppressor Cells	% Migration Inhibition	Percent Cytotoxicity
$C_{57}Bl/6$ anti-RLo1	RLo1	None	50	38
	RLo1	10% aCfT	-2	1
$C_{57}Bl/6$ anti-MSV	RBL-5	None	25	9
	RBL-5	10% aCfT	1	0

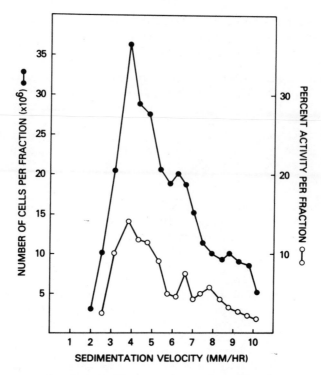

Fig. 2.   One g velocity sedimentation of cells from tumors induced by regressor MSV.   Profile of cytolytic activity (0) as percent activity per fraction.

Different patterns of results were obtained with cells from progressively growing tumors in conventional and nude mice.   Only one peak of cytolytic activity was found with cells from progressively growing tumors in conventional mice at 4 mm/hr (Fig. 3), even though the sedimentation profile of the macrophages from these animals, as measured by latex ingestion, was the same as that seen with macrophages from regressing tumors (data not shown).   No cytolytic activity was detected in the macrophages isolated from progressively growing tumors in nude mice (Fig. 4), and some of the subpopulations of macrophages, as determined by latex ingestion, were absent (data not shown).

To further examine the functional differences between macrophages of nude and conventional tumor-bearing mice, direct comparisons were made of the cytolytic and cytostatic activities of adherent PEC from normal or MSV injected animals and aCfT (Table V). aCfT and aPEC from tumor-bearing conventional animals were active in both the growth inhibition and cytolysis assays, while the aPEC from normal conventional mice had little activity.   In the first experiment with nude mice, no activity was detected in any of the

TABLE V

Comparison of Macrophage-Mediated Cytolysis and Cytostasis of Conventional and Nude
MSV Tumor-Bearing Mice

Exp	Strain	Effector Cells	Growth Inhibition[a]			Cytotoxicity[b]		
			10/1	5/1	2.5/1	200/1	100/1	50/1
1	C57Bl/6	aPEC (normal)	++	-	-	2.4 (1.6)	0.5 (1.3)	0.8 (0.7)
		aPEC (MSV)	+++	++	-	43.4 (1.6)	29.4 (1.3)	23.5 (1.0)
		aCfT (MSV)	+++	++	+	58.0 (0.6)	52.3 (1.2)	43.2 (0.6)
1	Swiss Nu	aPEC (normal)	++	-	-	7.9 (1.2)	NT[c]	NT
		aPEC (MSV)	++	-	-	5.0 (4.2)	-5.4 (1.3)	-2.5 (1.0)
		aCfT (MSV)	-	-	-	2.3 (0.8)	-1.3 (0.5)	-4.5 (0.9)
2	Swiss Nu	aPEC (normal)	+++	++	-	43.5 (3.3)	21.8 (3.4)	NT
		aPEC (MSV)	++	+	-	43.2 (3.4)	22.7 (1.0)	NT
		aCfT (MSV)	-	-	-	2.9 (2.7)	4.2 (2.2)	NT

[a]Effector cells were cultured with target cells (RBL-5) for 44 hrs. The cultures were pulsed
for 4 hrs with ^{3}H-thymidine and harvested. +++, 75–100% inhibition of ^{3}H-TdR uptake; ++, 50–75%,
+, 25–50%; - < 25%.

[b]Cytotoxicity was measured in an 18-hr ^{51}Cr release assay using RBL-5 target cells ($\pm$ standard
error).

[c]Not tested.

Peritoneal exudate cells (PEC) or cells from the tumor (CfT) were purified by adherence to
plastic Petri dishes and then tested for effector cell function, at various effector target
cell ratios, in the growth inhibition or cytotoxicity assay.

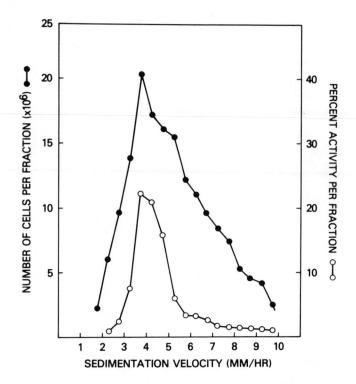

Fig. 3.   One g velocity sedimentation of cells from tumors induced by progressor MSV-H (60 days after injection).   Profile of cyto-lytic activity (O), as percent activity per fraction.

effector populations.   In a subsequent experiment, aPEC from normal and from tumor-bearing mice were active in both assays, but as with the first group of nude mice, the aCfT had no detectable activity. Hence, even when the macrophages in the PEC of the nude mice had been activated (perhaps through bacterial or viral infection), these activated macrophages did not find their way into the tumor.

From these results, several things can be concluded about the macrophages within the tumor and about their capacity to exert antitumor activity.   As measured by 1 g velocity sedimentation, these effector cells are heterogeneous, with several subpopulations evident in regressing tumors and only one in progressing tumors from conventional mice.   It is not clear whether these different size cells represent distinct populations of macrophages with separate differentiation pathways or whether they are macrophages at different stages of activation.   Studies are underway to clarify this point.   From the studies performed with the cells from the tumors induced by MSV in nude mice it is clear that activation of the macrophages to become cytolytic requires the

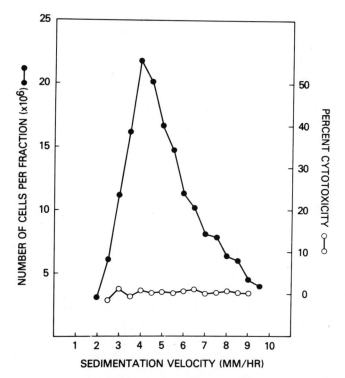

Fig. 4. One g velocity sedimentation of cells from MSV-
induced tumors in nude mice. Profile of cytolytic activity (0),
as percent cytotoxicity in each fraction.

presence of T lymphocytes. Grant et al. (4) had shown a similar
requirement for T cells in the activation of macrophages. However,
they reported that the T cells rendered normal macrophages
specifically growth inhibitory to target lymphoma cells while in
our studies, the T lymphocytes stimulate the macrophages to kill
the tumor targets nonspecifically.

SUMMARY

     In studies on the functional activity of macrophages isolated
from murine sarcoma virus (MSV)-induced tumors, we have found that
these cells may suppress immune responses as well as act as effect-
or cells against the tumor. Previously, we reported that macrophages from the tumor could inhibit the antitumor response by
suppressing proliferation-dependent immune functions. Here, we
demonstrate that macrophages can also suppress the production of
migration inhibition factor (MIF) and macrophage activation factor
(MAF), two lymphocyte activities that are independent of cell
proliferation. Conversely, we and others have found that macro-

phages from the tumor can exert an antitumor, cytolytic effect.
In this study, using 1 g velocity sedimentation separation techniques, we have been able to identify 2-3 subpopulations of cytolytic macrophages in regressing tumors but in progressing tumors,
only the smallest subpopulation of macrophages was active. T cells
appeared to be required for activation of macrophages within the
tumor, since MSV tumors induced in athymic, nude mice did not
contain cytolytic macrophages.

REFERENCES

1. Bloom, B. R., Gaffney, J. and Jimenez, L. J. Immunol. 109
    (1972) 1395.
2. Fossati, G., Holden, H. T. and Herberman, R. B. Cancer Res.
    35 (1975) 2600.
3. Gillespie, G. Y., Hansen, C. B., Hoskins, R. G. and Russell,
    S. W. J. Immunol. 119 (1977) 564.
4. Grant, C. K., Evans, R. and Alexander, P. Cell. Immunol. 8
    (1973) 136.
5. Herberman, R. B. Adv. in Canc. Res. 19 (1974) 207.
6. Holden, H. T., Haskill, J. S., Kirchner, H. and Herberman, R.
    B. J. Immunol. 117 (1976) 440.
7. Holden, H. T., Oldham, R. K., Ortaldo, J. R. and Herberman, R.
    B. J. Natl. Canc. Inst. 58 (1977) 611.
8. Holden, H. T., Kirchner, H. and Herberman, R. B. J. Immunol.
    115 (1975) 327.
9. Kirchner, H., Chused, T. M., Herberman, R. B., Holden, H. T.,
    and Lavrin, D. H. J. Exp. Med. 139 (1974) 1473.
10. Kirchner, H., Muchmore, A. V., Chused, T. M., Holden, H. T.
    and Herberman, R. B. J. Immunol. 114 (1975) 206.
11. Klein, E., Becker, S., Svedmyr, E., Jondal, M. and Vanky, F.
    Ann. N. Y. Acad. Sci. 276 (1976) 207.
12. Landolfo, S., Herberman, R. B. and Holden, H. T. J. Natl.
    Canc. Inst. 59 (1977) 1675.
13. Lavrin, D. H., Herberman, R. B., Nunn, M. and Soares, N. J.
    Natl. Canc. Inst. 51 (1973) 1497.
14. Oehler, J. R., Herberman, R. B. and Holden, H. T. Pharmacol.
    and Therapeut. A 2 (1978) 551.
15. Plata, F., MacDonald, H. R. and Sordat, B. Bibl. Hematol. 43
    (1976) 274.
16. Puccetti, P. and Holden, H. T. Intl. J. Canc. (1978) in press.
17. Ruco, L. P. and Meltzer, M. S. J. Immunol. 119 (1977) 889.
18. Russell, S. W., Gillespie, G. Y. and McIntosh, A. T. J. Immunol.
    118 (1977) 1574.

INVOLVEMENT OF PERITONEAL MACROPHAGES IN CELLULAR RESPONSES TO MASTOCYTOMA IN RESISTANT AND SUSCEPTIBLE MICE

P. FARBER[1], S. SPECTER[2], and H. FRIEDMAN[3]
[1]Dept. of Pathol., Temple Univ. School of Dental Med., Philadelphia, PA, [2]Dept. of Microbiology, Albert Einstein Med. Ctr. and Temple Univ. School of Med., Philadelphia, PA and [3]Dept. of Medical Microbiol., Univ. of South Florida College of Med., Tampa, FL (USA)

Murine mastocytoma cells have been extensively used in recent years for studying various aspects of tumor immunity, as well as cell mediated immunity systems in general (2,7,14). Many studies with these tumor cells have been concerned with T lymphocyte-mediated cytotoxicity using in vitro assays. Furthermore, recent studies have been performed describing ultrastructural changes of lymphocyte mediated cytolysis using scanning and transmission electron microscopy (9). The mastocytoma cell has a characteristic appearance by scanning electron microscopy (SEM) which facilitates its identity (8). In this regard, preliminary studies in this laboratory concerning the morphology of the peritoneal cellular response to mastocytoma cells in susceptible DBA/2 mice suggested that the macrophage was a major host cell type which developed following injection of the tumor cells (5). DBA mice are extremely susceptible to mastocytoma and succumb within 21 days following intraperitoneal injection of 10^6 tumor cells. Macrophages appear in large numbers in the peritoneal exudates within 24 hrs after injection of these tumor cells and increase in number rapidly during the first 4 days. Some of these cells could be observed attaching directly to tumor cells. As the tumor cells proliferated the numbers of macrophages declined so that by 12 days after injection of the mastocytoma, 95% of the peritoneal cells were characteristically tumor cells. Few, if any, lymphocytes were observed either attached to tumor cells or present in the peritoneal exudate cell population. In the present study the peritoneal cellular responses in mastocytoma resistant $C_{57}Bl/6$ mice was similarly examined to ascertain the cells involved in tumor rejection in comparison to the cellular response by susceptible DBA mice which succumb to the tumor.

METHODS AND MATERIALS

P815 mastocytoma cells, originally obtained from the American
Type Culture Collection, Rockville, Maryland, were maintained in
tissue culture or by biweekly intraperitoneal transfer of ascitic
cells into DBA/2 mice (Jackson Memorial Laboratories, Bar Harbor,
Maine). $C_{57}Bl/6$ mice and DBA/2 mice were inoculated at 6 weeks
of age with 10^7 tumor cells. At various times thereafter representative animals were sacrificed and peritoneal cells obtained by
lavage with 8.0 ml RPMI 1640 tissue culture medium (Grand Island
Biological Company, Grand Island, New York). The cells were washed
once in medium and cell numbers adjusted to 3×10^6/ml. The cells
were permitted to attach to poly-L-lysine coated glass coverslips
(Belco Glass, Inc., Vineland, New Jersey) using the method of
Mazia et al. (11) or to acid-cleaned untreated coverslips. Attachment was performed at 37 C in a volume of 1.0 ml medium in 30 mm
plastic petri dishes (Falcon Plastic Company, Oxnard, Georgia), for
30 min. Fixation of attached cells was accomplished at room
temperature using 1% alcohol dehydration and gluteraldehyde for
60 min. Coverslips were stained with Giemsa for examination by
the light microscope. For SEM examination coverslips were first
washed with phosphate buffered saline, dehydrated in a graded series
of alcohols and dried by the critical point method (1,3). The coverslips were attached to aluminum stubs (SPI Supply Co., West Chester,
P.A), coated with gold paladium and examined with an Etec autoscan
microscope operating at 20 kV (Etec Corporation, Haywood, CA).
Peritoneal cells, in suspension, were fixed in 1% gluteraldehyde,
post-fixed in 2% osmium tetroxide, dehydrated in ethanol and im-
bedded in epon for examination by transmission electron microscopy.
Thin sections were stained with 5% uranyl acetate and lead acetate
and examined with a Phillips microscope.

Experimental Results

Mastocytoma cells were evident in the peritoneum of the inoculated mice. The typical appearance of these tumor cells, as seen
by SEM, is illustrated in Fig. 1. These cells measured 6-8 µ in
diameter and were characterized by the presence of numerous short
surface microvilli. The cells readily attached to the glass
(Fig. 2). When grown in tissue culture medium the cells assumed
fusiform shapes (Fig. 3). Transmission electron microscopy of the
tumor cell revealed a highly villious surface, oval shaped nucleus
and various cytoplasmic organelles (Fig. 4).

Within 24-48 hr after injection of mastocytoma cells into the
peritoneum, large numbers of tumor cells were evident, as well as
a few macrophages, which appeared as flattened cells. Fig. 5
shows representative cells from DBA mice 48 hr after tumor cell

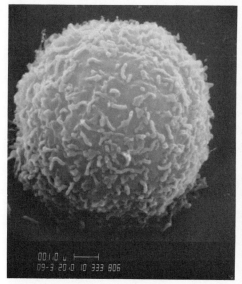 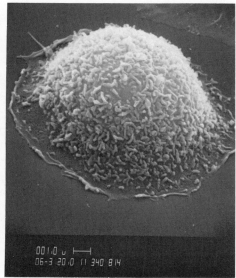

Fig. 1. Scanning electron photomicrograph of a mastocytoma
cell (9000X).

Fig. 2. Scanning electron photomicrograph of a mastocytoma
cell attaching to glass (6000X).

injection. The macrophage has a relatively smooth surface with
some shallow surface ridges and is surrounded by 4 tumor cells.
In contrast, peritoneal macrophages from $C_{57}Bl/6$ mice showed
highly ruffled membranes and many more cell surface folds (Fig. 6).
As the tumor growth progressed, the numbers of macrophages in the
peritoneum of $C_{57}Bl/6$ mice increased, with only an occasional
lymphocyte evident (Fig. 7). By the fourth day of tumor growth
in the peritoneum, many macrophages were seen to be attached to
the tumor cells. The cell in Fig. 7 shows both a lymphocyte,
as evident by its numerous microvilli, and a macrophage with
characteristic ruffled membrane and ridge-like profiles attached
to the tumor cell. Two other mastocytoma cells are present with
macrophages adhering to them.

Within four days after injection of the tumor cells into $C_{57}Bl$
mice, macrophages were much more numerous in the peritoneum of
these animals than in DBA mice. However, while the total
peritoneal cell count between the two strains did not differ
significantly, over 60% of the cells in the $C_{57}Bl/6$ mice appeared
to be macrophages, while fewer than 15% were of this cell class
in the peritoneum of the DBA/2 mice. As is evident in Fig. 8,

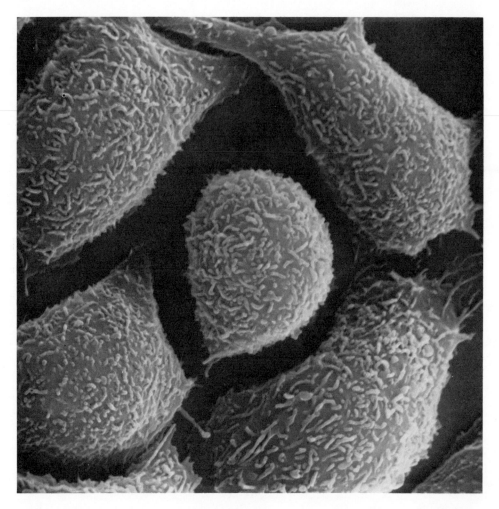

Fig. 3. Scanning electron photomicrograph of mastocytoma cells
grown in tissue culture (10,000X).

showing 5th day peritoneal cells stained by the Giemsa method,
many of the tumor cells are surrounded by macrophages. The dark
staining round cells are the mastocytoma. There is a predominance
of such cells in the peritoneum of the DBA mice. Cells in the
peritoneum of $C_{57}Bl/6$ mice were stained much more lightly and
appeared to be vacuolated macrophages.

When the peritoneal cells were permitted to incubate in tissue
culture for 48 hr, those from DBA/2 mice grew out almost a pure
culture of tumor cells. On the other hand, tumor cells failed to
proliferate from the peritoneal exudate of the $C_{57}Bl/6$ mice. Large

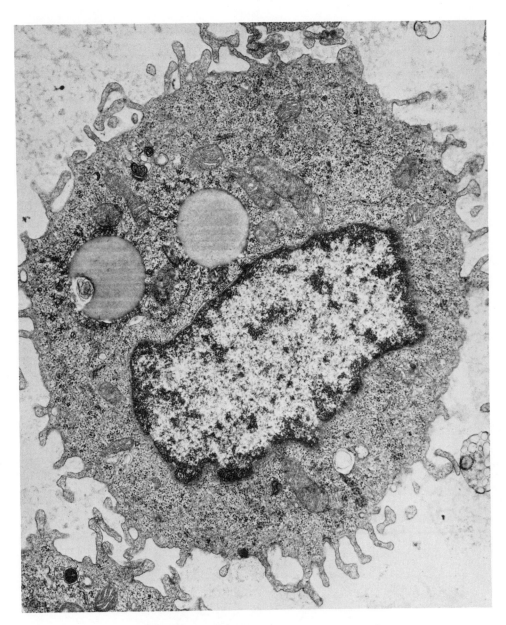

Fig. 4. Transmission electron photomicrograph of a mastocytoma cell (18,000X).

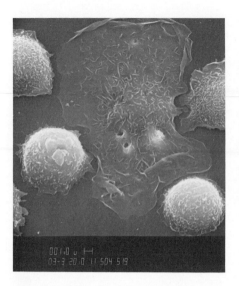

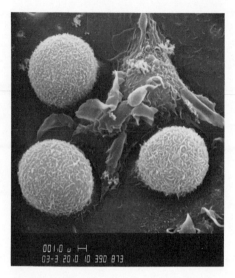

Fig. 5. Scanning electron photomicrograph of peritoneal
cells from a DBA mouse 48 hr
after infection. The cell in
the center is a macrophage
surrounded by four tumor
cells (3000X).

Fig. 6. Scanning electron photomicrograph of peritoneal cells
from a C_{57} mouse 72 hr after
infection. The macrophage has
numerous surface folds, the
three round cells are mastocytoma cells (3000X).

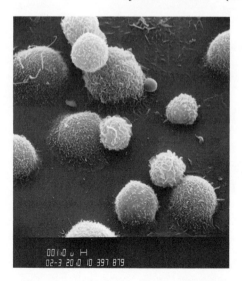

Fig. 7. Scanning electron photomicrograph of peritoneal cells
from a DBA mouse four days after infection. One lymphocyte and
four macrophages are seen attaching to tumor cells.

vacuolated macrophages were apparent, in addition to a few tumor
cells. SEM examination showed mastocytoma cells adhering to
macrophages during various stages of disintegration (Figs. 9 and
10). Some of the tumor cells showed numerous surface blebs
(Fig. 9), whereas others showed puncate lesions (Fig. 10). Transmission electron microscopy of $C_{57}Bl/6$ peritoneal cells, 5 days
after mastocytoma implantation showed contact between macrophage
and tumor cells (Fig. 11). Phagocytic vacuoles containing debris
from the attached mastocytoma cells were evident.

DISCUSSION

A number of previous studies from various laboratories have
shown that activated T lymphocytes are capable of destroying
mastocytoma cells in vitro. In the present study the effects of
peritoneal exudate cells in mastocytoma resistant and susceptible
mouse strains was examined in terms of microscopic structure in
order to assess the possible in vivo role of host effector cells
in tumor rejection. Although small numbers of lymphocytes were
observed following injection of the tumor cells into the peritoneum
of mice, the major host response in both resistant and susceptible
mouse strains appeared to be macrophages. These cells were most
prominent in the resistant $C_{57}Bl/6$ mice and the highly ruffled
surfaces suggested that these were more active than in the
relatively smoother-surfaced macrophages seen in the peritoneum of
DBA/2 mice injected with the same mastocytoma cells. Activated
murine macrophages have been shown to have prominent ridge-like
profiles and ruffled membranes (13). Incubation of PE cells in
vitro revealed that mastocytoma cells from the DBA mice were not
inhibited by the resident macrophages and the tumor cells continued
to proliferate. Conversely, the $C_{57}Bl/6$ macrophages were not able
to inhibit the tumor cells and lyse them in vitro.

The concept that macrophages constitute an important host
response to mastocytoma is supported by evidence from a number
of other laboratories. For example, Lohmann-Matthes et al.,
demonstrated that monolayers of sensitized macrophages were
capable of destroying mastocytoma cells (10). The importance
of macrophages in general, in tumor destruction, has been extensively studied in a number of systems (4). Despite relative
absence of lymphocytes among the peritoneal cells of the mouse
strains studied in this laboratory, the important role of
lymphocytes in stimulating macrophages through lymphokine production cannot be dismissed. Furthermore, the reasons for the
differential macrophage response to mastocytoma cells in DBA/2 and
$C_{57}Bl/6$ mice can only be conjectured at this point. The
vigorous response in $C_{57}Bl/6$ mice may be due to histocompatibility
antigens present on the DBA/2-derived tumor cells. Alternatively,
the tumor cells may secrete a factor which specifically inhibits

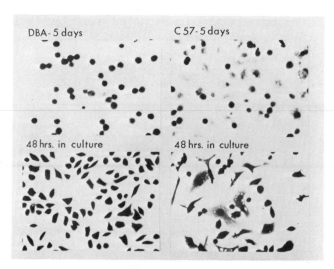

Fig. 8. Giemsa stained peritoneal cells from DBA and C_{57} mice five days after infection. The top panel shows cells after attachment to glass for 30 min and the bottom panel shows cells after 48 hr incubation in tissue culture.

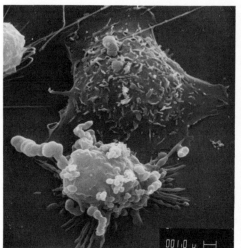

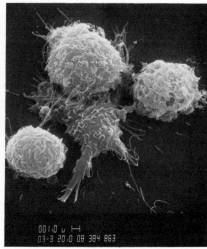

Fig. 9. Scanning electron photomicrograph of C_{57} peritoneal macrophage after 48 hr in tissue culture. The mastocytoma cell has lost its villi and has numerous surface blebs (4000X).

Fig. 10. Scanning electron photomicrograph of a C_{57} macrophage with three tumor cells, two cells have been lysed (3000X).

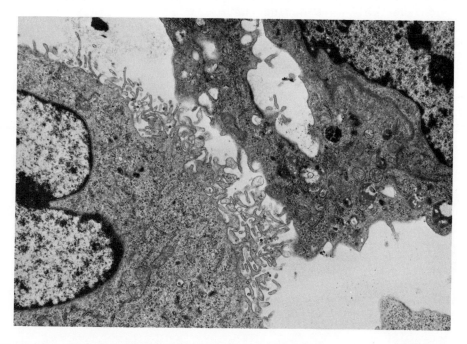

Fig. 11. Transmission electron photomicrograph of C_{57} peritoneal cells 72 hr after infection showing the attachment of a macrophage to a tumor cell. The macrophage has a phagocytic vesicle containing some of the villi from the mastocytoma cell (16,000X).

DBA/2 macrophages but not macrophages from $C_{57}Bl/6$ mice. Such factors produced by mastocytoma cells have been recently described but have been studied mainly in terms of humoral and not cellular immunity (6,12). It is apparent that further studies are warranted to examine in detail the mechanism of both progression and rejection of mastocytoma cells in genetically susceptible and resistant mouse strains.

SUMMARY

The involvement of peritoneal macrophages in rejection of mastocytoma cells in the $C_{57}BL/6$ mice was examined in comparison to similar cell responses in susceptible DBA/2 mice. By means of scanning and transmission electron microscopy it was found that macrophages constituted the major cell class responding to the mastocytoma cells in the peritoneum of both mouse strains. However, in the resistant mouse strain macrophages formed the predominant cell type during the course of tumor growth. Furthermore, tissue culture of peritoneal exudate cells from this resistant mouse strain injected with mastocytoma cells five days earlier failed to grow out tumor cells. On the other hand, macrophages decreased in number in the susceptible DBA/2 mouse strain and tumor cells did grow readily in vitro when peritoneal cells containing tumor cells and macrophages were cultured in vitro. These results indicate that macrophages constitute an important cell class in resistance of a mouse strain which is not susceptible to mastocytoma cells. The ultrastructural study provided some insight into the nature of the cell types involved and their interaction with the tumor cell.

REFERENCES

1. Anderson, T. F. Trans N. Y. Acad. Sci. 13 (1951) 130.
2. Chia, E. and Festenstein, H. Europ. J. Immunol. 3 (1973) 483.
3. Cohen, A. L., Marlow, D. P. and Garner, G. E. J. Microsc. 7 (1968) 331.
4. Evans, R. and Alexander, P. In: Immunobiology of the Macrophage (Ed. D. S. Nelson) Academic Press, Inc., New York, N. Y. (1976).
5. Farber, P. A., Chen, S.-Y., Geissler, R. H. and Friedman, H. Abst. Amer. Soc. Microbiol. (1977).
6. Friedman, H., Specter, S., Kamo, I. and Kateley, J. N. Y. Acad. Sci. 276 (1976) 417.
7. Hawrylko, E. J. Natl. Cancer Inst. 55 (1975) 413.
8. Knutton, S., Summer, M. C. B. and Pasternak, C. A. J. Cell Biol. 66 (1975) 568.
9. Liepins, A., Faanes, R. B., Lifter, J., Choi, Y. S., and de Harven, E. Cell Immunol. 28 (1977) 109.
10. Lohmann-Matthes, M. L., Schipper, H., and Fischer, H. Europ. J. Immun. 2 (1972) 45.
11. Mazia, D., Schatten, G. and Sale, W. S. J. Cell Biol. 66 (1975) 198.
12. Normann, S. J. J. Natl. Cancer Inst. 60 (1978) 1091.
13. Polliack, A. and Gordon, S. Lab Invest. 33 (1975) 469.
14. Thorn, R. M. and Henney, C. S. J. Immunol. 117 (1976) 2213.

SYNGENEIC ANTI-TUMOR GLOBULIN: SUPPRESSION OF MOUSE PLASMACYTOMA

BY THE IgG2 FRACTION

T. N. HARRIS and S. HARRIS

The Joseph Stokes, Jr., Research Institute of The
Children's Hospital of Philadelphia, and Department
of Pediatrics, School of Medicine, University of
Pennsylvania, Philadelphia, Pennsylvania (USA)

A substantial body of literature has indicated that anti-
tumor antibody can affect the rate of growth of experimental
tumors. In most of the experimental studies reported the effect
of passively administered antibody has been to enhance tumor
growth (4). However, a number of reports have indicated a suppressive effect of antibody on graft or tumor transplants in host
animals, and this difference has been ascribed to different experimental conditions (13), to different amounts or classes of the
antibodies injected (13), or to time of collection of serum relative to immunization (3).

Our data suggesting that differences in the class of antibody
could be involved in the enhancement or rejection of foreign
tissue were obtained in studies of the rejection of skin allografts exchanged between strains of inbred mice, in which alloantibodies injected into the grafted mice caused effects ranging
from accelerated rejection to prolonged retention of the grafts
(6). Alloantibody with relatively more of the IgG2 class was
associated with accelerated rejection of the allografts, and those
with more IgG1 class antibody, with prolonged retention (5). Since
similar mechanisms may well be involved in the rejection or enhancement of foreign tissues, both allogeneic tissue grafts and
tumors, a study was undertaken on the effects of anti-tumor antibodies on grafts of a transplanted tumor in a syngeneic host,
using antibodies produced in other syngeneic mice. Comparisons
were made between the original antibody-containing globulin and
IgG2 preparations of the same globulin pools. The latter were
by precipitation, or by anti-IgG1 immunoadsorbent, or by adsorption
to an elution from protein A-bearing staphylococci.

531

MATERIALS AND METHODS

Mice and tumors. Balb/c mice were from the Jackson Laboratory (Bar Harbor, Maine), or the Charles River Laboratories Inc.
(Wilmington, MA). A plasmacytoma, MOPC 315, was obtained from
Dr. Michael Potter of the NIH (Bethesda, MD) and propagated by
serial subcutaneous (s.c.) passage of small fragments of solid
tumor. For the experiments in tumor growth, cells were teased
from growing tumors, and injected intraperitoneally (i.p.) into
other Balb/c mice. Tumor cells thus obtained were washed and suspended at 6 x 10^6 cells/ml for the tumor growth experiments.

Balb/c anti MOPC 315 globulin. Balb/c mice, 2-3 months of
age, were given a priming injection of 1 x 10^7 MOPC 315 cells
treated with 0.1 M iodoacetate (1). Three weeks later they were
injected s.c. with 1 x 10^5 fresh MOPC 315 cells. A half week before the injection of the living cells and at one-week intervals
thereafter the mice received i.p. 0.5 ml of incomplete Freund's
adjuvant. Ascitic fluid was tapped on day 12 following the injection of the live tumor cells, and at intervals of 3-4 days
thereafter. The fluids were pooled by day of tapping, cleared
by centrifugation, stirred for 1 hr at 4 C with an equal volume
of fluorocarbon (Freon 113, DuPont Co., (Wilmington, Del) and
centrifuged for 30 min at 16,000 RPM. The aqueous, upper, phase
was treated with ammonium sulfate at 27% saturation to remove
fibrinogen. The supernate was brought to 50% saturation and kept
overnight at 4 C. The precipitate was then dissolved in half the
original volume and dialyzed overnight against phosphate buffered
saline.

Rabbit anti mouse IgG1 serum. This was prepared by inject-
ing papain digest of MOPC 21 tumor extracts, which had been passed
through anti-IgG2 columns. The rabbits were bled between 3 and 7
weeks and the sera were examined for absence of anti-IgG2 contamination by IDF as described elsewhere (7). Solid immunoadsorbent
of anti IgG1 serum was prepared by a modification of a method of
Axen et al. (2). A portion of the effluent was concentrated
4 times for examination against anti-IgG1 by IDF. A loss of
30-40% of IgG2 was incurred in this procedure.

Staphylococcal absorption and elution. The adsorbent was
prepared by growing Staphylococcus aureus, strain Cowan A., on
Trypticase soy agar in Blake bottles. After 24 hr the organisms
were harvested, washed twice, suspended and treated with formal-
dehyde at 0.5% for 3 hr at room temperature. After washing, the
organisms were placed at 85 C for 5 min and cooled. NaN$_3$ was
added at 0.2% and the suspension was stored at 4 C. For preparation of the eluates, anti-tumor globulin was treated with organisms
at levels known to be adequate to remove all IgG2a by IDF of a concentrated portion. After incubation the organisms were centrifuged,

washed, and suspended in glycine buffer 0.1 M, pH 2.8, for 30 min
at 0 C. The eluate was concentrated to the original volume of
the globulin treated and dialyzed versus RPMI 1640.

RESULTS

Original anti-tumor globulins. The anti-tumor globulins were
tested in vivo for their effect on growth of MOPC 315 cells. For
these tests, the cells were collected 7-9 days after intraperitoneal inoculation of 1 x 10^7 tumor cells. The cells harvested
were washed and suspended at 6 x 10^6/ml. Of this suspension,
0.2 ml was incubated for 30 min at 37 C with 1 ml of the globulin
solution, and 0.1 ml was injected subcutaneously at two sites into
Balb/c mice, in groups of 4. Tumor growth was measured as the
mean of two diameters of each tumor, at intervals of 2 or 3 days.
When the anti-tumor globulins, obtained between days 12 and 32
after the immunization described above were tested, it was found
that about one half of the 12-day globulins caused some decrease
in the growth rate and about one half of the later day globulins
(20-32 days) caused some enhancement of growth of the tumor.

Precipitation with rabbit anti-mouse IgG1 serum. Preliminary
titrations were done on several preparations of the later day globulins to determine the relative amount of anti-IgG1 necessary to
remove all evidence of IgG1 globulin. These were then treated
with the anti-IgG1 serum at the level indicated. After incubation
for 60 min at 37 C and overnight at 4 C, the precipitates were removed and the supernates were examined for their effect on growth
of MOPC 315 tumors, as in the experiments on the original globulins
described above. The results obtained with 5 typical preparations
are shown in Table I, where the mean tumor diameters on day 20 are
shown for the experimental group, over the control group in that
experiment. It can be seen that whereas the original globulins
(right side) showed either no effect or slight enhancement of
tumor growth, the anti-IgG1 treated preparations reduced the
tumor growth to between 8% and 25% of control tumors.

Anti-IgG1-column preparations. A larger number of experiments was done with anti-tumor globulins treated with an anti-
IgG1 absorption column. Globulin passed through an anti-IgG1
Sepharose 4B column showed loss of the IgG1, as determined by
IDF versus 4 times concentrated portions, but also a loss of
30-45% of IgG2 globulin, as determined by radial immunodiffusion
(11). The effluents were restored to the original volume of globulin and were examined without concentration to replace the IgG2
lost. Such experiments are summarized in Fig. 1. The growth of
control tumors caused by cells incubated with RPMI 1640, obtained
as an arithmetic mean of all experiments in which these column
preparations were tested, are shown by the solid circles connected

TABLE I

Effect on MOPC 315 Tumor Growth of Syngeneic Anti-Tumor Globulin:
Anti-IgG1 Precipitated and Original Globulin

Globulin from MOPC 315 Immuniz. No.	Anti-IgG1 Precipitated Preparations		Original Globulin	
	Exptl Group	Mean Control Diameters on Day 20: Exptl/Control mm	Exptl Group	Mean Tumor Diameters on Day 20: Exptl/Control mm
55	71B	5.8/14.6	56B	23.0/12.6
	78B	5.2/19.0	59B	21.0/17.0
56	71C	4.5/14.6	61B	26.0/15.6
	78C	1.7/19.0	66C	20.8/15.8
58	63C	7.3/25.0	68C	14.5/15.5
60	84B	6.9/20.0	86D	21.4/15.0
61	84C	6.5/20.0	81C	16.2/17.9

with solid lines. The anti-IgG1 column-treated preparations all
caused reduction in the rate of tumor growth, but in several
patterns. Of 32 tests, on 20 anti-IgG1 column preparations, derived from 13 immunizations, shown in this Fig., 11 showed complete suppression of growth over a 45-day period of examination.
Thirteen groups showed slight tumor growth, to a mean diameter
of less than 5 mm by day 45, and 8 others, a somewhat higher rate
of growth, to a mean tumor diameter between 5 and 10 mm by day
35, at which time occasional deaths of the mice terminated the
experiment. Control preparations from normal Balb/c globulin
passed through the anti-IgG1 column yielded the results shown by
the open circles (mean values from 4 experiments).

Specificity of the growth-suppressing anti-IgG1 column preparations. A pool of column preparations which showed such suppression of growth of MOPC 315 was absorbed with various preparations of MOPC 315 tumor, or other tumors, to determine the specificity of the growth suppression. Absorption of this anti-IgG1

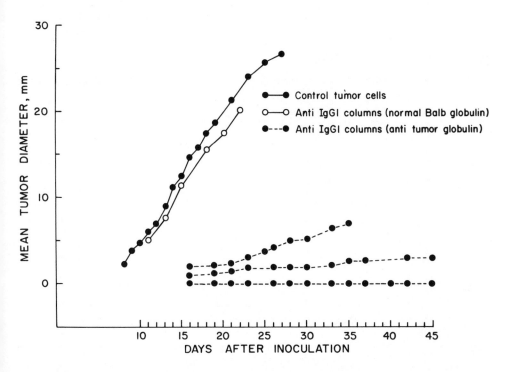

Fig. 1. Growth of MOPC 315 tumors following inoculation of tumor
cells treated with anti-tumor globulin which had been passed
through columns of anti-mouse IgG1 immunoadsorbent and control
material. Three typical patterns of tumor growth for the anti-
IgG1 treated anti-tumor globulin are shown (broken lines).

column pool, at 1:2, was done with 1×10^8 fresh MOPC 315 cells/
ml, or with lyophilized cell membrane fragments from this tumor.
As control materials cell membrane fragments of 2 unrelated
plasmacytomas, MOPC 31C and 173, were used for absorption, as
well as another tumor of Balb/c mice, a cultured brain tumor,
BBA. Table II shows the mean diameters of tumors in mice given
the control tumor cells, incubated only with RPMI 1640, and of
tumor cells incubated with the anti-IgG1 column pool to be used
for absorption. The untreated cells show the typical rapid growth
of the tumor, with deaths beginning after the 20-day measurement.
Tumor cells treated with the anti-IgG1 column pool show the typical suppression of growth, with tumors palpable only at day 18
and continuing to grow slowly to a mean diameter of 3.5 mm by day
32. Absorption of the pool with whole MOPC 315 cells caused

TABLE II

Mean Tumor Diameter (mm) Following Inoculation of MOPC 315 Cells Treated with
Various Preparations of Anti-Tumor Globulin

Tumor Cells Treated with:	No. of Groups	Day								
		11	13	15	18	20	22	25	27	29
RPMI 1640	6	4.6	7.9	11.5	15.3	19.4				
Anti-IgG1 column pools[a]	6	0	0	0	1.4	2.0	2.4	2.8	3.0	3.2
Same, absorbed with:										
MOPC 315 cells	2	10.0	11.3	15.4	20.2					
MOPC 315 membrane	3	2.1	4.6	9.2	15.1	18.9	20.5			
MOPC 31C membrane	2	0	0	0	0	0	0	1.2	1.4	1.8
MOPC 173 membrane	2	0	0	0	0	0	0	0	0	0
BBA tumor cells	2	0	0	0	1.7	4.0	5.5	6.5		

[a]Prepared from Balb/c anti MOPC 315 tumor globulin

reversal of the growth suppression, with unusually large tumors
from the early days of observation. After absorption with the cell
membrane fragments of MOPC 315 also, the pool did not cause suppression of tumor growth.

The results of the absorption with 3 unrelated tumors are
shown in the last 3 rows of the Table. Although there were different degrees of growth suppression, it can be seen that none of
these absorbed materials brought about loss of the suppressive
effect of the pool.

IgG2a fractions of anti-tumor globulin by elution from protein
A bearing staphylococci. As another test of the class of anti-
tumor globulin which suppresses the growth of MOPC 315, 3 preparations of Balb/c anti MOPC 315 globulin were absorbed with formalin-
fixed protein A bearing staphylococci and an eluate of each was prepared as described above, since it was shown by Kronvall et al. (10)
that staphylococcal protein A binds IgG2a of mouse globulin, but
not IgG1, 2b or 3. These eluates, returned to the volume of globulin treated, were incubated with MOPC 315 cells, as in the case
of the column effluents, and the cells were then injected into
Balb/c recipients to test for any effect on tumor growth. The
results of 3 experiments are shown in Table III. Again the mean
tumor diameters of the control groups of the 3 experiments are
shown in the first row. Tumor diameters obtained with cells treated
with the eluates are shown in the next 3 rows. In two cases no
tumor growth was observed. In one case there was a late growth of
tumors, the experiment being terminated by the death of one mouse
of this group after day 27. Control material of staphylococcal
eluates of normal Balb/c globulin produced tumor diameters quite
similar to those of the control tumor cells above (means of two
experiments).

DISCUSSION

In this study syngeneic anti-tumor globulins showed a range
of effects on growth of MOPC 315 tumors, from some suppression of
growth in about half of the early globulins, to some enhancement
in about half of the late globulins. The possibility that two
such effects could be caused by antibodies obtained at different
times, as well as earlier evidence that alloantibodies of IgG2 and
IgG1 class were involved in the rejection and enhanced retention
of skin grafts respectively (5), suggested the testing of fractions
of the anti-tumor antibody containing globulin of a single subclass,
especially IgG2. This was approached in three ways: by precipitation with anti mouse IgG1 serum, or passing through columns of
anti-IgG1 immunoadsorbents, or adsorbing to and eluting from protein A-bearing staphylocci.

TABLE III

Mean Tumor Diameter (mm) Following Inoculation of MOPC 315 Cells Treated with
Elutes from Staphylococcal Absorption of Anti-Tumor and Control Globulin

Tumor Cells Treated with:	Exp No.	Day										
		8	11	13	15	18	20	22	25	27	29	32
RPMI 1640[a]		2.6	5.3	9.1	11.6	15.8	19.2	21.4				
Eluates of staphylococcal absorption of anti tumor globulin	131C	0	0	0	0	0	0	0	0	0	0	0
	133E	0	0	0	0	0	1.3	2.7	5.1	6.3	0	0
	135E	0	0	0	0	0	0	0	0	0	0	0
Same, from normal Balb/c globulin	142F	0	4.8	7.1	10.6	13.3	14.7	16.7				

[a]Mean of control groups of these experiments.

The precipitation method yielded preparations which led to mean tumor diameters, on day 20 after the inoculation, usually less than one quarter of those of control tumors. Considerably more work was done with anti-tumor globulins prepared by passage through columns of anti-IgG1-Sepharose. These column preparations, whether from original 20-day globulins which showed no effect on tumor growth, or from those which enhanced the growth of MOPC 315 tumors, suppressed tumor growth to between one third and one tenth of the control tumor diameters, and in several cases caused complete suppression. Additional support for the IgG2 character of this antibody was given by the suppression of tumor growth by eluates from absorption of the anti-tumor globulin with protein A-bearing staphylococci. Anti MOPC 315 specificity was indicated by the fact that column preparations of the anti-tumor globulins which were absorbed with MOPC 315 cells or their cell membrane fragments were no longer able to suppress tumor growth, whereas similar treatment with cells of another Balb/c tumor or cell membrane fragments from unrelated plasmacytomas did not affect the suppression.

A number of factors have been suggested in the literature to explain the range of effects of antibodies, from enhancement of tumor growth to suppression. Among studies reported on tumor-growth suppression or inhibition by antibody, reviewed by Ting and Herberman (13), differences have been attributed to the class of antibodies involved. Thus, Rubinstein et al. (12) have suggested a role of IgG2 antibody because this subclass showed a synergistic effect with IgM class of antibody in suppressing tumor growth. On the other hand Johnson et al. (9) found suppression of tumor growth in preparations of globulin treated with staphylococcal protein A and therefore reflecting the IgG1 class. This effect was apparently dependent on collaboration with normal host cells.

The present studies were suggested by our earlier work with skin grafts, which, as indicated above, led to the association of accelerated rejection of allografts with IgG2-class, and of prolonged retention by IgG1-class antibody. In work on tumor growth we found that the IgG1 preparation of alloantibody-containing globulin led to enhanced growth of allogeneic tumors (8). In the present investigation the effect of the IgG2 class antibody has been examined with transplants of one plasmacytoma. The work was done in Balb/c mice, since the normal course of plasmacytoma in this strain is progressive growth of the tumor until death of the host. Three kinds of preparations which exhibited the effects of, or were restricted to, the IgG2 class of antibody led to suppression of growth of the tumor. Whether this is a direct effect of the antibody on the tumor cells or involves cooperation with cells of the host animal is being examined in current experiments.

ACKNOWLEDGEMENT

This investigation was supported by Grants Number CA 14487 and CA 17181, awarded by the National Cancer Institute, DHEW, and Grant IM 3C of the American Cancer Society.

REFERENCES

1. Apffel, C. A., Arnason, B. G., Peters, J. H., Nature, 209 (1966) 694.
2. Axen, R., Porath, J., Ernback, S., Nature, 214 (1967) 1302.
3. Baldwin, W. M., Cohen, N., Transplantation, 15 (1973) 633.
4. Feldman, J. D., Adv. Immunol., 15 (1972) 167.
5. Harris, T. N., Harris, S., Immunology, 25 (1973) 409.
6. Harris, T. N., Harris, S., Bocchieri, M. H., Farber, M. B., Ogburn, C. A., Transplantation, 14 (1972) 495.
7. Harris, T. N., Harris, S., Henri, E. M., J. Immunol. Methods, 8 (1975) 203.
8. Harris, T. N., Harris, S., Henri, E. M., Farber, M. B., J. Natl. Cancer Inst., 60 (1978) 167.
9. Johnson, R. J., Pastenack, G. R., Shin, H. S., J. Immunol., 118 (1977) 489.
10. Kronvall, G., Grey, H. M., Williams, R. C., Jr., J. Immunol., 105 (1970) 1116.
11. Mancini, G., Carbonara, A. O., Heremans, J. F., Immunochemistry, 2 (1965) 235.
12. Rubinstein, P., Decary, F., Streun, E. W., J. Exp. Med., 140 (1974) 591.
13. Ting, C. C., Herberman, R. B., International review of experimental pathology (Eds. G. W. Richter and M. A. Epstein), 15 (1976) 93.

MECHANISM OF RESISTANCE OF MICE TO SYNGENEIC METHYLCHOLANTHRENE

INDUCED FIBROSARCOMAS

D. S. NELSON, M. NELSON and K. E. HOPPER

Kolling Institute of Medical Research
Royal North Shore Hospital of Sydney
St. Leonards, (Australia)

There is abundant evidence to suggest that macrophages play important roles in the expression of immunity to many experimental tumors (2,4,12,17,31). Agents and procedures which increase or decrease the activity of the RES can increase or decrease resistance to tumors. Activated macrophages can selectively damage tumor cells in vitro. Macrophages are often present in tumors and there may be a relationship between their presence or activity and the outcome of the host-tumor confrontation. The experiments to be summarized here reflect three approaches to determining the role of macrophages in resistance to tumors. First, it was reasoned that if macrophages were important in vivo, treatment of mice with anti-macrophage agents (silica or carrageenan) would inhibit resistance and promote tumor growth. Second, if macrophages exert cytotoxic effects in vitro, the peritoneal cavity should provide an excellent source of effector cells for studies of anti-tumor cytotoxicity. Third, the demonstration that tumor cells secrete substances with anti-macrophage and anti-tumor activity suggested that the acquisition of tumor immunity might entail the development of mechanisms for overcoming what might be viewed as the tumor cell's own defenses.

MATERIALS AND METHODS

The tumors had been induced by s.c. injection of 1 mg of 3-methylcholanthrene in olive oil. Their biological and immunological behavior and maintenance (in vivo and in vitro) have been described in detail elsewhere (6,8,9,15,16,18-21,28). They included tumors designated C-1, C-4, C-9 and C-15 of CBA/J mice, H-1 and H-7 of CBA/H mice and A-1 and A-2 of A/J mice.

Most of the tumors elicited concomitant immunity. Mice bearing s.c. isografts of those tumors can resist the growth of a second tumor isograft in the footpad. Resistance occurs in two phases: an early, specific phase about 7 days after the primary isograft, in which there is resistance to challenge with 5×10^5 cells of the same tumor as that growing s.c.; and a later, nonspecific phase 14-21 days after the primary isograft, in which there is also resistance to other fibrosarcomas. Tumors inducing concomitant immunity do not metastasize in normal mice. In thymus-deprived mice those same tumors fail to elicit concomitant immunity but do metastasize.

One tumor (H-7, of CBA/H mice) does not elicit concomitant immunity but does elicit "sinecomitant" immunity. A s.c. injection of 2.5×10^4 cells does not give rise to a tumor but renders the mice specifically resistant to challenge in the footpad with 5×10^5 H-7 cells 1 to 4 weeks later.

The agents used to treat mice included silica (LiChroSorb, Merck), λ-corrageenan (kindly provided by Dr. Donald W. Renn, Marine Colloids, Inc.), niridazole ("Ambilhar", the gift of Ciba-Geigy, Australia Ltd.), reserpine ("Serpasil", Ciba-Geigy) and irradiation from a ^{60}Co source. Dosages are given in the footnotes to the Tables and full details elsewhere (19,20).

Winn assays (30) were carried out with splenic or peritoneal lymphocytes (non-adherent cells) from mice immune to H-7. The cells were mixed with target H-7 cells at a ratio of 7.5 to 1 and injected into the feet of irradiated (450 rad) non-immune CBA/H mice. Thy and Ly phenotypes of effector lymphocytes were determined with antisera kindly provided by Dr. I. F. C. McKenzie (24).

Cytotoxicity was assayed either (a) by measuring the release of ^{51}Cr from labeled target tumor cells after 4 to 22 hr incubation or (b) by measuring ^{125}I release from target cells labeled with ^{125}I-iododeoxyuridine after 48 hr incubation (16,27). Activity is expressed as percent specific lysis:

$$\frac{\text{counts released in test} - \text{spontaneous release}}{\text{total releasable counts} - \text{spontaneous release}} \times 100$$

Cells were separated on the basis of sedimentation velocity at 1 g essentially as described by Miller and Phillips (13), or on the basis of adherence to plastic Petri dishes (6×10^6 cells in 20% fetal calf serum and Hanks' solution for 3 hr at 37 C); adherent cells were recovered by treatment with 0.02% EDTA (26).

Macrophage mitosis was estimated by counting the proportion

of adherent, resident peritoneal cells incorporating tritiated thymidine (as shown by autoradiography) after brief incubation (14,18).

RESULTS

Effects of agents influencing macrophages and delayed-type hypersensitivity (19,20). Treatment with silica (0.2 mg i.v.) or carrageenan (0.5 mg i.p. daily for 4 days) promoted the initial growth of 5 out of 7 tumors in the footpads of non-immune mice. As also observed by Keller (10), however, growth promotion was critically dependent on the timing of the injections in relation to tumor challenge. Silica had little effect on the expression of concomitant or sinecomitant immunity. Carrageenan, however, tended to decrease immunity, i.e., to increase tumor growth in the footpads of immune mice. This effect was most pronounced in the case of H-7 (Table I).

Silica and carrageenan had, in these experiments, no effect on blood monocyte counts and little effect on peritoneal macrophage counts. Because of this it was thought that depression of

TABLE I

Effect of Carrageenan on Immunity to H-7 Tumor

Mice	Tumor Growth in Footpad 7 Days After Challenge (units of 0.1 mm, mean ± s.e.)
Normal	10.3 ± 1.1
Immune[b]	2.2 ± 0.2
Immune + carrageenan[c]	9.3 ± 2.0

[a]Data from ref. (20).

[b]Injected with 2.5×10^4 H-7 cells 18 days before challenge.

[c]0.5 mg of λ-carrageenan injected i.p. daily for 4 days before challenge.

immunity by carrageenan might reflect another of its pharmacological effects, depression of delayed-type hypersensitivity (DTH). The effect of other agents reported to depress DTH was therefore

examined. The reported depressive effect of sublethal irradiation, niridazole and reserpine was confirmed in experiments on
DTH to sheep erythrocytes. These agents were also found to depress not only sinecomitant immunity to H-7 (Table II) but also
concomitant immunity, including nonspecific concomitant immunity
(Table III). (Paradoxically, the growth of isografts in non-
immune mice tended to be reduced by similar treatment; the basis
of this phenomenon has not been further explored).

TABLE II

Effect of Agents Inhibiting Delayed-Type
Hypersensitivity of Immunity to H-7 Tumor[a]

Mice	Tumor Growth in Footpad 7 Days After Challenge (units of 0.1 mm, mean ± s.e.)
Normal	9.2 ± 2.0
Immune[b]	
no treatment	0.7 ± 0.2
irradiation[c]	6.0 ± 1.6
niridazole[c]	4.7 ± 1.6
reserpine[c]	3.8 ± 1.2

[a]Data from ref. (20).

[b]Injected with 2.5 x 10^4 H-7 cells 17 days before challenge.

[c]Irradiation: 500 rads 3 days before challenge.
Niridazole: 20 mg/kg orally 1 day before challenge.
Reserpine: 1 mg/kg i.v. on day of challenge and 3 days later.

Cells initiating tumor rejection. If DTH is involved in
immunity to these tumors one might picture tumor rejection
reactions as interactions between tumor antigens and specifically
committed lymphocytes, leading to a local accumulation of other
mononuclear cells which could serve as nonspecific effectors.
This view is consistent with an earlier finding that in Winn
(local passive transfer) assays of anti-tumor effector cells the
host contributes an immunologically uncommitted accessory cell
derived from a radiosensitive precursor in bone marrow (28). If
this is so, the cells initiating tumor rejection would be expected
to have Thy and Ly phenotypes typical of cells initiating DTH.
Splenic lymphocytes from mice immune to H-7 suppressed the growth

TABLE III

Effect of Agents Inhibiting Delayed-Type-Hypersensitivity
on Nonspecific Concomitant Immunity[a]

Mice	Tumor Growth in Footpad 11 Days After Challenge (units 0.1 mm, mean ± s.e.)
Normal	14.0 ± 3.4
Immune[b]	
no treatment	0.5 ± 0.3
irradiation[c]	8.5 ± 2.2
niridazole[c]	5.7 ± 3.2
reserpine[c]	4.7 ± 2.3

[a]Data from ref (19).

[b]Mice injected s.c. with 10^7 C-4 cells and challenged 14 days
later with 5×10^5 C-15 cells.

[c]See Table II for treatment schedules.

of H-7 in the feet of nonimmune CBA/H mice. This capacity was
abolished by treatment with anti-Thy-1.2 and complement, was much
reduced by treatment with anti-Ly-1.1 and complement but was un-
affected by treatment with anti-Ly-2.1 or anti-Ly-3.2 and complement. Thus, the specifically reactive lymphocytes are Thy-1[+],
Ly-2[−] and Ly-3[−], i.e., they have the markers characteristic of T
cells initiating DTH reactions (7,29).

Anti-tumor effector cells in mouse peritoneal cavities. Previous experiments had shown that spleens of tumor-bearing (concomitantly immune) mice contained anti-tumor effector cells detectable in visual microcytotoxicity assays (8). Effectors were
also detected in spleens and unstimulated peritoneal cavities in
assays ^{125}I release, over a 48 hr period, from ^{125} IUdR labeled
target cells, but not by means of ^{51}Cr release, over a 4 to 72 hr
period (16). As shown in Table IV, such cells were almost unde-
tectable (in ^{125}I release assays) in whole resident peritoneal
cell populations from normal, non-immune mice. If, however, exudates had been induced by proteose-peptone or by i.p. injection
with Salmonella enteritidis 11RX (1), the peritoneal exudates
contained effectors as active as those from mice bearing a tumor
(C-4). Furthermore, the cells in each case were active not only
against C-4 but also against another tumor (C-15) though not
against normal mouse fibroblasts.

Thus, both tumor carriage and nonspecific stimuli can lead to the appearance in mouse peritoneal cavities of cells which are slowly cytotoxic to target fibrosarcoma cells, discriminating between them and normal fibroblasts but lacking individual tumor

TABLE IV

Anti-Tumor Effector Cells in Mouse Peritoneal Cavities

Source of Peritoneal Cells	Percent Specific Lysis of ^{115}IUdR Labeled C-4 Target Cells at Effector: Target Ratio of 25:1
Normal resident	4 ± 2
Bearing C-4, resident	39 ± 11
Normal, proteose-peptone exudate	21 ± 2
Normal, S. enteritidis infected	32 ± 5

specificity.   Two approaches have been made towards characterizing these cells.   When peritoneal cells from mice bearing C-4 were separated according to their sedimentation velocity (Table V) activity was found in fractions containing medium-sized to large cells, many of which were Neutral Red-positive.   Medium sized cells were more active than the largest cells.   When the cells were separated on the basis of their adherence to plastic, non-adherent cells were essentially inactive.   Those adherent cells that were recovered were active, though not to the same extent as the original population (Table VI).   The effectors are, therefore, very tentatively identified, on the basis of size and adherence, as monocytes and macrophages.

Cell mobilization in tumor-bearing hosts.   Many tumors have been shown to produce substances which decrease macrophage mobility in vitro and reduce monocyte/macrophage entry into inflammatory reactions in vivo (3,21.25).   Despite this, macrophages enter growing tumors, and challenge tumors can be rejected by mechanisms which may well require the participation of macrophages (2,17).   Three classes of host responses could overcome this "anti-macrophage" barrier: the development of immunity to the substances produced by tumors - there seems to be little evidence for or against this; the development of a macrophage delivery system

TABLE V

Separation, by Sedimentation Velocity, of Peritoneal
Anti-Tumor Effector Cells from Mice Bearing C-4 Tumor for 7 Days

Fraction	Sedimentation Velocity,mm/h	Percent Cells Taking Up Neutral Red	Percent Specific Lysis of C-4 Target Cells at Effector:Target Ratio of 25:1
Whole		43	49 ± 3
1	0 - 3.6	0	16 ± 3
2	3.6 - 4.2	31	29 ± 1
3	4.2 - 5.0	59	52 ± 2
4	5.0 6.0	66	63 ± 4
5	6.0 - 8.4	77	48 ± 3
6	above 8.4	88	36 ± 2

TABLE VI

Adherence of Cytotoxic Effector Cells to Plastic

Population of Peritoneal Effector Cells[a]	Percent Specific Lysis of C-4 Target Cells at Effector:Target Ratio	
	12.5:1	25 : 1
Whole	41 ± 2	61 ± 1
Non-adherent	4 ± 1	6 ± 1
Adherent	27 ± 3	22 ± 1

[a]From mice concomitantly immune to C-4 7 days after s.c. injection of 10^7 C-4 cells.

sufficiently powerful to breach the barrier - DTH reactions might
serve such a purpose; and an increase in the numbers and activity
of mononuclear phagocytes.

There has long been good evidence for this third possibility.
In the classical experiments of Old et al.(23) increased clearance
of i.v. injected material provided evidence of macrophage stimulation. New monocyte production by the bone marrow can also be increased (5). Concomitant immunity can be accompanied by an increase
in macrophage-mediated resistance to Listeria infection (22). Mature macrophages resident in the peritoneal cavity normally show
little evidence of spontaneous proliferation, but can undergo quite
extensive mitosis in mice bearing tumors (18),(Table VII).

TABLE VII

Macrophage Stimulation in Tumor-Bearing Mice[a]

Mice (CBA/J)	Resident Peritoneal Macrophages Incorporating Tritiated Thymidine Maximum Percentage	Time After Tumor Graft
Normal	2.1 ± 0.3	–
With C-1 tumor	8.0 ± 1.6	7 days
With C-4 tumor	6.8 ± 0.6	7 days
With C-9 tumor	5.1 ± 1.1	12 days

[a]Data from ref. 18

Experiments were carried out to determine the extent to which
macrophages could be delivered to a site of tumor challenge in
concomitantly immune mice. Normal mice and mice bearing C-4 for
7 days were injected i.p. with 1 x 10^5 C-4 cells, 1 x 10^5 C-15
cells or saline. Their peritoneal cavities were washed out 24 hr
later and total and differential cell counts made. In the mice
bearing C-4 and injected with C-4 there was a significant increase
in the number of cells identified morphologically as macrophages
(Table VIII) but there was no such increase in macrophages in any
other group, nor in the numbers of other types of cell in any group.
Notably, the increase was specifically elicited by C-4 cells, which
is consistent with the specificity of this phase of concomitant
immunity. In another experiment, challenge with C-15 cells elicited an increase in macrophages in mice with nonspecific concomitant immunity after carriage of C-4 for 14 days.

TABLE VIII

Effect of Intraperitoneal Tumor Challenge On the
Macrophage Content of the Peritoneal Cavity

Mice Bearing Syngeneic Tumor	Intraperitoneal Injection	Macrophage Content of Peritoneal Fluid 24 hr later ($\times 10^{-3}$, mean ± s.e.)
None	saline	1122 ± 126
None	10^5 C-15 cells	2276 ± 499
None	10^5 C-4 cells	1605 ± 377
C-4, 7 days	saline	1742 ± 569
C-4, 7 days	10^5 C-15 cells	2342 ± 549
C-4, 7 days	10^5 C-4 cells	3604 ± 274

[a]Significantly different from all other groups, p<0.05 (t test)

DISCUSSION

The results of these experiments provide material for an
outline picture of the relationship between host mice and the
transplanted methylcholanthrene-induced tumors studied. By virtue
of nonspecific anti-tumor effector cells, perhaps monocytes and
macrophages, which it can mobilize into sites of inflammation the
host offers some natural resistance to the initial growth of an
isograft. This resistance is overcome by anti-macrophage, anti-
inflammatory factors produced by the tumor cells. One immune
response of the host to the growing tumor is the development of
T cells, of the class mediating DTH, reactive with tumor-specific
antigens. The host also responds in a fashion which appears to be
immunologically nonspecific, increasing the number and activity of
its monocytes and macrophages, including cells with nonspecific
anti-tumor effects. At the site of a challenge isograft a DTH
reaction occurs in which the interaction between specifically
reactive T cells and tumor antigen triggers the delivery of nonspecific anti-tumor effector cells, which are drawn in turn from
an enlarged and more active pool. These cells exert a slow cytotoxic effect on the target tumor cells. If they are delivered
in adequate numbers and if the number of cells they are called
upon to destroy is not too large, the outcome will be suppression of the challenge isograft. In the case of a primary isograft, however, the rate of growth of the tumor, vis-à-vis the
rate at which DTH reactivity develops and the rate at which

effector cells destroy target tumor cells, may be such that, in "a simple numbers game" (11), the tumor is almost certain to win. The paradox of concomitant immunity can be explained in this way.

The reason for the failure of these tumors to elicit the formation of highly efficient cytolytic T cells in syngeneic hosts is not known, but it has been suggested that the nature of the association between tumor-specific antigens and components of the major histocompatibility complex may be a determining factor.

Whatever the plausibility of the arguments above, several vital problems remain. It is not known how generally valid this picture may be, especially when human tumors are considered. The nonspecific effector cells have not been identified with complete certainty as monocytes or macrophages; and if or when such an identification is made the place of the most active anti-tumor effectors within the spectrum of heterogeneous mononuclear phagocytes is still to be determined. Most notable to a biologist, however, is the ignorance and confusion still prevailing over the ways in which the tumor cells are recognized and selectively destroyed; and most challenging to those concerned with human patients is the search for ways in which this knowledge can be applied to the control of cancer.

SUMMARY

Mice become resistant to challenge with certain fibrosarcomas when bearing a tumor graft (concomitant immunity) or after injection of a low, non-tumorigenic dose of cells (sinecomitant immunity). Resistance to footpad challenge was depressed or abolished by treatment with carrageenan, niridazole or reserpine, or by sublethal irradiation, all of which also depressed delayed-type hypersensitivity (DTH) reactions. Immune lymphocytes initiating tumor-suppressive reactions in the feet of non-immune mice were Thy-1$^+$, Ly-1$^+$, Ly-2$^-$ and Ly-3$^-$. Injection of tumor cells into the peritoneal cavities of immune mice specifically elicited an influx of macrophages. There was evidence of macrophage stimulation in tumor-immune mice. In vitro, anti-tumor effector cells lacking individual tumor specificity could be detected among the resident peritoneal cells of tumor-immune mice and among peritoneal exudate cells of non-immune mice. The expression of acquired resistance to some tumors may involve reactions akin to DTH in which a specific reaction triggers an accumulation of nonspecific effectors.

ACKNOWLEDGEMENTS

This work was carried out in part pursuant to Research

Contract NO1-CB-63973 with the U . S. National Cancer Intitute
and was supported in part by the Australian National Health and
Medical Research Council. We thank Drs. R. V. Blanden, I. D.
Gardner, R. Kearney and I. F. C. McKenzie for collaboration and
Jannis Harrison, Julia Henderson and Paul Wood for assistance.

REFERENCES

1. Ashley, M. P. and Hardy, D., Aust. J. Exp. Biol. Med. Sci.
    51 (1973) 801.
2. Evans, R. and Alexander, P. In: Immunobiology of the Macro-
    phage (Ed. D. S. Nelson), Academic Press, New York, (1976)
    535.
3. Fauve, R. M., Hevin, B., Jacob, H., Gaillard, J. A. and Jacob,
    F., Proc. Natl. Acad. Sci. 71 (1974) 4052.
4. Fink, M. A., The Macrophage in Neoplasia, Academic Press,
    New York (1976).
5. Fisher, B., Taylor, S., Levine, M., Saffer, E. and Fisher,
    E. R.,Cancer Res. 34 (1974) 1668.
6. Hopper, K. E. and Nelson, D. S. (1978)(submitted for publi-
    cation).
7. Huber, B., Devinsky, O., Gershon, R. K. and Cantor, H.,J. Exp.
    Med. 143 (1976) 1534.
8. Kearney, R., Basten, A. and Nelson, D. S., Int. J. Cancer 15
    (1975) 438.
9. Kearney, R. and Nelson, D. S., Aust. J. Exp. Biol. Med. Sci.
    51 (1973) 723.
10. Keller, R. J.,Natl. Cancer Inst. 57 (1976) 1355.
11. Klein, G.,Natl. Cancer Inst. Monograph 44 (1976) 135.
12. Levy, M. H. and Wheelock, E. F., Adv. Cancer Res. 20 (1974)
    131.
13. Miller, R. G. and Phillips, R. A., J. Cell Physiol. 73 (1969)
    191.
14. More, D. G., Penrose, J. M., Kearney, R. and Nelson, D. S.,
    Int. Arch. Allergy Appl. Immunol. 44 (1973) 611.
15. Nelson, D. S., Transplant. Rev. 19 (1974) 226.
16. Nelson, D. S., Hopper, K. E., Blanden, R. V., Gardner, I. D.
    and Kearney, R., Cancer Lett. (1978) (in press)
17. Nelson, D. S., Hopper, K. E. and Nelson, M. In: The Hand-
    book of Cancer Immunology (Ed. H. Waters) Garland STPM
    Press, New York 3 (1978).
18. Nelson, D. S. and Kearney, R.,Brit. J. Cancer 34 (1976) 221.
19. Nelson, M. and Nelson, D. S..Aust. J. Exp. Biol. Med. Sci.
    56 (1978) 211.
20. Nelson, M. and Nelson, D. S.,Cancer Immunol. Immunother.
    (1978) in press.
21. Nelson, M. and Nelson, D. S.,Immunology 34 (1978) 277.
22. North, R. J., Kirstein, D. P. and Tuttle, R. L.,J. Exp. Med.
    143 (1976) 574.

23. Old, L. J., Benacerraf, B., Clarke, D. A., Carswell, E. A. and Stockert, E.,Cancer Res. 21 (1961) 1281.
24. Pang, T., McKenzie, I. F. C. and Blanden, R. V.,Cell. Immunol. 26 (1976) 153.
25. Pike, M. C. and Synderman, R.,J. Immunol. 117 (1976) 1243.
26. Rabionowitz, Y.,Blood 23 (1964) 811.
27. Seeger, R. C., Rayner, S. A. and Owen, J. J. T.,Int. J. Cancer 13 (1974) 697.
28. Simes, R. J., Kearney, R. and Nelson, D. S.,Immunology 29 (1975) 343.
29. Vadas, M. A., Miller, J. F. A. P., McKenzie, I. F. C., Chism, S. E., Shen, F.-W., Boyse, E. A., Gamble, J. R. and Whitlaw, A. M. , J. Exp. Med. 144 (1976) 10.
30. Winn, H. J. , J. Immunol. 86 (1961) 228.
31. Yashphe, D. J. In: Immunological Parameters of Host-Tumor Relationships (Ed. D. S. Weiss) Academic Press, New York, (1972) 90.

OPSONIZATION OF ANTITUMOR REACTIVE LYMPHOCYTES IN SJL/J MICE BEAR-

ING SPONTANEOUS OR TRANSPLANTED RETICULUM CELL SARCOMAS (RCS)

I. V. HUTCHINSON, J. ROMAN and B. BONAVIDA

Department of Microbiology and Immunology

UCLA School of Medicine, Los Angeles, California (USA)

SJL/J ($H-2^s$) mice suffer a high incidence of spontaneous reticulum cell sarcoma (RCS) (11). Several lines of transplantable
and cultured cell lines have been developed from the spontaneous
neoplasms in our laboratory, some of which have been described
elsewhere (13). These cells express neoantigens which strongly
cross-react with (and may be identical to) alloantigens present
on Balb/c ($H-2^d$) and $C_{57}Bl/6$ ($H-2^b$) lymphocytes both in serological
(immunofluorescence and complement-mediated lysis) tests and in
cell-mediated cytotoxicity assays (18). RCS cells from all sources
(spontaneous, transplantable and cultured) stimulate proliferation
of syngeneic lymphocytes in vitro (14,9,15) and transplantable
cells have been shown to stimulate lymphocyte proliferation in
vivo (17,2). It is not clear whether the proliferation stimulating antigens are identical to the determinants detected in
serological and cellular assays.

Since the tumor cells are antigenic and immunogenic, and are
susceptible to both antibody and cell-mediated lysis it is
surprising that they are not rejected in vivo, especially since
SJL/J mice appear to be fully immunocompetent by many criteria
(12,1,16). One possible explanation is that a specific active
suppressor mechanism is operative in tumor-bearer mice. Of the
several specifically suppressive mechanisms known, immunolgoical
enhancement is an attractive candidate because at least some
tumor-bearing animals produce antibody reactive with RCS cells
(unpublished data).

Antigen-reactive cell opsonization (ARCO), a mechanism of
immunological enhancement, has been described and studied in both
xenogeneic (3) and allogeneic (4,5,6) models. According to the

553

ARCO hypothesis, specific antigen reactive lymphocytes can bind
free antigenic determinants in antigen-antibody complexes while
the Fc region of the antibody in the complexes is bound by the
Fc receptor on macrophages. Thus, antigen-reactive cells are
specifically opsonized in a manner entirely analogous to opsonization of any antibody-coated cell or particle (Fig. 1).

    Our present experiments were designed to investigate the pos-
sible role of ARCO in the survival of RCS tumors in SJL/J mice and
this paper is a report of our preliminary findings.

MATERIAL AND METHODS

    <u>Mice</u>. Female mice of the SJL/J ($H-2^S$) inbred strain (ages 6
weeks to 15 months) and male mice of the Balb/c ($H-2^d$), $C_{57}Bl/6$
($H-2^b$) and C_3H/HeJ ($H-2^k$) inbred strains were used in these
experiments.

    <u>RCS tumors and tumor cell lines</u>. SJL/J mice greater than 6
months of age are regularly screened for the appearance of
spontaneous neoplasm. The transplantable RCS line, LA-6 derived
from a spontaneous tumor, is maintained by passage of 1×10^8 cells
i.p. every 7-10 days into young (6-8 weeks) tumor-free syngeneic
recipients.

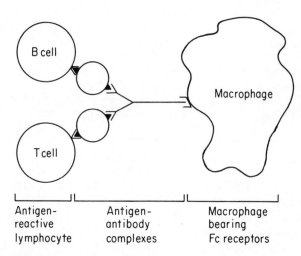

Fig. 1. Antigen-reactive cell opsonization. Antigen-reactive
lymphocytes specifically bind free antigenic determinants in antigen-antibody complexes. Specific cells and antibody need not recognize the same determinant. The complex is taken up by macrophages bearing Fc receptors. Consequently, specific antigen-
reactive cells are opsonized and destroyed by macrophages of the host.

Preparation of radiolabelled antigen-reactive cells (*ARC).
Anti-LA-6 *ARC were prepared by immunization of young SJL/J mice
with 10^8 mitomycin C treated LA-6 i.p. followed by a single dose
of 20 µCi ^{125}I-iododeoxyuridine (^{125}IUdR) given i.p. 3 days after
tumor cells to label dividing cells. The spleen cells harvested
from these mice on day 4 are referred to as anti-LA-6 *ARC.

Anti-C_{57}Bl/6 and C_3H/HeJ *ARC were prepared similarly by
immunizing SJL/J mice with 10^8 allogeneic spleen cells i.p., followed by ^{125}IUdR on day 3. Anti-Balb/c *ARC were prepared after two
immunizations (days 0 and 14) followed by 20 µCi ^{125}IUdR on days
16 and 17 and were harvested on day 18.

Preparation of radiolabelled normal cells. Spleen white cells
from young unimmunized SJL/J mice were labelled with ^{51}Cr as described elsewhere (8).

Nylon wool fractionation of spleen cells. Spleen cells were
fractionated by nylon wool adherence as described by Julius et al.
(7). Eluted cells were routinely less than 4% surface Ig positive
by indirect immunofluorescence.

Preparation of tumor-bearer sera (TBS). Groups of young SJL/J
mice injected with 1 x 10^8 LA-6 cells i.p. were bled at intervals
after tumor injection, the sera were pooled and stored at -20 C.
The sera were not heat-inactivated.

Antisera. Normal SJL/J mouse serum (NMS) and hyperimmune
Balb/c anti-SJL/J, SJL/J anti-Balb/c, Balb/c anti-C_{57}Bl/6, and
C_{57}Bl/6 anti-Balb/c allo-antisera were prepared in our laboratory
by immunization 4-6 times with 1 x 10^8 allogeneic spleen cells
i.p. Sera were prepared from bleeds taken 10 days after immunization. The C_{57}Bl/6 anti-Balb/c and Balb/c anti-C_{57}Bl/6 reagents
were absorbed extensively with normal SJL/J spleen cells to remove
all activity on SJL/J cells detectable by cytotoxicity or indirect
immunofluorescence.

Goat anti-mouse immunoglobulin (anti-Ig) was obtained from
Kallestad Laboratories (Minneapolis, MN). AKR anti-C_3H serum
(anti-Thy 1.2) was obtained from Litton Bionetics Incorporated
(Kensington, MD).

Opsonization assays. Two variations of the in vivo liver
diversion assay (10) were used:

a) opsonization of cells in tumor bearing mice: 0.2 ml of
radiolabelled cells 1 x 10^8 cells/ml were injected intravenously
into groups of 3-4 mice either injected with 1 x 10^8 LA-6 cells
i.p. 4-10 days previously or into mice bearing spontaneous RCS.
Ninety min later the mice were killed and their spleens and livers

were removed for gamma counting. The following calculations were
performed:

Opsonization Ratio (OR) = $\dfrac{\text{Cpm liver}}{\text{Cpm spleen}}$ (for each mouse)

$\overline{\text{OR}}$ = mean O.R. in each group of mice.

Localization Index (LI) = $\dfrac{\overline{\text{OR}} \text{ of tumor bearer group}}{\text{OR of normal group}}$

b) opsonization of cells by various antisera: Various sera
including NMS, anti-SJL/J, anti-Ig, anti-Thy 1.2, and batches
of LA-6 TBS, were used in this assay. Volumes (50 or 100 µl) of
antiserum were added to 1 ml aliquots of radiolabeled cells at
H 10^8 cells/ml in MEM. The cell-serum mixtures were incubated
at room temperature for 30 min then 0.2 ml volumes were injected
i.v. into normal SJL/J mice. After 90 min, spleens and livers
were removed for gamma counting and the calculations outlined
above were performed. In this case:

Localization Index (LI) = $\dfrac{\text{OR (antiserum group)}}{\text{OR (NMS group)}}$

In most opsonization experiments the radiolabelled cell suspensions were 10:1 mixtures of ^{125}I-labelled *ARC and ^{51}Cr-labelled
normal spleen cells. The radioactivity due to each isotope in a
sample can be determined and since the presence of either the
normal or immune cells does not affect opsonization of the other
cell type, opsonization of both normal and immune cells can be
assessed under identical conditions in the same animal.

RESULTS

Cell surface phenotype of *ARC. The antigens expressed on
anti-LA-6 and anti-Balb/c *ARC were detected by incubating cells
in various antisera then performing a liver diversion assay as
described above.

It was found that only T cells were labelled in SJL/J mice
immunized with Balb/c splenocytes. In contrast, both B cells and
T cells were labelled in LA-6 immunized mice. Since we were
interested mainly in T cell opsonization in tumor-bearer mice all
subsequent experiments with anti-LA^{-6} *ARC were performed with
nylon wool fractionated normal and immune cells. This procedure
was not performed with the anti-Balb/c *ARC because of the absence
of labelled immunoglobulin positive B cells.

Opsonization of anti-LA-6 *ARC in LA-6 tumor-bearer mice.   Nylon wool fractionated anti-LA-6 *ARC were diverted to the liver
of mice injected with LA-6, 7 or 8 days previously but not 4 days
after tumor injection (Table I).   In neither group of tumor-bearing
mice was localization of normal T cells different from localization
in normal tumor-free animals.

TABLE I

Opsonization of Anti-LA-6 *ARC in LA-6 Tumor-Bearer SJL/J Mice

Group	Localization Indices Normal T Cells[a]	Anti-LA-6 *ARC[b]
Normal	1.00 ± 0.06[c]	1.00 ± 0.01
LA-6 mice day 4	0.82 ± 0.03	0.71 ± 0.01
LA-6 mice day 7	1.08 ± 0.20	2.40 ± 0.02 ($p < 0.05$)

[a]Nylon wool fractionated ^{51}Cr-labelled SJL/J splenocytes.
[b]Nylon wool fractionated ^{125}IUdR-labelled SJL/J anti-LA-6
  antigen-reactive splenocytes.
[c]Localization index $\pm$ standard error.

Specificity of *ARC opsonization in LA-6 tumor-bearer mice.
Day 8 LA-6 tumor-bearer SJL/J mice were injected i.v. with
2×10^7 nylon wool fractionated *ARC from SJL/J mice immunized
with mitomycin C inactivated LA-6, C57Bl/6 or C3H splenocytes.
The localization of these cells in tumor-bearer mice was compared
with their localization in normal SJL/J mice.   The anti-LA-6 *ARC
were strongly opsonized in tumor-bearer animals, anti-C57Bl/6 *ARC
showed some liver diversion while anti-C3H *ARC showed a normal
localization pattern in LA-6 bearing animals (Table II).

Opsonization of anti-LA-6 *ARC by tumor-bearer sera.   Anti-LA-6
*ARC T cells incubated in day 7 TBS were opsonized in normal
syngeneic recipients.   This serum activity was absent in day 4
serum (Table III).   Normal T cells were not affected.   We are
currently investigating the kinetics of appearance of the serum
"ARCO factors" in tumor-bearer mice.

Opsonization of anti-Balb/c *ARC in mice bearing spontaneous
RCS tumor and by serum from the same mice.   Anti-Balb/c *ARC were
injected i.v. into six old SJL/J mice (ages 8-14 months) bearing
spontaneous neoplasms to assess *ARC opsonization.   In a parallel

TABLE II

Specificity of *ARC Opsonization in LA-6 Tumor-Bearer Mice

Cells Injected	Mice	Localication Index
Normal[a]	Normal	1.00 $\pm$ 0.26
	d8 LA-6[c]	1.00 $\pm$ 0.36
anti-LA-6 *ARC[b]	Normal	1.00 $\pm$ 0.03
	d8 LA-6	3.57 $\pm$ 0.35
anti-C$_{57}$B1/6 *ARC[b]	Normal	1.00 $\pm$ 0.12
	d8 LA-6	1.37 $\pm$ 0.08
anti-C$_3$H *ARC[b]	Normal	1.00 $\pm$ 0.08
	d8 LA-6	1.13 $\pm$ 0.03

[a]Nylon wool fractionated ^{51}Cr-labelled normal SJL/J, nylon wool
 fractionated splenocytes.
[b]Nylon wool fractionated ^{125}IUdR-labelled immune SJL/J splenocytes
 (see text.
[c]SJL/J mice injected 8 days earlier with 2 x 10^8 LA-6 cells i.p.

TABLE III

Opsonization of Anti-LA-6 *ARC By Tumor-Bearer Serum

Serum[a]	Localization Indices Normal T Cells[b]	Anti-LA-6 *ARC[c]
NMS	1.00 $\pm$ 0.02	1.00 $\pm$ 0.16
anti-SJL/J	3.31 $\pm$ 0.29	3.06 $\pm$ 0.32
anti-Ig	0.95 $\pm$ 0.25	0.97 $\pm$ 0.25
anti-Thy 1.2	1.23 $\pm$ 0.28	1.32 $\pm$ 0.08
d4 TBS	0.93 $\pm$ 0.05	0.90 $\pm$ 0.06
d7 TBS	1.02 $\pm$ 0.03	1.60 $\pm$ 0.07
d11 TBS	0.95 $\pm$ 0.21	1.35 $\pm$ 0.04

[a]For details of sera see text.
[b]See footnote a, Table I.
[c]See footnote b, Table I.

experiment, anti-Balb/c *ARC were incubated in serum taken from
these mice two days previously to assay for circulating "Arco factors." After removal of the spleens and livers from the tumor bearer animals, samples of tumor from mesenteric lymph nodes were
removed and prepared as single cell suspensions. The presence of
SJL/J, Balb/c, and C_{57}Bl/6 antigens on the tumor cells was examined
by indirect immunofluorescence using Balb/c anti-SJL/J serum, and
the SJL/J absorbed C_{57}Bl/6 anti-Balb/c and Balb/c anti-C_{57}Bl/6,
respectively.

Anti-Balb/c *ARC were opsonized only in those mice with Balb/c
positive tumors and the opsonization in these mice could be correlated to brightness of fluorescence of the tumors with the anti-
Balb/c serum (Table IV). The presence of C_{57}Bl/6 antigens was not
related to opsonization of anti-Balb/c *ARC. Serum from the mice
with "Balb/c positive" tumors caused opsonization of the anti-Balb/c

TABLE IV

Opsonization of SJL/J Anti-Balb/c *ARC in Tumor Bearing
SJL/J Mice

Group	Ag[1]	Ab[2]	L.I. + S.E.[3]	p[4]	SJL/J[5]	Balb/c[5]	C_{57}Bl/6[5]
1	−	−	1.00 +	−			
2	+	−	0.99 + 0.18	−			
3	−	+	1.03 + 0.21	−			
4	+	+	1.39 + 0.06	0.005			
T1[6]			1.52		++	+	+[7]
T2			1.76	0.01	++	++	+
T3			2.08	0.00001	++	+++	−
T4			1.24	N.S.	++	−	−
T5.			1.81	0.0001	++	+++	+
T6			1.73	0.001	++	+++	+

[1]10^8 Balb/c spleen cells.

[2]10 μl SJL anti-Balb/c serum.

[3]Localization index ± standard error.

[4]Significance of difference from group 1.

[5]Antigens detected by indirect immunofluorescence (see text).

[6]Tumor-bearing mice T1-6

[7]Strength of reaction +++ = bright fluorescence to − = no visible
fluorescence.

*ARC but was weak and, in the case of animal 1, not significant (data not presented).

In a control experiment anti-Balb/c *ARC were injected into normal SJL/J mice or mice injected i.v. 3 hr previously with 10^8 Balb/c spleen cells, 10 ul of SJL/J anti-Balb/c serum or a preincubated mixture of Balb/c spleen cells plus antiserum.

DISCUSSION

Our results show that tumor-reactive T lymphocytes injected into tumor-bearing SJL/J mice have an abnormal homing pattern and are diverted to the liver. This is true whether the mice have been injected with a syngeneic RCS neoplasm or have spontaneous neoplasms. Furthermore, the liver diversion of immune cells is specific since a) T cells from mice immunized with non-cross-reactive antigens (i.e., anti-C_3H *ARC) are not opsonized in LA-6 injected animals (Table II) and b) anti-Balb/c *ARC are only opsonized in mice with "Balb/c positive" spontaneous tumors (Table IV). It is of interest that anti-$C_{57}Bl/6$ *ARC, but not anti-C_3H *ARC, are opsonized to some degree in LA-6 tumor-bearer mice (Table II), an observation consistent with detection of $C_{57}Bl/6$ but not C_3H antigens on LA-6 by indirect immunofluorescence.

Serum from tumor-bearer mice contains "ARCO factors" which cause opsonization of antitumor *ARC in normal mice (Table III). We are currently examining the kinetics of appearance of these factors in tumor-bearer mice and attempting to characterize them. Thus far we have found that the active component(s) in day 7 TBS is fully precipitated by addition of polyethylene glycol to 3.5% (w/v), suggesting that the "ARCO factors" in this serum contain IgM or are immune complexes containing IgM and/or IgG. Gel filtration of the precipitated material on AcA 22 in 6M urea yielded two peaks, one in the void volume (M.Wt. greater than 10^6 daltons), the other eluting where IgM might be expected.

The opsonization of *ARC in tumor-bearer animals and by tumor-bearer serum is analogous to specific opsonization of anti-donor ARC in rats bearing enhanced renal allografts and by serum from the same animals (4,5). The present paper is the first report of antigen-reactive cell opsonization (ARCO) in a syngeneic system.

ARCO could account for survival of antigenic and immunogenic RCS tumors in SJL/J mice since immunization with RCS cells leads to early B cell proliferation. Complexes between antigen shed from the growing tumor and endogenously produced antibody could act as "ARCO factors" provided that there are free antigenic determinants in these complexes (See Fig. 1). It has been proposed that complexes in tumor-bearing hosts act as "blocking factors" (19) although there is no direct in vivo evidence of such a function. Our in vivo experiments suggest another way in which immune complexes would regulate antitumor immunity, namely, specific destruction of antitumor reactive T cells by Fc receptor-bearing cells in the presence of antigen-antibody complexes. The present experiments implicate the reticuloendothelial system (RES) in immune suppression and suggest that the macrophage plays a major role. However, this is not to deny that K-cell killing (ADCC) may also be important in some situations.

We speculate, on the basis of our findings, that the macrophage may be of paramount importance in tumor etiology in some systems, particularly when the tumor is highly antigenic. Clinical use of RES stimulating agents in tumor immunotherapy without concommitant attempts to suppress antibody formation might lead to increased suppression of T cell-mediated immunity, while the opposite approach, RES suppression, could allow expression of existing antitumor potential. Our future experiments will be aimed at greater understanding of the interaction of complexes and macrophages with immune cells, and the development of an immunotherapy model based on RES suppression.

SUMMARY

Radiolabelled antitumor reactive T lymphocytes (*ARC) were prepared in vivo by immunization of SJL/J mice with mitomycin C inactivated syngeneic LA-6 tumor cells followed by injection of ^{125}IUdR to label dividing cells. These *ARC were specifically diverted to the liver when injected i.v. into LA-6 tumor-bearer SJL/J hosts or when incubated in LA-6 tumor-bearer serum and injected i.v. into normal SJL/J mice. Likewise, SJL/J anti-Balb/c *ARC were diverted to the liver of SJL/J mice bearing spontaneous reticulum cell sarcomas (RCS) carrying Balb/c cross-reactive antigens but not in mice with Balb/c negative neoplasms. Mice with Balb/c positive tumors also had circulating *ARC opsonizing factors.

These results suggest a mechanism for the survival of antigenic tumors involving macrophages and ARC opsonizing (ARCO) factors. A novel approach to immunotherapy is discussed.

ACKNOWLEDGEMENT

Supported by Grant NCI CA19753 and Damon Runyon-Walter Winchell Grant DRG-241-F.

REFERENCES

1. Carswell, E. A., Waneto, J. H., Old, L. J. and Boyse, E. A.
   J. Natl. Cancer Inst. 44 (1970) 1281.
2. Hutchinson, I. V. and Bonavida, B. (In preparation).
3. Hutchinson, I. V. and Zola, H. Cell Immunol. 36 (1978) 161.
4. Hutchinson, I. V. and Zola, H. Transplant. Proc. 9 (1976) 961.
5. Hutchinson, I. V. and Zola, H. Transplant. 23 (1977) 464.
6. Hutchinson, I. V. and Bonavida, B. Transplant. Proc. 10 (1978)
   31.
7. Julius, M. H., Simpson, E. and Herzenberg, L. A. Eur. J.
   Immunol. 3 (1973) 645.
8. Kedar, E. and Bonavida, B. J. Immunol. 115 (1975) 1301.
9. Lerman, S. P., Chapman, J. M., Carswell, E. A. and Thorbecke,
   G. J. Int. J. Cancer 14 (1977) 808.
10. Marin, W. J. and Miller, J. F. A. P. Int. Arch. Allergy 35
    (1969) 163.
11. Murphy, E. D. Proc. Amer. Assoc. for Cancer Res. 4 (1963) 46.
12. Murphy, E. D. J. Natl. Cancer Inst. 42 (1969) 797.
13. Owens, M. H. and Bonavida, B. Cancer Res. 37 (1977) 4439.
14. Owens, M. H. and Bonavida, B. Proc. Amer. Assoc. Cancer Res.
    16 (1975) 162.
15. Owens, M. H. and Bonavida, B. (1978) (Submitted).
16. Owens, M. H. and Bonavida, B. Cancer Res. 36 (1976) 1077.
17. Ponzio, N. M., David, C. S., Shreffler, D. C. and Thorbecke,
    G. J. J. Exp. Med. 147 (1977) 132.
18. Roman, J. M., Owens, M. H. and Bonavida, B. In: Immune
    System: Genetics and Regulation. (Eds. E. E. Sercarz, L. A.
    Herzenberg and C. F. Fox) Academic Press, (1977) 639.
19. Sjogren, H. O., Hellström, I., Bansal, S. C. and Hellström, K.
    E. Proc. Nat. Acad. Sci. USA 68 (1971) 1372.

ANTI-INFLAMMATORY CONSEQUENCES OF TRANSPLANTED TUMORS

S. J. NORMANN,[1] E. SORKIN,[2] and M. SCHARDT[2]

[1]Department of Pathology, University of Florida, College
of Medicine, Gainesville, Florida (USA)
[2]Schweizerisches Forschungsinstitut, Medizinische
Abteilung, Davos (Switzerland)

It seems well established in vitro that activated macrophages
possess growth regulating activities over cancer cells (5,6,7).
For instance, macrophages obtained from the peritoneal cavities of
animals injected with BCG kill neoplastic but not normal cells in
culture (6). Furthermore, macrophages may inhibit cell proliferation by a mechanism not involving cytotoxicity (7). However, in
vivo this tumor-host relationship may involve reciprocal tumor
generated elements which impair effector activity. Among these is
the capacity of the tumor bearing host to compromise monocyte
inflammation. Three aspects of this phenomenon have been documented. a) Patients with malignancy often have decreased in vitro
chemotactic activity of their circulating monocytes (1,19). This
impairment has been observed with a diversity of tumors and is
improved significantly by surgical resection of the tumor. b) Animals bearing transplanted tumors have an anti-inflammatory effect
directed against macrophages but not (polymorphonuclear neutrophiles)
which is systemic and demonstrable both in subcutaneous tissues and
in the peritoneal cavity (8,9,10,20). It occurs despite adequate
levels of blood monocytes and in animals whose tumors contain
relatively few macrophages, and c) Supernates from cultured tumor
cells (11) or cell-free homogenates (21) of tumors inhibit macrophage chemotaxis in vitro and inflammation in vivo. While such
products decrease the influx of macrophages in response to transient
stimuli, they do not alter the total number of macrophages which
accumulate in response to persistent stimuli (10).

One critical factor for efficient macrophage growth control
in vitro is the ratio of macrophages to tumor cells (5,17). This
insures close contact between effector and target cells necessary
for killing. Could it be that by compromising monocyte chemotaxis

and decreasing macrophage accumulation in inflammatory foci, a growing tumor alters the ratio of macrophages to tumor cells, decreases the probability of close contact, and escapes growth control by macrophages?

This attractive hypothesis presupposes several unproven conditions. For example, is tumor infiltration by macrophages compromised concurrently with the systemic defect in inflammation? How does the defect relate to the number of tumor cells? Does the anti-inflammatory effect actually compromise chemotaxis of either monocytes or macrophages? Questions such as these form the basis for the current report.

EXPERIMENTS AND RESULTS

Correlation between anti-inflammation demonstrable at remote sites and macrophage infiltration of the tumor. We have used two methods to measure macrophage inflammation. First, we quantitated the number of macrophages washed from the peritoneal cavity 3 days after the i.p. injection of proteose peptone. Second, we developed a test for macrophage inflammation applicable to subcutaneous tissues which employs a small disk cut from an 0.2 µ pore size nitrocellulose filter (12). The filter is placed under the skin for variable lengths of time and is then removed, stained, and the macrophages adherent to the filter counted under an oil immersion objective. Fig. 1 presents data on the rate of macrophage accumulation on filters in normal and tumor-bearing animals. Tumor-bearing animals had been transplanted with a 7, 12 dimethylbenz(a) anthracene (DMBA) induced fibrosarcoma 16 days prior to filter insertion. In contrast to controls, tumor-bearing animals had a pronounced depression in macrophage inflammation. This macrophage inflammation test (MIT) has been used successfully to measure macrophage responsiveness repetitively in the same animal during tumor progression (13).

The cellular composition of tumors was determined as follows (18). The tumor mass was excised, necrotic debris removed, and the viable tumor mass divided into two parts. The weights of the total tumor as well as each part were recorded. One part was homogenized and used for DNA determinations (23). The total number of cells in the tumor was calculated by dividing the DNA content of the tumor by the amount of DNA contained in a known number of cells extracted from the tumor. The second part was used for cell extraction. The tumor was minced finely and digested for 30 mins at room temperature with a mixture of 0.25% trypsin in Medium 199 containing 20 mg DN'ase and 20 mg collagenase per g tumor. After digestion, the cells were passed through a 70 mesh screen to remove large aggregates, centrifuged, and washed. Differential cell counts

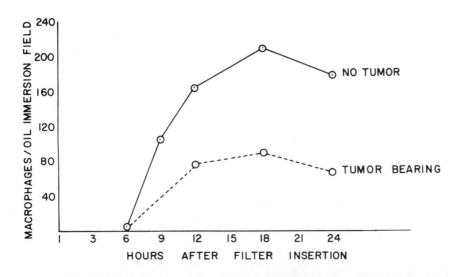

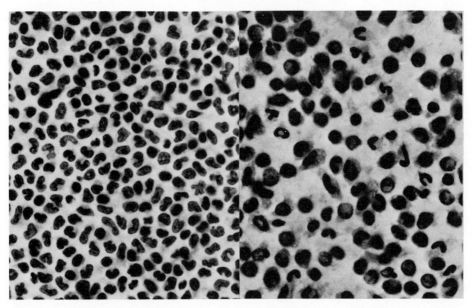

Fig. 1. Tumor-bearing inhibits macrophage accumulation on subcutaneous filters. Data for a DMBA-induced tumor transplanted to
syngeneic DA rats 18 days after challenge. The photomicrographs
contrast macrophages on filters of normal rats (lower left) with
tumor-bearing rats (lower right).   250X.

were made on slides prepared using a cytocentrifuge. In addition,
macrophages were recognized by their content of nonspecific esterase,
adherence to plastic tissue culture dishes, and by their capacity
for phagocytosis. The data were used to compute the total number
of cells within the tumor as well as the tumor to macrophage
(T/M) ratio.

During growth of a DMBA induced fibrosarcoma transplanted to
syngeneic DA strain rats, we measured concurrently the degree of
inhibition in macrophage inflammation (MIT), the number of macrophages within the tumor, and the T/M ratio. Fig. 2 presents the
results. During early tumor growth and for up to about 12 days
after tumor transplantation, there was no significant inhibition
in MIT and macrophages readily entered the tumor. This was
reflected by a stable T/M ratio, indicating that macrophage infiltration of the tumor was keeping pace with tumor growth. Beyond
12 days, however, progressive tumor growth was associated with
marked impairment of MIT. Concurrently macrophages failed to
continue accumulating within the tumor and the T/M ratio rose
dramatically. As observed in Fig. 2, the rising T/M ratio paralel-

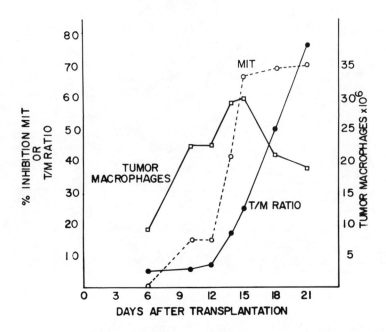

Fig. 2. Inhibition in macrophage inflammation test (MIT) correlat-
es with an inhbition in macrophage infiltration of the tumor and
a rising tumor to macrophage (T/M) ratio. Data for a DMBA-induced
tumor transplanted to syngeneic DA rats.

ed the degree of inhibition in macrophage inflammation as measured
by MIT. We have observed a similar correlation between inhibition
of inflammation distant to the tumor and an increasing T/M ratio
in P-815 mastocytoma syngeneic with DBA/2 mice and methylcholanthrene induced fibrosarcomas transplanted to $C_{57}Bl/6$ mice (14,12)

Anti-inflammation requires relatively large numbers of tumor
cells. We have determined the number of tumor cells necessary to
inhibit macrophage inflammation in three tumors in two animal species.
These tumors were the DMBA-induced fibrosarcoma in DA strain rats,
a methylcholanthrene induced fibrosarcoma (designated PC-8) syngeneic with $C_{57}Bl/6$ mice, and the P-815 mastocytoma syngeneic with
DBA/2 mice. At various days after tumor transplantation, the number
of tumor cells was determined and related to the presence or
absence of demonstrable inhibition in macrophage inflammation. Three
points emerge from the results presented in Table I. First, the
degree of inhibition for a given tumor size as measured by MIT
was slightly less than that based upon peritoneal macrophage yields.
This conclusion derives from data presented for the DMBA-induced
tumor in rats and is consistent with our previous observation that
peritoneal exudative macrophages are more sensitive to tumor growth.
Second, the approximate number of tumor cells required to produce
anti-inflammation was as follows: 1.5×10^9 for the fibrosarcoma
in rats, greater than 2×10^8 for the fibrosarcoma in C57Bl/6·mice,
and greater than 5×10^6 mastocytoma cells in the DBA/2 mice. Thus,
the number of tumor cells necessary to inhibit inflammation was
large and variable between different tumors in different animal
species. Third, different tumors had different T/M ratios at the
onset of anti-inflammation. This is consistent with the generally
held notion that the content of tumor macrophages is variable
between tumors (4). The data show also that the T/M ratio rose
concurrently with inhibition in systemic inflammation. Since anti-
inflammation required relatively large numbers of tumor cells, it
can be concluded that macrophage infiltration of emerging tumors
is unimpaired and proportional to tumor growth.

Rats bearing transplanted tumors do not have decreased monocyte or macrophage chemotactic responsiveness. Blood monocytes
were obtained from DA rats bearing a transplanted fibrosarcoma.
Blood from two rats were pooled, diluted 1:1 with saline, and
layered onto a Ficoll-Paque column (Pharmacia Fine Chemicals). The
column was centrifuged at 400 g for 30 mins in order to separate
the red cells and PMNs from the mononuclear cells. The latter
cells were collected, washed, and suspended in Medium 199 containing
1% bovine serum albumin. Chemotaxis was performed using 2×10^6
monocytes and heated rat serum as attractant (16). The two
compartments of the chemotaxis chamber were separated by a
Sartorius filter of 8.0 µ pore size. Incubation time was 5 hrs
and the tests were performed at a pH of 7.1. Only cells which

TABLE I

Anti-Inflammation Directed Against Macrophages Required Relatively Large Numbers of Tumor Cells[a]

Tumor Type and Animal	Days After Transplant	Number of Tumor Cells x 10^6	Anti-Inflammation		
			Percent Inhibition Peritoneal Exudate	Percent Inhibition MIT	Tumor/ Macrophage Ratio
DMBA fibrosarcoma DA rats, s.c.	6	400	None	None	5
	10	1500	63	15	6
	14	5000	70	62	17
PC-8 fibrosarcoma C57Bl/6 mice, s.c.	14	203	11	--	25
	24	730	53	--	42
P-815 mastocytoma DBA/2 mice, i.p.	5	4	None	--	3
	7	22	82	--	8

[a] For P-815 mastocytoma, the tumor/macrophage ratio has been corrected for the resident cells. Peritoneal exudates were measured 3 days after i.p. proteose peptone injection.

migrated completely through the filter were counted in evaluating chemotaxis.

DA rat monocytes were less responsive in chemotaxis tests than macrophages obtained from the same animal population. Surprisingly, monocyte chemotactic activity increased with tumor-bearing even when when macrophage inflammation was severely compromised (Table II). For instance, animals bearing advanced malignancies showed a 44% decrease in macrophage inflammatory accumulation on subcutaneous filters at the same time that their circulating monocytes had increased chemotactic activity by 451%. Accordingly, there was no demonstrable defect in chemotactic activity of circulating monocytes sufficient to account for their failure to accumulate in inflammatory foci.

The chemotactic activity of exudative macrophages induced at various times during tumor-bearing also was examined. The data presented in Table III support the following conclusions. First, resident peritoneal macrophages were chemotactically a poorly responding cell population. Their numbers were not altered by tumor-bearing. Second, proteose peptone induced peritoneal macrophages[a] were chemotactically active cell population. Third, tumor bearing decreased the yield of exudate induced macrophages and decreased the overall chemotactic activity of the harvested peritoneal cells. But, when chemotactic activity was computed to reflect only the exudate population undiluted by resident cells, there was no defect in macrophage chemotactic activity associated with progressive cancer growth. This conclusion (but not the data) differs from that reached by Stevenson and Meltzer (23) or Snyderman et al. (22). This difference is explained by the fact that these investigators did not correct their data for the anti-inflammatory effect of tumor-bearing or for the poorly responding population of resident cells.

DISCUSSION

A significant point which now emerges is that the tumor related anti-inflammatory effect directed against macrophages is not restricted to any particular site or type of inflammatory stimulus. During tumor-bearing, a defect in macrophage inflammation has been documented in the peritoneal cavity and pleural space to transient irritants (8,20) in the subcutaneous tissues to persistent foreign body stimulants (10) and in the tumor itself (14,15). Indeed, the onset and severity of the anti-inflammatory defect presages a failure of tumor macrophage accumulation to keep race with neoplastic growth. By increasing the T/M ratio, the defect could compromise the growth regulating activities of macrophages and provide conditions favorable to metastasis (2).

TABLE II

Tumor-Bearing Concurrently Depresses Macrophage Inflammation but Increases Circulating Monocyte Chemotaxis[a]

Days After Transplant	Number of Rats	Mean Tumor Wt g	MIT Macrophages per OIF	Chemotaxis Monocytes per 20 OIF	MIT Percent Change	Monocyte Chemotaxis Percent Change
0	7	--	178 + 10	75 + 19	--	--
10	7	3.2 + .2	170 + 4	127 + 20	0	+69
16	6	17.0 + .9	111 + 8	153 + 42	-38	+104
20	6	23.2 + .8	99 + 10	413 + 96	-44	+451

[a]Inbred DA rats were transplanted with a syngeneic DMBA induced fibrosarcoma. Data reported as mean + 1 standard error. OIF = Oil immersion field. MIT = macrophage inflammation

TABLE III

Tumor-Bearing Inhibits Peritoneal Macrophage Inflammation Without a Defect in Exudate Macrophage Chemotaxis[a]

Days After Transplant	Number of Rats	Macrophages Total x 10^6	Percent Inhibition[b]	Chemotaxis Macrophages[c] /4 HPF	Cells Applied to Chamber		
					Exudate Macrophages x10^4	Resident Macrophages x10^4	Chemotaxis Exudate Macrophages[d] /4 HPF
0 unstimulated	6	8.3 ± 0.9	–	58 ± 4	– –	200	– –
0 stimulated	10	36 ± 3.4	0	426 ± 49	154	46	536
4	5	31 ± 4.9	18	525 ± 78	126	64	804
10	6	13 ± 1.2	83	266 ± 59	72	128	636
16	6	11 ± 4.9	90	189 ± 62	50	150	582

[a]Data for DA rats bearing a syngeneic DMBA induced fibrosarcoma. Exudate induced animals (stimulated) were injected with 10 ml of sterile proteose peptone i.p. 3 days before harvest of peritoneal exudate cells. Data reported as mean ± strd. error. HPF = high power field.

[b]Percent inhibition = 100 – (macrophage yield – 8.3)/27.7.

[c]All chemotaxis chambers contained 2 x 10^6 macrophages. Attractant was heated rat serum.

[d]Chemotaxis exudate macrophages = $\dfrac{\text{observed chemotaxis} - \left[\dfrac{\text{resident macrophages}}{2 \times 10^6} \cdot 58\right]}{\dfrac{2 \times 10^6 \text{ exudate macrophages}}{\text{phages}}}$

However, the defect does not appear to arise soon enough to compromise host surveillance. When the defect ensues from a transplanted tumor, it generally develops late in tumor growth approximately midway between transplantation and death. Therefore, the number of tumor cells necessary to produce the defect varies often as a function of the rate of tumor proliferation. More malignant tumors inhibit inflammation with fewer tumor cells than less malignant ones. Further, it is noteworthy that in some tumors the defect does not develop at all. Also no defect occurs when P-815 mastocytoma cells are transplanted subcutaneously in contrast to the intraperitoneal route of challenge (14). Consequently, it can be concluded that the anti-inflammatory effect requires a threshold number of transplanted tumor cells which varies between tumors in different animals and with the same tumor in different sites.

The possibility, of course, exists that transplanted tumors are not analogous to spontaneous ones. With respect to monocytes, it has been observed that transplanted tumors frequently produce a bloo monocytosis which is not a general feature of spontaneous tumors of either animals or man (8). Then too, monocyte chemotaxis is often depressed in human patients with malignancy (1,19) as opposed to normal or augmented chemotactic activity of monocytes recovered from animals bearing transplanted tumors. As yet, a monocyte specif ic anti-inflammatory defect has not been demonstrated during evolution of spontaneous malignancies. Until such studies have been performed, the true relationship of the defect to cancer emergence remains enigmatic.

In animals bearing transplanted tumors, the defect clearly arises as a consequence of tumor progression. It can be distinguished from the counter-irritant effect (9) by the fact that macrophage accumulation during early tumor growth is not associated with any inflammatory abnormality and by the fact that the defect occurs in monocytes but not PMNs (8). While sizable numbers of macrophages are present within the tumor at the time the abnormality develops, there is no clear association between the number of tumor associated macrophages and the presence or absence of the defect. These observations together with the generalized nature of the defect with its concordant paralysis of both macrophage accumulation in the tumor and at remote sites argue against the defect being due solely to sequestration or movement of macrophages into the tumor.

At issue is the nature of the inflammatory abnormality. Curiously, it does not appear to result from an intrinsic abnormality in chemotactic responsiveness. Using a different system of chemotactic measurement in vitro and passive transfer of labeled monocytes in vivo, Eccles (3) concluded that the defect is both acquired and not due to a demonstrable chemotactic deficiency. Paradoxically, cultured tumor cells (21) and cell-free homogenates of tumors (11) possess factors selectively inhibitory to macrophage chemotaxis. Surely inhibition of chemotaxis could impair monocyte inflammation, but it may not be the only or even significant mechanism of tumor associated anti-inflammation. In support of the latter hypothesis, we have observed that tumor bearing can markedly enhance in vitro monocyte chemotaxis at the same time the cells fail to accumulate in foci of inflammation. By understanding the mechanism involved in this selective paralysis of monocyte inflammation, new approaches might be developed to favorably influence the tumor host relationship.

SUMMARY

Rats and mice bearing transplanted chemically induced neoplasms have defective macrophage infiltration of inflammatory sites distant to the tumor. The defect limits concurrently accumulation of macrophages within the tumor, raising dramatically the tumor to macrophage cell ratio. The defect may not compromise host surveillance because it requires relatively large numbers of tumor cells. The abnormality does not appear to result from circulating monocyte depletion, defective monocyte chemotaxis, or the traffic of monocytes into the tumor.

ACKNOWLEDGEMENTS

Supported by grant CA 22517 from the National Cancer Institute, Grant 3 '13.77 from the Swiss National Science Foundation, and in part   the Florida Division, American Cancer Society (Tumor Biology Unit Publication No. 141)

REFERENCES

1. Boetcher, D. A. and Leonard, E. J. J. Natl. Canc. Inst. 52 (1974) 1091.
2. Eccles, S. A. and Alexander, P. Nature 250 (1974) 667.
3. Eccles, S. A. In: Macrophages and Noeplasia (Eds. K. James, B. McBride and A. Stuart) Econoprint, Edingurgh (1977) 308.
4. Evans, R. Transpl. 14 (1972) 468.
5. Hibbs, J. B. In: The Macrophage and Neoplasia (Ed. M. A. Fink) Academic Press (1976) 83.
6. Hibbs, J. B. J. Reticuloendothel. Soc. 20 (1976) 223.
7. Keller, R. In: Immunobiology of the Macrophage (Ed. D. S. Nelson) Academic Press, New York (1976) 487.
8. Normann, S. J. and Sorkin, E. J. Natl. Canc. Inst. 57 (1976) 135.
9. Normann, S. J. and Sorkin, E. In: Perspectives in Inflamma-

tion (Ed. D. A. Willoughby, J. P. Giroud and G. P. Velo) MTP Press Ltd, London (1977) 303.

10. Normann, S. J. and Schardt, M. J. Reticuloendothel. Soc. In press.
11. Normann, S. J. and Sorkin, E. Cancer Res. 37 (1977) 705.
12. Normann, S. J. and Schardt, M. J. Reticuloendothel. Soc. 23 (1978) 153.
13. Normann, S. J., Schardt, M. and Sorkin, E. In: The Macrophage and Cancer (Eds. K. James, B. McBride and A. Stuart) Econoprint, Edinburgh, (1977) 247.
14. Normann, S. J. and Cornelius, J. Cancer Res. (1978) In press.
15. Normann, S. J. J. Natl. Canc. Inst. 60 (1978) 1091.
16. Normann, S. J. and Sorkin, E. J. Reticuloendothel. Soc. 22 (1977) 45.
17. Russell, S. W., Doe, W. F. and McIntosh, A. T. J. Exp. Med. 146 (1977) 1511.
18. Russell, S. W., Doe, W. F., Hoskins, R. G. and Cochrane, C. G. Int. J. Canc. 18 (1976) 322.
19. Snyderman, R. and Stahl, C. In: The Phagocytic Cell in Host Resistance (Eds. J. A. Bellanti and D. H. Bayton) Raven Press, New York (1975) 267.
20. Snyderman, R., Pike, M. C., Blaylock, B. L. and Weinstock, P. J. Immunol. 116 (1976) 585.
21. Snyderman, R. and Pike, M. C. Science 192 (1976) 370.
22. Snyderman, R., Pike, M. C., Blaylock, B. L. and Weinstein, P. J. Immunol. 116 (1976) 585.
23. Stevenson, M. M. and Meltzer, M. S. J. Natl. Cancer Inst. 57 (1976) 847.

PARTICIPANTS

ABRAMOFF, P.
Marquette University
Milwaukee, Wisconsin

ADES, E.
Comprehensive Cancer Center
University of Alabama
Birmingham, Alabama

ADLER, A.
Hadassah Medical School
Hebrew University
Jerusalem, Israel

AKSAMIT, R.
National Cancer Institute, NIH
Bethesda, Maryland

ARONSON, M.
Sackler School of Medicine
Tel Aviv University
Tel Aviv, Israel

BABNIK, J.
J. Stefan Institute
Ljubljana, Yugoslavia

BAR-ELI, M.
Hadassah Medical School
Hebrew University
Jerusalem, Israel

BARTH, R. F.
Mount Sinai Medical Center
Milwaukee, Wisconsin

BASIC, I
Faculty of National Sciences
and Mathematics and Central
Institute for Tumors and Allied
Health Diseases
Zagreb, Yugoslavia

BATTISTO, J. R.
Cleveland Clinic Foundation
Cleveland, Ohio

BENDINELLI, M.
University of Pisa
Pisa, Italy

BENNEDSEN, J.
Statens Seruminstitut
DK-2300, Copenhagen S, Denmark

BERTOK, L.
National Research Institute
for Radiobiology and
Radiohygiene
Budapest, Hungary

BERTOLI, F.
Via Donzelle No 1
Bologna, Italia

BLIZNAKOV, E. G.
New England Institute
Ridgefield, Connecticut

BOEHME, D. H.
Veterans Administration Hospital
East Orange, New Jersey

BOLTZ-NITULESCU, G.
Institute of General and
Experimental Pathology
University of Vienna
Vienna, Austria

BONAVIDA, B.
University of California at
Los Angeles
Los Angeles, California

CASS, I. M.
79 Old Forest Hill Road
Toronto, Canada

CEGLOWSKI, W. S.
Pennsylvania State University
University Park, Pennsylvania

CHAUVET, G.
Centre de Physiologie
et d' Immunologie Cellulaires
Inserm U. 104
CNRS et Ass. Cl. Bernard
Hospital St-Antoine
Paris Cedex 12
France

CLOUGH, J. D.
Cleveland Clinic Foundation
Cleveland, Ohio

COHN, D. A.
York College
City University of New York
Jamica, New York

COOPER, D. A.
Department of Immunology
St. Vincent's Hospital
Sydney, Australia

DAMAIS, C.
Immunotherapie Experimentale
Institut Pasteur
Paris, France

DAVIES, W. A.
Prince of Wales Children's Hosp.
Randwick, N. S. W.
Australia

DE HALLEAUX, F.
Brocades Belga
Blvd. General Jacques, 26
Brussels, Belgium

DELVILLE, J.
School of Public Health
Universite Catholique de Louvain
1200 Brussels, Belgium

DI LUZIO, N. R.
Tulane University School of
Medicine
New Orleans, Louisiana

DIXON, J.
University of Southern Californi
School of Medicine
Los Angeles, California

DRATH, D.
Harvard Medical School
Boston, Massachusetts

DUBROFF, L. M.
Hahnemann Medical College
Philadelphia, Pennsylvania

EISENSTEIN, T. K.
Temple University School of
Medicine
Philadelphia, Pennsylvania

ESCOBAR, M. R.
Medical College of Virginia
Richmond, Virginia

FABIAN, I.
Sackler School of Medicine
Tel Aviv University
Tel Aviv, Israel

FIDLER, I. J.
Frederick Cancer Center
Frederick, Maryland

FILKINS, J. P.
Loyola University Medical Center
Maywood, Illinois

FRANK, M.
National Institutes of Health
Bethesda, Maryland

FLEMMING, K. B. P.
University of Freiburg
Freiburg, Germany

FORD, P. M.
Queen's University
Kingston, Ontario
Canada

FORSTER, O.
Institute of General and
Experimental Pathology
University of Vienna
Vienna, Austria

FRIEDMAN, H.
University of South Florida
College of Medicine
Tampa, Florida

GABIZON, A.
The Weizmann Institute of
Science
Rehovot, Israel

GHAFFAR, A.
Department of Microbiology and
Immunology
University of South Carolina
Columbia, South Carolina

GILLET, J.
School of Public Health
Universite Catholique de Louvain
1200-Brussels, Belgium

GINSBURG, H.
Technicon University
School of Medicine
Haifa, Israel

GINSBURG, I.
Hadassah School of
Dental Medicine
Hebrew University
Jerusalem, Israel

GLOBERSON, A.
Hadassah Medical School
Hebrew University
Jerusalem, Israel

GOLDBLUM, N.
Hadassah Medical School
Hebrew University
Jerusalem, Israel

GOLDMAN, R.
Weizmann Institute
Rehovot, Israel

GOLUB, S. H.
Department of Surgery
University of California
at Los Angeles
Los Angeles School of Medicine
Los Angeles, California

GORCZYNSKI, R. M.
Ontario Cancer Institute
Toronto, Ontario   Canada

GORELICK, E.
Hadassah Medical School
Hebrew University
Jerusalem, Israel

GREENBLATT, C.
Hebrew University
Jerusalem, Israel

HALL, J. M.
Proctor Foundation
University of California
San Francisco, California

HAMBURGER, J.
Hadassah Medical School
Hebrew University
Jerusalem, Israel

HANNA, M. G., Jr.
Frederick Cancer Center
Frederick, Maryland

HARAN, Ghera, J.
Tel Aviv University
Tel Aviv, Israel

HARRIS, S.
The Children's Hospital of
Philadelphia and School
of Medicine
University of Pennsylvania
Philadelphia, Pennsylvania

HARRIS, T. N.
University of Pennsylvania
Children's Hospital
Philadelphia, Pennsylvania

HAYASHI, T.
Fukushima Medical College
Fukushima, Japan

HELLMAN, A.
National Cancer Institute
Bethesda, Maryland

HEMSTREET, G. P.
University of Alabama at
Birmingham
Birmingham, Alabama

HENSEN, E.
Department of Immunohematology
University Hospital
Leiden, The Netherlands

HERBERMAN, R. B.
National Cancer Institute
Bethesda, Maryland

HERMAN, F.
School of Public Health
Universite Catholique de Louvain
1200-Brussels
Belgium

HERSCOWITZ, H. B.
Georgetown University
Medical Center
Washington, D. C.

HIBBS, J. B., Jr.
Veterans Administration Hospital
and University of Utah
Medical College
Salt Lake City, Utah

HOFFMAN, M. K.
Memorial Sloan-Kettering
Cancer Center
New York, New York

HOLDEN, H. T.
Laboratory of Immunodiagnosis
National Cancer Institute
Bethesda, Maryland

HOLY, H. W.
Technicon International
Division S. A.
12-14 Chemin Rieu
1208 Geneva
Switzerland

HOOGHE, R.
Weizmann Institute of Science
Rehovot, Israel

ISAKOV, N.
Department of Cell Biology
Weizmann Institute of Science
Rehovot, Israel

JACQUES, P. J.
Catholic University of Louvain
Brussels, Belgium

JAKAB, G.
Department of Environmental
Health Sciences
Johns Hopkins University
Baltimore, Maryland

JANICKI, B. W.
National Institutes of Health
Bethesda, Maryland

KAGAN, E.
Department of Pathology
Georgetown University
Medical Center
Washington, D. C.

KALTER, S. S.
Southwest Foundation for
Research and Education
San Antonio, Texas

KAMPSCHMIDT, R. F.
S. R. NObel Foundation
Ardmore, Oklahoma

KAPLAN, A. M.
Medical College of Virginia
Richmond, Virginia

KAPLOW, L. S.
Veterans Administration Hospital
West Haven, Connecticut

KIESSLING, R.
Karolinska Institute
Stockholm, Sweden

KFIR, S.
Hebrew University of Jerusalem
Jerusalem, Israel

KLEIN, M.
Temple University Medical School
Philadelphia, Pennsylvania

KODITSCHEK, L. K.
409 Highland Avenue
Upper Montclair, New Jersey

KOJIMA, M.
Fukushima Medical College
Fukushima, Japan

KOPITAR, M.
J. Stefan Institute
Ljubljana, Yugoslavia

KOREN, H. S.
Division of Immunology and
Department of Pathology
Duke University
Durham, North Carolina

KRAKAUER, R. S.
Departments of Dermatology
and Immunology
Cleveland Clinic Foundation
Cleveland, Ohio

KRIPE, M.
Frederick Cancer Center
Frederick Maryland

LA VIA, M.
Medical University of
South Carolina
Charleston, South Carolina

LEFLER, A. M.
Jefferson Medical College of
Thomas Jefferson University
Philadelphia, Pennsylvania

JEJEUNE, F. J.
Institut Jules Bordet
Universite Libre de Bruxelles
Brussels, Belgium

LEONARD, E. J.
National Institutes of Health
Bethesda, Maryland

LESPINATS, G.
Institute for Cancer Research
Villejuif, France

LICHTER, W.
University of Miami School of
Medicine
Miami, Florida

LINNA, T. J.
Temple University School of
Medicine
Philadelphia, Pennsylvania

LONAI, P.
Weizmann Institute
Rehovot, Israel

LOOSE, L. D.
Institute of Comparative
and Human Toxicology
Albany Medical College
Albany, New York

LOWELL, G. H.
Walter Reed Army Institute
Washington, D. C.

LOWY, I.
Immunotherapie Experimentale
Institut Pasteur
75015 Paris, France

LUCAS, D. O.
Department of Microbiology
University of Arizona
Tucson, Arizona

LUMB, J. R.
Atlanta University
Atlanta, Georgia

MADDISON, S. E.
Parasitology and
Pathology Divisions
Center for Disease Control
Atlanta, Georgia

MARSHALL, N. B.
Department of Hypersensitivity
Diseases
The Upjohn Company
Kalamazoo, Michigan

MEKORI-FELSTEINER, T.
Rambam Medical Center
Haifa, Israel

MELTZER, M. S.
National Cancer Institute
Bethesda, Maryland

MOORE, M.
Paterson Laboratories
Christie Hospital and
Hold Radium Institute
Manchester M20 9BX
England

MORRELL, R. M.
Neurology Service
Veterans Administration Hospital
Allen Park, Michigan

MYRVIK, Q. N.
Bowman Gray School of Medicine
Winston-Salem, North Carolina

NACHTIGAL, D.
Weizmann Institute
Rehovot, Israel

NAJJAR, V. A.
Tufts University
Boston, Massachusetts

NELSON, D. S.
Kolling Institute of
Medical Research
Sydney, Australia

NELSON, M.
Kolling Institute of
Medical Research
Royal North Shore Hospital
Sydney, Australia

NGUYEN, B. T.
Service Microbiologie
Clinique Universitaire Saint Luc
Universite de Louvain
Brussels 1200
Belgium

NORMANN, S. J.
University of Florida
Gainesville, Florida

NOWOTNY, A.
Temple University Medical School
Philadelphia, Pennsylvania

OMURA, Y.
Fukushima Medical College
Fukushima, Japan

OPPENHEIM, J. J.
National Institute of
Dental Research
Bethesda, Maryland

PARANT, M.
Immunotherapie Experimentale
Institut Pasteur
Paris, France

PATRIARCA, P.
University of Trieste
Trieste, Italy

PELED, A.
Department of Chemical
Immunology
Weizmann Institute of Science
Rehovot, Israel

PENNY, R.
St. Vincent's Hospital
Sydney, Australia

PITT, J.
Columbia University College of
Physicians and Surgeons
New York, New York

PLUZNIK, D. H.
Bar-Ilan University
Ramat-Gan, Israel

POLAKOW
Hadassah Medical School
Hebrew University
Jerusalem, Israel

POUPON, M.
Institute for Cancer Research
Villejuif, France

PRIBNOW, J. F.
Proctor Foundation
University of California
San Francisco, California

PRESANT, C.
Jewish Hospital
of St. Louis
St. Louis, Missouri

QUASTEL, M.
Soroka Medical Center
Beer-Sheba, Israel

RABINOWITZ, R.
Hadassah Medical School
Hebrew University
Jerusalem, Israel

RACHMILEWITZ, M.
Hebrew University
Hadassah Medical School
Jerusalem, Israel

REGELSON, W.
Department of Medicine
Medical College of Virginia
Virginia Commonwealth University
Richmond, Virginia

REICHARD, S. M.
Medical College of Georgia
Augusta, Georgia

ROMEO, D.
University of Trieste
Trieste, Italy

ROOS, D.
Netherlands Red Cross Blood
Transfusion Service
The Netherlands

ROSENBERG, R.
Accurate Chemical Scientific Corp
New York, N. Y.

ROSENBERG, S. A.
National Cancer Institute
National Institutes of Health
Bethesda, Maryland

ROSENSTEIN, M. M.
Department of Zoology
and Physiology
Rutgers University
Newark, New Jersey

ROSENTAHL, A. S.
National Institute of Allergy
and Infectious Diseases
Bethesda, Maryland

ROSSI, F.
University of Trieste
Trieste, Italy

RUPOLD, H.
Heitzinger Hauptstr. 18 A 16
Vienna, Austria

RUN, R.
Hadassah Medical School
Hebrew University
Jerusalem, Israel

RUTTER, V.
Weizmann Institute of Science
Rehovot, Israel

SALEM, H.
Cannon Lab, Inc.
Reading, Pennsylvania

SAMAK, R.
Chemotherapy Unit
University of Paris
XIII. CHU Bobigny
93000 France

SAUDER, D. N.
Department of Dermatology
and Immunology
Cleveland Clinic Foundation
Cleveland, Ohio

SCHECHTER, G.
Veterans Administration
Hospital and George Washington
University Medical Center
Washington, D. C.

SCHILDT, B. E.
University of Linkoping
Regional Hospital
S-581 85 Linkoping
Sweden

SCHIRRMACHER, V.
Institute of Immunology and
Genetics
Deutsches Krebsforschungszentrum
Heidelberg, Federal Republic
of Germany

SCHLESINGER, M.
Hebrew University
Jerusalem, Israel

SCOTT, M. T.
The Wellcome Research
Laboratories
Beckenham, Kent
England

SEGAL, S.
The Weizmann Institute of
Science
Department of Cell Biology
Rehovot, Israel

SIECK, R. K.
University of Heidelburg
Heidelburg, Germany

SIEDHI, B.
Hadassah Medical School
Hebrew University
Jerusalem, Israel

SIEGEL, B. V.
University of Oregon
Medical School
Portland, Oregon

SIEGEL, J. I. M.
University of Oregon Health
Sciences Center
Portland, Oregon

SIGEL, M. M.
University of South Carolina
School of Medicine
Columbia, South Carolina

SILKWORTH, J.
Institute of Comparative
and Human Toxicology
Albany Medical College
Albany, New York

SILVERSTEIN, E.
State University of New York
Downstate Medical Center
Brooklyn, New York

SOROUDI, M.
5360 Rural Ridge
Anaheim, Canada

SYNDERMAN, R.
Duke University
Durham, North Carolina

SOLOMON, J. B.
University of Aberdeen
Aberdeen, Scotland

STERN, K.
Bar-Ilan University
Tel Aviv, Israel

STIFFEL, C.
Curie Foundation
Institute of Radium
Paris, France

STINNETT, J. D.
University of Cincinnati
Medical Center
Cincinnati, Ohio

STRAUSS, R. R.
Albert Einstein Medical Center
Philadelphia, Pennsylvania

STRAUSSER, J. L.
National Cancer Institute
National Institutes of Health
Bethesda, Maryland

STUART, A. E.
University of Edenburgh
Eidenburgh, Scotland

SULITZEANU, D.
Dept. of Immunology
Hadassah Medical School
Hebrew University of Jerusalem
Jerusalem, Israel

TAL, C.
Hadassah Medical School
Hebrew University
Jerusalem, Israel

TAUB, R. N.
Medical College of Virginia
Richmond, Virginia

TIMAR, M.
Chemical-Pharmaceutical
Research Institute
Vitan 112 Bucuresti 4
Romania

TRAININ, N.
Weizmann Institute
Rehovot, Israel

UETSUKA, A.
Laboratory of Medical Mycology
Department of Infectious Diseases
Institute of Medical Science
University of Tokyo, Japan

URBASCHEK, R.
Institute of Hygiene and
Medical Microbiology
University of Heidelberg
Heidelberg, Germany

VERCAMMEN-GRANDJEAN, A.
Institut Jules Bordet
Centre des Tumeurs
de l'Universite
libre de Bruxelles
Brussels, Belgium

WARD, H. A.
Department of Pathology
and Immunology
Monash Medical School
Victoria, Australia

WEEKS, B. A.
University of South Carolina
Columbia, South Carolina

WERTHEIM, G.
Hebrew University of Jerusalem
Jerusalem, Israel

WHEELOCK, E. F.
Thomas Jefferson University
Philadelphia, Pennsylvania

YOFFEY, J.
Hadassah Medical School
Hebrew University of Jerusalem
Jerusalem, Israel

ZIEGLER, J.
Prince of Wales Hospital
Randwick, Australia

ZLOTNIK
Hadassah Medical School
Hebrew University
Jerusalem, Israel